Advances in Neurosurgery 19

W. J. Bock · Ch. Lumenta
M. Brock · M. Klinger (Eds.)

Intracranial Angiomas

Neurosurgical Intensive Care

Supratentorial Tumors in Children

With 101 Figures

Springer-Verlag
Berlin Heidelberg New York London Paris
Tokyo Hong Kong Barcelona Budapest

Proceedings of the 41th Annual Meeting of the
Deutsche Gesellschaft für Neurochirurgie
Düsseldorf, May 27–30, 1990

Prof. Dr. Wolfgang Joachim Bock
Prof. Dr. Christianto Lumenta
Neurochirurgische Universitätsklinik
Moorenstraße 5, W-4000 Düsseldorf 1, FRG

Prof. Dr. Mario Brock
Neurochirurgische Klinik und Poliklinik
Universitätsklinikum Steglitz, Freie Universität Berlin
Hindenburgdamm 30, 1000 Berlin 45, FRG

Prof. Dr. Margareta Klinger
Neurochirurgische Klinik der Universität Erlangen-Nürnberg
Schwabachanlage 6 (Kopfklinikum), W-8520 Erlangen, FRG

ISBN 3-540-53311-7 Springer-Verlag Berlin Heidelberg New York
ISBN 0-387-53311-7 Springer-Verlag New York Berlin Heidelberg

Library of Congress Cataloging-in-Publication Data. Deutsche Gesellschaft für Neurochirurgie. Tagung (41st : 1990 : Düsseldorf, Germany) Intracranial angiomas ; Neurosurgical intensive care ; Supratentorial tumors in children / W. J. Bock . . . [et al.] (eds.). (Advances in neurosurgery ; 19) "Proceedings of the 41st Annual Meeting of the Deutsche Gesellschaft für Neurochirurgie, Düsseldorf, May 27–30, 1990"–T. p. verso. Includes bibliographical references. Includes index. ISBN 3-540-53311-7.– ISBN 0-387-53311-7 1. Intracranial angiomas–Surgery–Congresses. 2. Supratentorial brain tumors in children–Surgery–Congresses. 3. Surgical intensive care–Congresses. I. Bock, Wolfgang Joachim. II. Title. III. Title: Neurosurgical intensive care. IV. Title: Supratentorial tumors in children. V. Series. [DNLM: 1. Critical Care–congresses. 2. Hemangiomas–congresses. 3. Nervous System–surgery–congresses. 4. Supratentorial Neoplasms–in infancy & childhood–congresses. W1 AD684N v. 19 / WL 100 D486i 1990] RD594.D49 1990 616.99'281–dc20, 91-4614 CIP

11/3130-543210 – Printed on acid-free paper

Contents

President's Opening Remarks
W.J. Bock 1

Coordination of Neurosurgical Training in the Europe of the 1990s
R. Fahlbusch, R. Braakman, M. Brock. C. Brocklehurst,
L. Calliauw, and Y. Keravel (With 1 Figure) 5

Winning Poster Presentations

Perioperative Monitoring of Subarachnoid Hemorrhage:
Transcranial Doppler Sonography and
Somatosensory Evoked Potentials
R. Laumer, R. Steinmeier, F. Gönner, R. Fahlbusch, J. Schramm,
M. Mück, B. Hinkelmann, and M. Purrucker (With 2 Figures) . . . 17

Mechanisms of K^+-induced Glial Swelling
H. Weight, F. Staub, O. Kempski, J. Peters, F. v. Rosen,
and A. Baethmann 20

Effects of Anesthetic Agents on Brain Edema and
Cerebral Blood Flow from a Focal Cold Lesion in Rabbit Brain
R. Murr, L. Schürer, S. Berger, R. Enzenbach, and A. Baethmann . 24

Single-Stage Neuro-rhinosurgical Operation and Management
of Malignant Tumors of the Anterior Cranial Skull Base
U. Neubauer, R. Fahlbusch, M.E. Wigand, and M. Weidenbecher
(With 1 Figure) 29

Vascular Malformations of the Brain

Diagnostic and Interventional Neuroradiology
of Brain Arteriovenous Malformations:
Implications on Angioarchitecture for Embolization
A. Valavanis and W. Müller-Forell 35

Embolization Techniques in the Treatment
of Cerebral Arteriovenous Malformations
B. Richling and G. Bavinzski (With 3 Figures) 41

Results of Combined Endovascular and Surgical Treatment
of Intracranial Arteriovenous Malformations
D. Wijnalda and T.G. Tjan (With 3 Figures) 46

Indications, Technique, and Results of Microsurgical Treatment
of Intracranial Arteriovenous Malformations
Ch. Lumenta, M. Bettag, A. Bertels, and W.J. Bock
(With 1 Figure) 50

Surgical Problems in Partially Embolized Angiomas
J.M. Gilsbach and M. Schumacher (With 3 Figures) 55

Arteriovenous Malformations of the Brain:
What is the Best Way to Treat Them?
J. Brotchi, O. Dewitte, A. Vandesteene, G. Rodesch,
D. Baleriaux, and J. Noterman (With 3 Figures) 61

Arteriovenous Malformations of the Medial Surface
of the Parieto-occipital Region and the Basal Ganglia
G.H. Spincemaille 66

Considerations on the Coexistence
of Intracranial Arteriovenous Malformations and Aneurysms
J.A. Grotenhuis and J.A.N. van der Spek 70

Follow-up After Treatment for
Intracranial Arteriovenous Malformations
H.M. Mehdorn, S.P. Müller, D. Koch, and W. Grote
(With 4 Figures) 74

Posterior Fossa Arteriovenous Malformations:
Angioarchitecture in Relation to Hemorrhagic Episodes
G. Rodesch, R. Garcia Monaco, H. Alvarez, A. Goulao,
and P. Lasjaunias 81

Clinical and Radiological Prognostic Factors
in Cerebral Arteriovenous Malformations
H.-G. Höllerhage, K.-M. Dewenter, and H. Dietz 84

Venous Angiomas: Experience with Surgical and Nonsurgical Management
J.C. Tonn, U. Schuchard, C.R. Hornig, A.L. Agnoli, and K. Roosen (With 2 Figures) 90

Intracranial Venous Angiomas
C. Plets, G. Wilms, J. Goffin, and Y.S. Ho (With 4 Figures) 94

Congestive Cardiac Manifestations from Cerebrocranial Arteriovenous Shunts
G. Rodesch, R. Garcia Monaco, D. Devictor, C. Mann, A. Hannedouche, K. Terbrugge, and P. Lasjaunias 100

Neuropsychological Abnormalities in Patients with Cerebral Arteriovenous Malformations: A Pilot Study
N. Muik, U. Zoworka, B. Kimmig, E. Irle, and B. Wowra (With 4 Figures) 103

Cerebral Cavernous Hemangiomas: Treatment and Surgical Decisions
M. Westphal, D. Winkler, G. Nowak, R. Schwachenwald, H. Arnold, and H.-D. Herrmann (With 3 Figures) 110

Microsurgery of Cavernous Angiomas of the Brain with Special Reference to Cerebral Midline Localizations
V. Seifert and D. Stolke (With 3 Figures) 116

667 Histologically Verified Cavernous Hemangiomas of the CNS: Review of Localization, Symptoms, and Signs, Diagnosis, and Results of Operative Treatment
M. Hahn, A. Aschoff, and S. Kunze (With 4 Figures) 122

Asymptomatic Cryptic Vascular Malformations
C. Gilliard, P. Laloux, C. Thiran, and S. Mourin (With 3 Figures) 127

Supratentorial Tumors in Childhood

Pediatric Brain Tumors
R.W. Oberbauer (With 1 Figure) 135

Multidisciplinary Approach to the Treatment of Supratentorial Tumors in Children
J.J.A. Mooij, J.H. Begeer, R. le Coultre, J. Leeuw, R. Tamminga, A. Kingma, D.M. Mehta, and L. Vencken (With 1 Figure) 141

Treatment and Course of Malignant Supratentorial Brain Tumors in Childhood
A.M. Messing, Ch. Lumenta, W. Otten, R. Schober, and U. Göbel (With 1 Figure) 146

Interstitial Irradiation of Supratentorial Cerebral Gliomas in Childhood with Permanently Implanted Iodine 125: Preliminary Results
J. Voges, H. Treuer, W.J. Schlegel, O. Pastyr, and V. Sturm (With 2 Figures) 151

Radiological Results of Intracavitary Brachytherapy of Cystic Craniopharyngioma in Childhood and Adolescence
G. Blaauw and J.H. van den Berge (With 3 Figures) 158

Long-Term Results of Combined Surgery and Radiotherapy of Pilocytic Astrocytomas in the Middle Cranial Fossa
F. Rauhut, V. Reinhardt, H. Wiedemayer, and V. Budach (With 4 Figures) 163

Discussion: PNET – A Melting-Pot of Unspecified Tumors?
W. Wechsler 168

Prognosis of Supratentorial Gliomas in Children
J. Pospiech, R. Kalff, W. Kocks, and W. Grote 171

Proliferative Activity of Pilocytic Astrocytomas: Examination Using Monoclonal Antibody Ki-67
R. Schröder and K. Bien (With 1 Figure) 176

Immunohistochemical Investigations with a Monoclonal Anti-Epidermal Growth Factor Receptor Antibody in Supratentorial Tumors in Children
J. Behnke, H. Ludwig, G.A. Luckenbach, B. Rama, and E. Markakis 180

Neurosurgical Intensive Care

Neurosurgical Intensive Care – An Interdisciplinary Field
A. Encke 187

Neurosurgical Intensive Care: General Considerations
W.J. Bock, J. Piek, and C. Sprick (With 4 Figures) 189

Prognostic Value of Motor Evoked Potentials
in Traumatic and Nontraumatic Coma
V. Rohde and J. Zentner (With 4 Figures) 194

The Temporal Structure of Information Processing in Patients
Following Diffuse Head Injuries: Electrophysiological Studies
B.M. Reuter, D.B. Linke, and M. Kurthen (With 1 Figure) 201

TCD, SEPs and ICP: Comparative Analysis
in Severe Head Injury
M. Lorenz, G. Dorfmüller, W.-P. Sollmann, and M.R. Gaab
(With 5 Figures) 205

Parenteral Nutrition in Patients
with Spontaneous Intracranial Hemorrhages
J. Piek and W.J. Bock (With 2 Figures) 211

Susceptibility to Infection
During Continuous Thiopentone Therapy
J. Nadstawek, D. Moskopp, M. Fischer, M. Födisch,
and A. Bartsch (With 3 Figures) 217

Infection Rate and Bacterial Spectrum in 413 Patients
of a Neurosurgical Intensive Care Unit:
Results of a 2-year Prospective Study
A. Feldges, R. Kalff, E. Rosenthal, and W. Grote
(With 3 Figures) 222

Risk During the First Hours After Severe Head Injury
R.A. Frowein, U. Stammler, R. Firsching, G. Friedmann,
and F. Thun (With 4 Figures) 228

Disturbances of Water-Electrolyte Regulation
After Surgery of the Hypothalamus and Pituitary Region
G. Hildebrandt and H.W. Mueller (With 1 Figure) 234

CBF Dynamics During Hyperventilation Therapy
for Intracranial Hypertension
J. Meixensberger, A. Brawanski, M. Holzschuh,
I. Danhauser-Leistner, and W. Ullrich (With 3 Figures) 240

THAM in Traumatic Brain Swelling:
A Comparative Experimental and Clinical Study
M.R. Gaab, K. Seegers, R.J. Smedema, H.E. Heissler,
and C. Goetz (With 4 Figures) 245

Effects of the Antihypertensive Drug Ketanserin
on Intracranial Pressure in Patients with Head Trauma
L. Heytens, J. Verlooy, C. De La Porte, M. Van Vyve,
P. Selosse, and L. Bossaert 255

A Comparison Between Mannitol and Glycerol Therapy
for Intracranial Hypertension
R.J. Smedema and M.R. Gaab (With 4 Figures) 259

Decompressive Craniectomy After Severe Head Injury:
Useful Therapy in Pathophysiologically Guided Indication
M. Rittierodt, M.R. Gaab, and M. Lorenz (With 4 Figures) 265

Safety of Fraxiparine Administration
in Neurosurgical Patients: Preliminary Report
F. Martens, T. Bruyns, T. Vandekerckhove, J. Caemaert,
O. Kalala, and L. Calliauw (With 2 Figures). 274

Subject Index 277

List of Contributors

Agnoli, A.L. 90
Alvarez, H. 81
Arnold, H. 110
Aschoff, A. 122
Baethmann, A. 20, 24
Baleriaux D. 61
Bartsch, A. 217
Bavinzski, G. 41
Begeer, J.H. 141
Behnke, J. 180
Berge, J.H. van den 158
Berger, S. 24
Bertels, A. 50
Bettag, M. 50
Bien, K. 176
Blaauw, G. 158
Bock, W.J. 1, 50, 189, 211
Bossaert, L. 255
Braakman, R. 5
Brawanski, A. 240
Brock, M. 5
Brocklehurst, C. 5
Brotchi, J. 61
Bruyns, T. 274
Budach, V. 163
Caemaert, J. 274
Calliauw, L. 5, 274
Coultre, R. le 141
Danhauser-Leistner, I. 240
De La Porte, C. 255
Devictor, D. 100
Dewenter, K.-M. 84
Dewitte, O. 61
Dietz, H. 84
Dorfmüller, G. 205
Encke, A. 187
Enzenbach, R. 24
Fahlbusch, R. 5, 17, 29
Feldges, A. 222
Firsching, R. 228
Fischer, M. 217
Födisch, M. 217
Friedmann, G. 228
Frowein, R.A. 228
Gaab, M.R. 205, 245, 259, 265
Garcia Monaco, R. 81, 100
Gilliard, C. 127
Gilsbach, J.M. 55
Göbel, U. 146
Goetz, C. 245
Goffin, J. 94
Gönner, F. 17
Goulao, A. 81
Grote, W. 74, 171, 222
Grotenhuis, J.A. 70
Hahn, M. 122
Hannedouche, A. 100
Heissler, H.E. 245
Herrmann, H.-D. 110
Heytens, L. 255
Hildebrandt, G 234
Hinkelmann, B. 17
Ho, Y.S. 94
Höllerhage, H.-G. 84
Holzschuh, M. 240
Hornig, C.R. 90
Irle, E. 103
Kalala, O. 274
Kalff, R. 171, 222
Kempski, O. 20
Keravel, Y. 5
Kimmig, B. 103

Kingma, A. 141
Koch, D. 74
Kocks, W. 171
Kunze, S. 122
Kurthen, M. 201
Laloux, P. 127
Lasjaunias, P. 81, 100
Laumer, R. 17
Leeuw, J. 141
Linke, D.B. 201
Lorenz, M. 205, 265
Luckenbach, G.A. 180
Ludwig, H. 180
Lumenta, Ch. 50, 146
Mann, C. 100
Markakis, E. 180
Martens, F. 274
Mehdorn, H.M. 74
Mehta, D.M. 141
Meixensberger, J. 240
Messing, A.M. 146
Mooij, J.J.A. 141
Moskopp, D. 217
Mourin, S. 127
Mück, M. 17
Mueller, H.W. 234
Muik, N. 103
Müller, S.P. 74
Müller-Forell, W. 35
Murr, R. 24
Nadstawek, J. 217
Neubauer, U. 29
Noterman, J. 61
Nowak, G. 110
Oberbauer, R.W. 135
Otten, W. 146
Pastyr, O. 151
Peters, J. 20
Piek, J. 189, 211
Plets, C. 94
Pospiech, J. 171
Purrucker, M. 17
Rama, B. 180
Rauhut, F. 163
Reinhardt, V. 163
Reuter, B.M. 201
Richling, B. 41
Rittierodt, M. 265
Rodesch, G. 61, 81, 100
Rohde, V. 194
Roosen, K. 90
Rosen, F. v. 20
Rosenthal, E. 222
Schlegel, W.J. 151
Schober, R. 146
Schramm, J. 17
Schröder, R. 176
Schuchard, U. 90
Schumacher, M. 55
Schürer, L. 24
Schwachenwald, R. 110
Seegers, K. 245
Seifert, V. 116
Selosse, P. 255
Smedema, R.J. 245, 259
Sollmann, W.-P. 205
Spek, J.A.N. van der 70
Spincemaille, G.H. 66
Sprick, C. 189
Stammler, U. 228
Staub, F. 20
Steinmeier, R. 17
Stolke, D. 116
Sturm, V. 151
Tamminga, R. 141
Terbrugge, K. 100
Thiran, C. 127
Thun, F. 228
Tjan, T.G. 46
Tonn, J.C. 90
Treuer, H. 151
Ullrich, W. 240
Valavanis, A. 35
Van Vyve, M. 255
Vandekerckhove, T. 274
Vandesteene, A. 61
Vencken, L. 141
Verlooy, J. 255
Voges, J. 151
Wechsler, W. 168

Weidenbecher, M. 29
Weigt, H. 20
Westphal, M. 110
Wiedemayer, H. 163
Wigand, M.E. 29
Wijnalda, D. 46
Wilms, G. 94
Winkler, D. 110
Wowra, B. 103
Zentner, J. 194
Zoworka, U. 103

President's Opening Remarks

W. J. Bock[1]

In 1990 we celebrate the 40th anniversary of the founding of the Deutsche Gesellschaft für Neurochirurgie, which in 1950 became the spiritual and scientific home of all German-speaking neurosurgeons. Originally it was to have been founded in 1939. This plan was thwarted, however, by the course of history and delayed by 11 years. After these 11 years of building up, a painful separation was enforced by the effects of political developments. One section of the membership was forced to resign and found its own society. Although the society's statutes were sacrificed to social structures, both scientific messages and human relations were kept alive. They have been preserved and extended over time.

The exciting events of recent months enable us to meet again openly and without reserve, and to show to those once shut out: "We belong together again."

It is a special pleasure to have neurosurgeons from the Société Belge de Neurochirurgie – Belgische Wetenschappelijke Vereniging voor Neurochirurgie and Nederlandse Vereniging van Neurochirurgie participating in this annual meeting, which is thus a joint meeting. The preparation period has shown us how many aspects we have in common, where further harmonization is required, and how much more important a European community of science is than all national frontiers knowing East and West, North and South only as geographical terms. With this in mind Düsseldorf, this centrally situated, open-minded city where we meet, has acquired a new significance which was not thought of when it was first selected.

As early as 1947 the then responsible city, together with the Academy of Medicine, in wise foresight and prompted by the then holder of the chair of internal medicine and neurology, Prof. Bodechtel, established a position for a neurosurgeon within the Department of Surgery. This was held by Hans Kuhlendahl from the summer of 1947, and by January 1960, 30 years ago, neurosurgery had achieved a department of its own with a Chair of Neurosurgery. For this reason I am particularly pleased to welcome in person Hans Kuhlendahl, who will be 80 in a few weeks.

During the years of my chairmanship, there is one line of thought which has preoccupied me in a particular way. At no previous time have there been such changes of staff in one field. No less than 14 Chairs and 5 positions as Head of De-

[1] Direktor der Neurochirurgischen Universitätsklinik, Moorenstr. 5, W-4000 Düsseldorf 1, FRG

Advances in Neurosurgery, Vol. 19
W. J. Bock, Ch. Lumenta, M. Brock, M. Klinger (Eds.)

partment were or are on offer. Thus the second and third generation of neurosurgeons is following or is about to follow the pioneers for 1950. This will give rise to further integration of the subject of neurosurgery, with its ability to encompass related fields through its preoccupation with brain, spinal cord, and the peripheral nervous system, into the field of medical science and the teaching of students.

Neurosurgery's period of growth and expansion is about to come to an end. Nonetheless, it still appears necessary to point out that the unbalanced and biased support often received from the administrative side does not always meet requirements. Such decisions and actions, however, originate from the organ which is our daily interest as neurosurgeons, the brain. I therefore call upon young neurosurgeons to follow developments critically, to take up the task of being valiant scientists of their field, and to carry the burden of this work. This commitment will in the end result in pleasure and contentment with our profession.

One present burden is a tremendous shortage of nursing staff. In stark contrast to the number of junior doctors available – some are even out of work – there is a staffing disaster in the nursing profession in Germany. The German hospital system, from university department to community hospital, is in danger. Staff shortages are rapidly leading towards total collapse of the inpatient system. Half-empty nursing schools indicate that the peak of this problem is still ahead. This year or 1991 at the latest will see even emergencies not being adequately attended to, and regular treatment will become very limited. All this foreseeable future, rather than calculated pessimism. In order to overcome this social emergency in German hospitals steps to be taken rapidly are: training programmes for those out of work and recruitment of staff who have left the profession; better timing of working shifts; but, above all, better pay for the nursing profession. It is our duty as physicians here and now to counteract the decline of a profession by acknowledging the outstanding achievements of our working colleagues.

We have at present been forced to close down beds, thereby transferring controversies to the last participant of the chain of events, namely, the patient. This is indeed evidence of the ignorance of twentieth-century man. In addition, with respect to space available and technical equipment, many university departments figure below community and Church-supported hospitals, a situation which may also interfere with speedy recovery.

Last year I discussed the approbation act with reference to neurosurgery. This year one further factor is to be added. Since January 1, 1990, a European training act is in force which incorporates a 6-year course with an additional period of 2 years as a doctor-in-training, this model largely corresponding to our present procedure. This European concept is being opposed by those in Germany who would attempt to modify the approbation procedure to a 5-year course and a 3-year doctor-in-training period. I must emphasize that the scientific study of medicine, with the ever-increasing amounts of knowledge about biological interactions on the one hand and the increasing importance of psychological and social factors for the definition of health and disease on the other, will not allow a reduction of the course of studies. I would like to remind you of Stefan Zweig who spiritually prepared the way for the mutual understanding of the nations and civilizations of Europe and who is rightly called a great European. His admonition is that the present can only be understood if the traces of the past are followed. Understanding the past will point to the path we should take in the future. To him intellectual work was pure joy and personal freedom, the highest pleasure on earth, as he put it. This noble spirit may be a measure for discussion on a European level and the selfishness of some individual groups should give way before it.

German science, founded on humanist tradition, will contribute considerably to this European process of integration. And thus I return to where I started from. The historic sites of humanist learning such as Weimar, Leipzig, and the Berlin of Humboldt have become accessible once again to all of us and will contribute their values towards the edifice of European science about to be set up, as will the technical know-how of the Federal Republic. This noble task lies ahead in our field of neurosurgery as well. To follow the spirit of Karl Jaspers, who in his inaugural lecture in 1949 said: "University is only possible in the living communication of the men of research, of *universitas* in the cosmos of sciences, in *studium generale*," a broad scientific spectrum is required for universal well-balanced learning.

Jaspers looks at medicine as a cornerstorne of the university and at the physician as the down to earth philosopher. The physician's role does not at first sight appear to be very attractive. Looking at this formal training, however, one cannot help noticing that, increasingly, in addition to matters scientific, those from the fields of letters and social sciences have found their way there. Thus, a synthesis of various areas of science collectively influences the physician's thinking. Putting this into practice, however, he encounters a rigid course of work ordered according to the needs of an oganization. The pressure thus built up is frequently countered by the devious means of material compensation. The fascinating European task ahead of reviewing all aspects of life on our continent will also stimulate the role of the physician.

If in conclusion I quote Erasmus of Rotterdam, who I consider one of the great European thinkers, I do so because he set standards both in synthetical and analytical thinking. He who far-sightedly freed the philosophical, theological and scientific discoveries of his time from narrow selfishness also stated that the defective working of a single man's brain may create unrest in the whole world. In his lecture in praise of medicine he continues, "Care for this science with all your soul, give yourself with all your strength." Four centuries later we neurosurgeons take this to heart in our fateful manipulations of the brain.

The great responsibility of our profession towards the individual must be founded on a concept of humanity based on humanist ideals. We are thus closer than ever to the realization of Erasmus' idea of the dissolution of controversies in a spirit of justice, in nations united by a community of civilization.

Let us therefore offer our neurosurgical contribution to this magnificent edifice of science in Europe.

Coordination of Neurosurgical Training in the Europe of the 1990s

Round Table discussion, summarized by R. Fahlbusch[1]

Participants: R. Fahlbusch (moderator) FRG; R. Braakman, Netherlands; M. Brock, FRG; C. Brocklehurst, UK; L. Calliauw, Belgium; Y. Keravel, France

Introduction

It was the desire of the officers of the three societies to discuss the topic "Coordination of Neurosurgical Training in the Europe of the 1990s." Our guests from Belgium were represented by Luc Calliauw and those from the Netherlands by Rainer Braakman. The host country was represented by Mario Brock. All participants have considerable experience of work in neurosurgery at the European level: Luc Calliauw as the present secretary of the European Association of Neurosurgical Societies (EANS), Rainer Braakman as the chairman of the committee of the European board examination, and Mario Brock as the former chairman of the EANS training committee.

When the trade boundaries in the European Community go down on the first day of 1993, there will be 12 member countries, not just three. For this reason Wolf Bock – Chairman of the Deutsche Gesellschaft für Neurochirurgie – also invited C. Brocklehurst from Hull. He is the President designate of the joint meeting to be held by the Society of British Neurological Surgeons and the Deutsche Gesellschaft für Neurochirurgie in 1992 in Hull. Further, Yves Keravel, President of the French Neurosurgical Society, also participated in the discussion. This limitation of representatives from different countries was intended to achieve greater efficiency. "EANS is more than the Common Market" [2]. We all know, at least since the end of the last year, that Europe means more than this: it includes the EFTA group as well as the eastern European countries, especially the GDR.

Rudolf Fahlbusch was asked to moderate because of his position as Chairman of the National Training Committee of the FRG, the members of which are Profs. Eckard Halves, Hamburg; Norfrid Klug, Cologne; Rüdiger Lorenz, Frankfurt; Johannes Schramm, Bonn; and Wolf-Ingo Steudel, Frankfurt. Rudolf Fahlbusch is also the German delegate to the EANS Training Committee.

Political Background

In the night of December 31, 1992, the internal European market will come into being. The highest European institution, the European Commission with its presi-

[1] Neurochirurgische Universitätsklinik, Schwabachanlage 6 (Kopfklinikum), W-8520 Erlangen, FRG

Advances in Neurosurgery, Vol. 19
W. J. Bock, Ch. Lumenta, M. Brock, M. Klinger (Eds.)

dent Jacques Delors, has decided that the structure of the European Common Market should be completed by 1993. This is based on four freedoms: unhindered exchange of products, of services, of capital, and of manpower. Jacques Delors has the futuristic idea that by the mid-1990s about 80% of all regulations on economic and social life of 325 million Europeans will be decided in Brussels. The spirit of 1993 will be: elimination of all border control of products and persons within the EC; no discrimination on grounds of nationality; and liberation and freedom of movement for all dependent and independent members of the labor force – including neurosurgeons. There are two possibilities for harmonization: either uniformity and unification at a European level, which would mean minimizing the standard in all fields, including neurosurgery, or preserving local qualifications in a federalist manner. For us this could be mean an optional European Board examination.

For physicians the European Common Market has been a reality for 15 years. Since the recommendations of 16 June 1975 and 30 October 1989 by the European Council – on which all countries are represented at ministerial level – the legal framework has been in place. This means that there is mutual recognition of diplomas, examinations, and approbations. However, no detailed guidelines are given about the practice of medicine. There are minimum guidelines for the study of medicine, which is set at 6 years or 5500 hours.

Chapter 4 of the guidelines says that acceptance of physicians in EC countries other than their country of origin is only possible in medical disciplines which already exist in the former. There are 11 disciplines, including neurosurgery, which are generally accepted by all states of the European Community. However there are 36 other disciplines which are only accepted in some countries. For example, an EC neurosurgeon can practice in Germany because neurosurgery is an official discipline there. However, a pediatric neurosurgeon from Italy is not allowed to practice pediatric neurosurgery in Germany, because this subdiscipline is not officially accepted.

Supranational Organizations of Physicians in Europe

The permanent Committee of European Physicians (CP) receives suggestions and advice from other groups (Fig. 1). Two of the most important ones are the AEMH and the UEMS. In the AEMH (Association Européenne de Médecins Hôpitaux) the medical heads of hospitals are represented; representatives from countries outside the EC such as Austria and Switzerland are members of this body. The second body, the UEMS (Union Européene de Médecins Spécialists or European Union of Medical Specialists) is the Commission for harmonization. Its chairman is Dr. Schydlo, a pediatric psychiatrist in Düsseldorf.

After the opening of the internal market Europe will have about 100000 unemployed physicians. Two hundred physicians from other EC countries work in the FRG. Four hundred German physicians work in Great Britain. Insurance systems must be accepted in Section 3 of the European Commission (chaired by Bangemann). The present EC principle in this section is liberalization with a minimum of

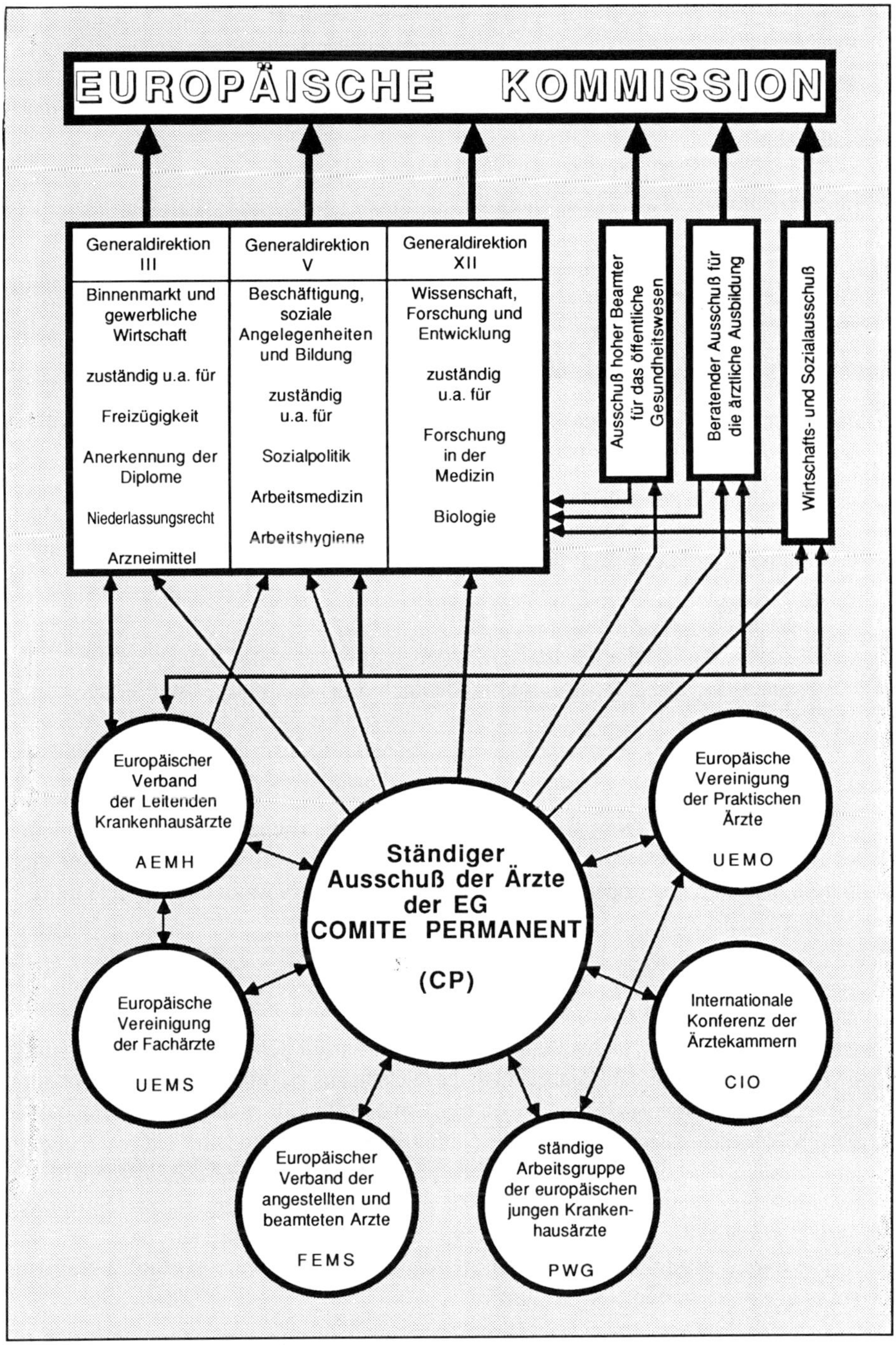

Fig. 1. The most important supranational medical bodies in the European Committee. Modified from [1]

centralization. The UMS (Union Européenne of Médical Spécialists) has an influence on this section. The neurosurgical representative is Prof. Verbiest, Netherlands. The German representative is Wolfgang Bock by his position as First Chairman. This committee has not met for the last 5 years. Professor Kuttner, Berlin, is Chairman.

On May 25, 1990, the German urologists organized a meeting on "Physicians in Europe 1993" in Brussels, although with German participants only [10].

Facilities and Service Requirements in Neurosurgery

Minimum Requirements for Neurosurgical Units

Following the EANS conclusions [3] there was general agreement that the following are the minimum requirements for any neurosurgical unit:

- 40 Neurosurgical beds
- A 24-h service for elective and emergency procedures
- Two operating theatres, at least one exclusively for neurosurgery
- 250 Major operations per year
- An intensive care unit
- Full-time access to diagnostic facilities including computed tomography
- Adequate operating theatre equipment including operating microscope and bipolar diathermy
- Presence on staff of an anesthetist wich special responsibility for neuroanesthesia
- Full inclusion of neurotraumatology and pediatric neurosurgery in the unit

In addition to the above, functional neurosurgery, a scientific library, and neurosurgical laboratories are required [3]. The neuropathologist with facilities for rapid histological diagnosis need not necessarily be absolutely limited to a single unit.

Minimum Requirement for Training in Basic Neurosurgery

According to the EANS resolutions [3] the minimum period of training should be 6 years. Among the 12 countries of the EC this is accepted by all except three (Greece, Italy, Spain). However, only 16 of the 25 full member countries of the EANS have accepted this [5]. The Netherlands, Spain, and the United Kingdom have limited the number of trainees per year. The selection of candidates will also be a problem in future. The subject of prospective neurosurgical manpower is a very important one and will be come even more so in the future (Brock).

The 6-year minimum period should always include 4 years in clinical neurosurgery. The other periods are facultative:

- 1 Year in surgical fields other than neurosurgery
- 6 Months in medial neurology

– 6 Months in related disciplines such as neuroradiology, neuropathology, intensive care

There is no clear agreement on the length of this optional period, which could vary. All participants agree that trainees should keep – as in Germany – a logbook of operating experience in the near future. This should include as a minimum the following operations performed by the candidate himself: 30 operations on intracranial tumors, 30 spinal operations, 30 operations for cranial trauma, 10 operations for hydrocephalus, 50 miscellaneous operations including for pain and vascular surgery.

Examinations (in European Countries)

A final examination before completion of neurosurgical training is desirable. However, to date this occurs only in Germany, in the form of an oral test. The qualification as *Facharzt* (specialist) is certified by the various *Landesärztekammer* (State Chambers of Physicians), not by an institution of the government. In other countries, the neurosurgical qualification is awarded at national level by the central government. It was generally felt that all European countries would wish to have a final examination at the end of the training and that some assessment of operative ability should be made either at this stage or when the neurosurgeon is in practice. Mario Brock proposed that a standard neurosurgical operation should be part of the examination. Luc Calliauw argued that it is ethically untenable to do this on patients, as the examiners have to accept that the physician being examined has the right to fail.

It is intended that these minimum requirements for facilities and service and for training in basic neurosurgery should be introduced in each European country. The final goal is a European Board (see below).

Neurosurgical Training Activities

Local Activities in Different Countries

In the Netherlands compulsory training courses are held twice a year, each lasting 2 days. There are lectures on one particular topic and detailed discussions with the trainees.

Since 1982 there has been an annual neurosurgical training course in Germany comparable to the annual courses of the EANS. The whole cycle of courses is 6 x 1 annual 2 day course, which covers all important topics in neurosurgery.

In the United Kingdom the annual training program deals mainly with basic neurosciences. Regional training is held in France. For the relatively small number of neurosurgeons in Belgium there is local training every month for about 2 h.

EANS Training Courses

Of particular interest to those concerned with neurosurgical education are the European Courses in Neurosurgery [8]. The first EANS Training Course was held in Brussels in 1974. The activities of the Training Committee of the EANS had the following aims [5]:

1. To ascertain the current situation with regard to postgraduate training in neurosurgery in the member countries of the EANS.
2. To reach agreement on neurosurgical training of the different member countries and societies and to reach basic and minimal recommendations.
3. To influence the national societies and member countries to assume these minimal recommendations for training in neurosurgery endorsed by the EANS.
4. To continue and to systematically carry out the Postgraduate Course in Neurosurgery (very well organized by M. Brock during his chairmanship of the EANS Training Comittee).
5. To extend neurosurgical teaching outside Europe.
6. To examine the feasibility and usefulness of a European Certification Assessment in Neurosurgery.

Other EANS Training Activities (Calliauw)

Other training activities of the EANS include publications in an official journal of the EANS (*Acta Neurochirurgica*) and in *Advances and Technical Standards in Neurosurgery*. Other activities are an annual winter symposium (Vice-presidents' meeting) including coverage of a particular neurosurgical topic and the presentation of the European lecture, given by an outstanding European neurosurgical personality. Since 1985 advanced seminars in neurosurgical research have been held annually. The neurosurgical training activities also include courses for the Pan-Arab Union of Neurosciences every 2 years.

European Board of Neurosurgery (Braakman)

European Examination Practice

After completing a 5-year cycle of the European training courses, an oral examination – combined since a year ago with multiple choice questions – can be taken on a voluntary basis and successful candidates are then certificated.

Future Examination Practice

Science 1988, a committee consisting of seven neurosurgeons from different EANS countries has worked out proposals, which are to be discussed and, hopefully, accepted by the Administrative Council of the EANS during its meeting in September 1990, during the European Course in Neurosurgery in Jerusalem. A two-part examination has been proposed:

Part 1: A primary multiple choice examination which can be taken by any trainee in an official program in a European country, provided that this program is an officially accredited program for neurosurgery, that the trainee is in the 3rd year of training or later, and that the program director has consented to the trainee's taking the examination. Qualified neurosurgeons may also take this examination.

Part 2: If the first examination is passed successfully, a candidate may apply after a period of at least 18 months for a final, oral examination lasting 3 x 1 h, during which diagnostic procedures and the surgical management of specific cases will be discussed. This examination can only be taken 2 years or more after certification as a neurosurgeon by the appropriate national neurosurgical society (or other authorized institution). A survey of the operative experience gained during 1 continuous year of neurosurgical practice has to be presented and to be accepted as sufficient by the official examination board.

This examination is not compulsory but *voluntary*. It is not a substitute for the national license, but is intended rather to set a standard at the highest level. It is more a prize than a license. Generally speaking, the level of the diploma obtained by this examination will be higher than the level represented by a national license.

Neurosurgeons will not be the first physicians to introduce European examinations (Fahlbusch). European anesthesiologists have had good experience with European Board Examinations for several years [6].

The American Board of Neurosurgery also holds a voluntary examination; at present about 80% of American neurosurgeons have successfully passed it. It is a long procedure, but in contrast with the European position, an operative logbook is not obligatory. The examination is not obligatory and it is quite possible to start a practice without having passed it; however, at present it is almost impossible to obtain a position in the larger American hospitals without this diploma (E. Laws, personal communication).

Other Considerations for the Future

Rotating in Europe, as requested by Brihaye et al. [3] is not easy at present. Financial support from the Erasmus program, for example, is available only for teachers and medical students, not for neurosurgical residents.

It was recognized that exchange of neurosurgeons at various levels of training is theoretically possible. Where posts are advertised, discrimination among applicants on the basis of nationality can be eliminated. However, emphasis was placed more on prearranged exchanges between units as part of each country's training program.

Looking forward, the "European spirit" in neurosurgery [2] in the year 2000 would be: to keep the standard and to introduce it into eastern countries as well (Calliauw), better integration of the United Kingdom into the European Community (Brocklehurst), more integration and more compatibility (Keravel), and European Certification (Brock). There was general agreement about subspecialization [7] so as to resist the tendency to split into small groups, which would mean isolation. All specialists should receive a solid general training in neurosurgery and with only few exceptions should practice within an organized clinical framework. Personality is an important role in neurosurgical training, in the trainee as well as the teacher (Brock). The following personal characteristics are required: surgical ability, good character, integration of knowledge, decisive personality, manual skill.

Finally, there is an open discussion as how to influence the European Commission. "The EANS is not a university and has no legal status" [2]. For this reason, the European Commission can only be influenced via the Permanent Committee of European Physicians (CP) and the European Union of Medical Specialists (UEMS). Their members should meet as soon as possible. It would be wise to see the administrative mechanisms to present the views of neurosurgeons set up in the European Community before less informed regulations are drawn up (Brocklehurst).

References

1. Bammel E (1990) Die wichtigsten überregionalen Ärzteorganisationen in der EG aus der Sicht der Europäischen Vereinigung der leitenden Krankenhausärzte. Arzt und Krankenhaus 5:130–132
2. Brihaye J (1989) The European Spirit and the European Association of Neurosurgical Societies. (Tenth European Lecture.) Acta Neurochir (Wien) 99:1–10
3. Brihaye J, Brock M, Isamat F, Garfield J, Vigouroux R (1983) Assessment of neurosurgical departments and training in neurosurgery. Conclusions of a symposium of the EANS in Brussels, 1981. Acta Neurochir (Wien) 68:171–174
4. Guidetti B (1987) European courses of neurosurgery and other training and postgraduate education activities of the European Association of Neurosurgical Societies. Acta Neurochir (Wien) 85:115–128
5. Isamat F (1984) European neurosurgical education: report of the Chairman of the Training Committee of the EANS. Acta Neurochir (Wien) 71:317–330
6. Josten KU (1986) DEAA – Diploma of the European Academy of Anaesthesiology – Erfahrungen und Aussichten. Anasth. Intensivmed. 27:173–75
7. Mosberg WH, Castillo R, Acevedo CA, Asenjo A, Dinning TAR, Gonzalez-Monteagudo O, Kristiansen K, Pia HW, Ramamurthi B, Schurmann K (1982) Worldwide survey of neurosurgical training requirements and certifying mechanism: report of the Committee on Neurosurgical Eduation of the World Federation of Neurosurgical Societies. Neurosurgery 10:390–400
8. Rossi GF (1988) Subspecialisation in neurosurgery. (Ninth European lecture.) Acta Neurochir (Wien) 94:1–9

9. (1990) Der Arzt in Europa '93: Symposium der Urologen in Brüssel. Dt Ärztebl 24: C–1193
10. (1983) Europäisches Diplom für Anästhesiologie der Europäischen Akademie für Anästhesiologie. Anasth Intensivmed 11:378

EC Guidelines Relating to Neurosurgery

- Richtlinien des Rates
  für die gegenwärtige Anerkennung der Diplome, Prüfungszeugnisse und sonstigen Befähigungsnachweises des Arztes und für Maßnahmen zur Erleichterung der tatsächlichen Ausübung des Niederlassungsrechts und des Rechts auf freien Dienstleistungsverkehr. Richtlinie.
  Amtsblatt der Europäischen Gemeinschaften
  (= ABL) Nr. L 167/30.6.1975
- Richtlinien des Rates 75/363/EWG ABL. Nr. 167, 1975
- Richtlinien des Rates 8 2/76/EWG ABL. Nr. 43, 1982
- Richtlinien des Rates 89/594/EWG ABL. Nr. L 341/19 1989

Winning Poster Presentations

Perioperative Monitoring of Subarachnoid Hemorrhage: Transcranial Doppler Sonography and Somatosensory Evoked Potentials

R. Laumer, R. Steinmeier, F. Gönner, R. Fahlbusch, J. Schramm, M. Mück, B. Hinkelmann, and M. Purrucker[1]

Transcranial Doppler Sonography (TCDS) is a well-established method for detecting changes in flow velocities in basal cerebral arteries following subarachnoid hemorrhage. However, conclusions on cerebral blood flow cannot be directly drawn from such TCDS findings. In addition, recent investigations have shown further restrictions because of discrepancies between Doppler findings and patients' neurological status [1–3].

The usefulness of somatosensory evoked potentials (SEP) during aneurysm surgery has been reported in several studies and is widely accepted. Especially during temporary clipping of main branches of the basal cerebral arteries, the advantage of SEP monitoring is obvious. Descriptions of the perioperative use of this form of monitoring are contradictory [1, 4–6]. The present study aimed to evaluate the advantage of investigations combining TCDS and SEP monitoring.

Patients and Methods

In a prospective study, the relationship between SEPs, TCDS findings and clinical status was compared in 35 patients with subarachnoid hemorrhage.

Using TCDS (EME 3-D; Eden Medizinische Elektronik, Überlingen, FRG), the mean, systolic and diastolic velocities in the middle cerebral, anterior cerebral and internal carotid arteries were measured. The data relating to SEPs (Nicolet Pathfinder I; Nicolet Biomedical Instruments, Medusa, USA) were central conduction time (CCT) and the N20/N14 amplitude ratio after stimulation of the median nerve. The findings of serial combined SEP investigations and TCDS at 1- to 3-day intervals until discharge or death were compared to the neurological status.

Results

TCDS proved to be of very restricted reliability in the prediction of neurological deficits. Nine patients had mean velocities over 200 cm/s and systolic velocities over 300 cm/s without any concurrent signs of clinical deterioration. In these pa-

[1] Neurochirurgische Klinik mit Poliklinik, Universität Erlangen-Nürnberg, Schwabachanlage 6, W-8520 Erlangen, FRG

Advances in Neurosurgery, Vol. 19
W. J. Bock, Ch. Lumenta, M. Brock, M. Klinger (Eds.)

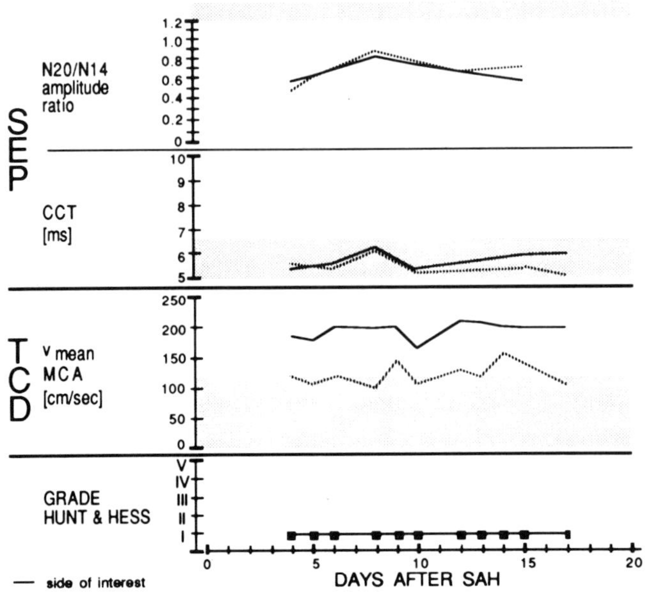

Fig. 1. A 26-year-old woman, operated on for an aneurysm of the right middle cerebral artery: constant Hunt and Hess grade I. While TCD indicated severe vasospasm on the affected side, with flow velocities around 200 cm/s, stable values for central conduction time and N20/N14 amplitude ratio seem to indicate good compensation

tients, stable CCT and N20/N14 amplitude ratios seemed to indicate adequate compensatory circulation (Fig. 1).

In Hunt and Hess grade IV patients, a normalization of increased flow velocities did not allow any prognostic conclusions. Simultaneous prolongation of CCT and decrease in amplitude, however, was found to correlate positively with poor outcome (Fig. 2).

Conclusion

TCDS is a sensitive and noninvasive method for detecting vasospasm patients with subarachnoid hemorrhage. However, its prognostic value in regard to delayed ischemic deficits is limited. Even high flow velocities, over 200 cm/s are not necessarily associated with deficits.In such cases, simultaneous SEP monitoring seems to be able to detect adequate compensation and improves the prognostic capacity of TCDS. In patients whose condition was Hunt and Hess grade IV or V, a normalization of flow velocities as detected by TCDS seemed to indicate that improvement was imminent although clinically the condition of the patients deteriorated. In such patients SEP monitoring can be used prognostically, since continuous prolongation of central conduction time and a reduction in the N20/N14 amplitude ratio was found to be in positive correlation to poor outcome.

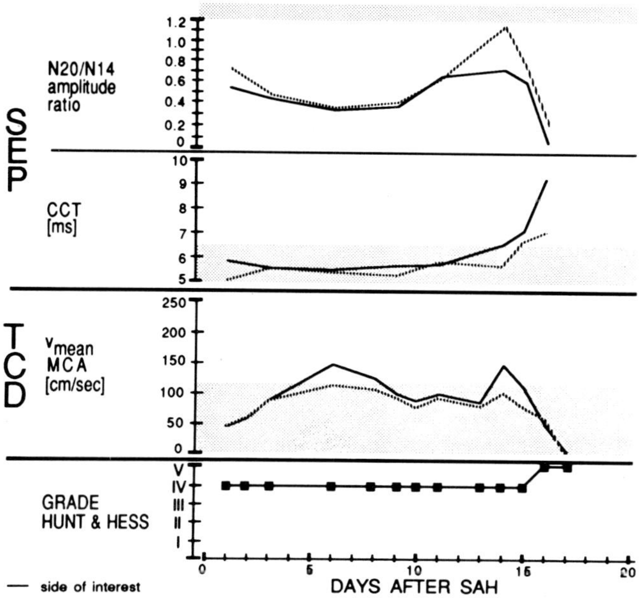

Fig. 2. A 42-year-old man, operated on for an aneurysm of the right internal carotid artery; deteriorated from Hunt and Hess grade IV to V. While TCD showed decreasing flow velocities, a continuous increase in central conduction time and decrease in N20/N14 amplitude ratio could be used to predict a poor outcome

References

1. Symon L, Compton J, Redmond S et al. (1988) Bedside monitoring in subarachnoid hemorrhage: Evoked responses, hemispheral blood flow, and flow velocity measurements. In: Wilkins RH (ed) Cerebral vasospasm. Raven, New York, pp 73–78
2. Laumer R, Steinmeier R, Priem R, Gönner F, Hinkelmann B, Purucker M. Schramm J (1988) Perioperative monitoring of aneurysmal subarachnoid hemmorhage by transcranial Doppler sonography and somatosensory evoked potentials. Preliminary report on the 2nd international conference of transcranial Doppler sonography, Salzburg, 27–30 Nov 1988
3. Laumer R, Steinmeier R, Vogtmann T, Gönner F, Mück M (1989) Stellenwert der transcraniellen Dopplersonographie beim Management der Subarachnoidalblutung. Nervenheilkunde 8:297–303
4. Suzuki A, Yasui N, Ito Z (1982) Brain dysfunction following vasospasm evaluated by somatosensory evoked potentials. Acta Neurochir 63:53–58
5. Symon L, Wang AD, Costa e Silva I, Gentili F (1984) Perioperative use of somatosensory evoked responses in aneurysm surgery, J Neurosurg 60:269–275
6. Wang AD, Cone J, Symon L, Costa e Silva IE (1984) Somatosensory evoked potential monitoring during management of aneurysmal SAH. J Neurosurg 60:264–268

Mechanisms of K^+-induced Glial Swelling*

H. Weigt, F. Staub, O. Kempski, J, Peters, F. v. Rosen, and A. Baethmann[1]

Abstract

The effect of high extracellular K^+ (K^+_e) on glial swelling was analyzed in vitro employing C6 glioma cells or astrocytes obtained from primary culture. The cells were suspended in an incubation chamber with continuous control of pH, temperature, and PO_2. Cell swelling was quantified by flow cytometry. After a control period, the K^+_e level in the suspension medium was increased to 30 m*M*, with maintenance of isotonicity and normal pH. Elevation of K^+_e led to an increase in cell volume by 7%–10% within 12 min. This was followed by spontaneous normalization of volume although K^+_e remained increased. The K^+-induced glial swelling was prevented by ouabain or by inhibition of glycolysis using iodoacetate. The findings indicate that cell swelling from high K^+_e results from intracellular accumulation of this ion secondary to activation of Na^+/K^+-ATPase. Cell swelling under these conditions is supported by enhanced intracellular formation of lactic acid resulting from K^+_e-induced stimulation of anaerobic metabolism.

Introduction

An important manifestation of ischemic brain edema is swelling of glial cells and of dendrites, i.e., cytotoxic brain edema [1, 7]. The underlying mechanisms resulting in ischemic brain edema are far from understood, perhaps because in ischemia many processes become simultaneously activated in a particularly complex tissue. Assessment of the molecular mechanisms underlying ischemic cell swelling and cell demage is therefore rather difficult. Accumulation of K^+ ions in the extracellular compartment is regularly observed in cerebral ischemia. It has been shown that interstitial K^+ concentrations in cerebral cortex may rise as high as 80 m*M* [9]. Therefore, it is conceivable that this phenomenon is involved in cytotoxic cell swelling, possibly damaging astrocytes and neurons.

In vitro conditions permit a high level of control, so that the significance of a single pathophysiological factor such as high K^+_e can be analyzed in isolation as to its function in the induction of cell swelling. C6 gliomas, which are employed in a variety of studies on glial function, have been used for this purpose [2, 8]. Many

---

* Supported by Deutsche Forschungsgemeinschaft ba 452/6–7

[1] Institut für Chirurgische Forschung, Klinikum Großhadern, Ludwig-Maximilians-Universität, Marchionistr. 15, W-8000 München 70, FRG

Advances in Neurosurgery, Vol. 19
W. J. Bock, Ch. Lumenta, M. Brock, M. Klinger (Eds.)

findings obtained using that cell line have been confirmed in experiments using astrocytes from primary culture [6].

Materials and Methods

C6 glioma cells [2] were cultivated as monolayers in Petri dishes using Dulbecco's modified minimal essential medium (DMEM) with 25 m*M* bicarbonate. The medium was supplemented with 10% fetal calf serum (FCS) and 100 IU/ml penicillin G and 50 µg/ml streptomycin. The cells were grown in a humidified atmosphere of 5% CO_2 and 95% room air at 37°C. Glial cells from primary culture were prepared from 3-day-old DB9 rats according to a method modified from the procedure described by Frangakis and Kimelberg [3]. The culture conditions were identical with those described above. For the experiments only confluent cultures were used. The cells were harvested with 0.05% trypsin-0.02% EDTA in phosphate-buffered saline and then washed twice. After resuspension in serum-free medium the glial cells were transferred to a plexiglas incubation chamber supplied with electrodes for control of pH, temperature, and pO_2. A gas-permeable silicon rubber tube in the chamber provided the suspended cells with a mixutre of O_2, CO_2, and N_2. Sedimentation of the cells was prevented by a magnetic stirrer. Further details of the in vitro model have been published elsewere [5, 6].

Cell volume was determined by flow cytometry using an advanced Coulter system with hydrodynamic focusing [4]. The effect of high K^+_e on the volume of the glial cells was analyzed by increasing K^+ in the suspension medium to 30 m*M* after a control period with a normal K^+ concentration. In additional experiments 1 m*M* ouabain or 2.5 m*M* iodoacetate were administered during the control period (15 min) prior to increasing the K^+ level in the medium.

Results

Table 1. Volume response of C6 glioma cells or astrocytes to increasing the K^+ concentration in the suspension medium to 30 m*M*. Means ± SEM of cell volume in 6 experiments as percentage of control

	Control			K^+_e = 30 m*M*					
Time (min)	–15	–10	–5	1	7	12	20	40	60
C6 glioma cells									
volume (%)	99.81	100.27	100.14	101.60	104.53	106.52	102.90	101.42	100.44
SEM	0.26	0.23	0.34	0.73	0.62	0.49	0.57	0.44	0.94
Primary culture									
volume (%)	100.12	100.04	99.84	101.20	107.85	109.97	106.21	104.75	103.04
SEM	0.30	0.27	0.55	0.91	1.93	2.09	1.58	1.90	1.39

Raising the K^+ concentration in the medium to 30 m*M* led to a volume increase of C6 glioma cells to 104.53 ± 0.62% (mean ± SEM) within 7 min ($p < 0.01$, Table 1). The maximum cell swelling was reached at 12 min, with an increase in cell volume to 106.52 ± 0.49% of control. This was followed by spontaneous volume normalization, although the extracellular K^+ level remained high. After 60 min, cell volume had completely recovered to normal (Table 1). A similar biphase volume response to raised K^+_e level was obtained in astrocytes from primary culture. Cell swelling was significant within 3 min ($p < 0.01$) after raising extracellular K^+ to 30 m*M*. Again a maximum was seen after 12 min, reaching 109.97 ± 2.09% of control. Cell volume normalized subsequently to 103.04 ± 1.39% within 60 min.

Additional experiments were performed to analyze the mechanisms of K^+-induced glial swelling. Inhibition of Na^+/K^+-ATPase by ouabain had no effect on cell volume during the control period [6]. However when, the K^+ concentration was elevated to 30 m*M*, cellular swelling was almost completely inhibited ($p < 0.01$). Similar re-sults were obtained by addition of iodoacetate to inhibit anaerobic glycolysis in the presence of 30 m*M* K^+. Then, cell volume of C6 glioma remained normal for about 20 min ($p < 0.01$), but it increased slightly during the following observation period. The viability of the glial cells was not adversely affected by any experimental condition during exposure to elevated K^+ concentrations in the medium.

Discussion

The data indicate that the mechanisms causing glial swelling and subsequent recovery from high K^+ concentrations are complex. A function of glial cells is clearance of K^+ ions from the extracellular space once their level exceeds the normal concentration [10]. Cellular uptake of K^+ involves Na^+/K^+-ATPase and thereby activates the energy metabolism. As shown, inhibition of the Na^+/K^+-ATPase by ouabain prevented swelling of the glial cells in response to high K^+ levels in the medium. Since uptake of K^+ ions is associated with a discharge of intracellular Na^+, however, activation of this process including Na^+/K^+-ATPase may still not suffice to explain the K^+-induced glial swelling. The activation of the ion pump results in an increased consumption of metabolic energy, which stimulates aerobic and anaerobic metabolism. Consequently, respiration and glycolysis increase, leading to enhanced formation of CO_2 and lactic acid. CO_2 associates with H_2O, forming H_2CO_3. The resulting carbonic acid decays into H^+- and HCO_3 ions, which are eliminated by the Na^+/H^+- and Cl^-/HCO_3^- antiporters, causing intracellular accumulation of Na^+ and Cl^-ions [6]. The activation of anaerobic glycolysis by supranormal K^+ levels in the medium may lead to intracellular accumulation of lactic acid; this can be concluded from the experiments conducted with the addition of iodoacetate to inhibit formation of lactic acid, in which the K^+-induced cell swelling was largely prevented. Finally, the spontaneous normalization of the cell volume after initial swelling from high K^+ levels requires a possible discharge of osmotic active solutes from the cells. The solutes may be lactate anions, which can leave the glial cells by utilizing specific transport mechanisms [11]. In conclusion, the present results support the idea that glial swelling induced by higher than normal K^+ levels in the culture medium reflects a homeostatic control function of these cells. The increase in cell volume may be the price paid for activation of a vital mechanism allowing reestablishment of the normal extracellular K^+ levels necessary for maintenance of neuronal function.

Acknowledgements. The excellent technical and secretarial assitance of Helga Kleylein, Dennise Linke, and Barbara Kempski is gratefully acknowledged.

References

1. Baethmann A (1978) Pathophysiological and pathochemical aspects of cerebral edema. Neurosurg Rev 1:85–100
2. Benda P, Lightbody J, Sato G, Levine L, Sweet W (1968) Differentiated rat glial cell strain in tissue culture. Science 161:370–371
3. Frangakis MV, Kimelberg HK (1984) Dissociation of neonatal rat brain by dispase for preparation of primary astrocyte cultures. Neurochem Res 9:1689–1698
4. Kachel V, Glossner E, Kordwig G, Ruhenstroth-Bauer G (1977) Fluvo-Metricell, a combined cell volume and cell fluorescence analyzer. J Histochem Cytochem 25:804–812
5. Kempski O, Chaussy L, Gross U, Zimmer M, Baethmann A (1983) Volume regulation and metabolism of suspended C6 glioma cells: an in vitro model to study cytotoxic brain edema. Brain res 279:217–228
6. Kempski O, Staub F, v Rosen F, Zimmer M, Neu A, Baethmann A (1988) Molecular mechanisms of glial swelling in vitro. Neurochem Pathol 9:109–125
7. Klatzo I (1967) Neuropathological aspects of brain edema. J Neuropath Exp Neurol 26:1–14
8. Pfeiffer SE, Betschart B, Cook J, Mancini P, Morris R (1977) Glial cell lines. In: Fedoroff S, Hertz L (eds) Cell, tissue, and organ cultures in neurobiology, Academic, New York, pp 287–346
9. Siemkowicz E, Hansen AJ (1981) Brain extracellular ion composition and EEG activity following 10 minutes ischemia in normo- and hyperglycemic rats. Stroke 12:236–240
10. Walz W, Hertz L (1984) Intense furosemide-sensitive potassium accumulation in astrocytes in the presence of pathologically high extracellular potassium levels. J Cereb Blood Flow Metabol 4:301–304
11. Walz W, Mukerji S (1988) Lactate release from cultured astrocytes and neurons: a comparison. Glia 1366–370

Effects of Anesthetic Agents on Brain Edema and Cerebral Blood Flow from a Focal Cold Lesion in Rabbit Brain*

R. Murr[1], L. Schürer[2], S. Berger[2], R. Enzenbach[1], and A. Baethmann[2]

Introduction

Brain edema is a major cause of morbidity and mortality in patients with severe head injury. Anesthetic agents, which often have to be administered in these patients for diagnostic or operative procedures, usually decrease cerebral metabolism [7]. On the other hand, inhalation anesthetics may increase cerebral blood flow (CBF) by vasodilation of brain vessels [1]. Therefore, anesthesia may either protect the injured brain by reduction of metabolism, or contribute to the spread of brain edema by cerebral hyperemia. To date, little information is available about the effect of anesthetic agents in traumatized brain. We therefore carried out experimental investigations to analyze the influence of isoflurane, fentanyl, thiopental, and α-chloralose on regional cerebral blood flow (rCBF) and formation of brain edema from a focal injury to the brain.

Materials and Methods

Four groups of six New Zealand White rabbits each were studied. In all groups, anesthesia was induced with thiopental. After tracheotomy and the start of artificial ventilation (30% O_2/70%, N_2, PCO_2 = 35–37 mmHg), the following anesthetic agents were administered: isoflurane (I) 1 minimal alveolor concentration (MAC) (in rabbits 2.1 vol%), fentanyl (F; per kg b.w.: 5 µg bolus, 90 min 1 µg/min, thereafter 0.5 µg/min), thiopental (T; 32.5 mg/kg b.w. per hour), and α-chloralose (C; 50 mg/kg b.w.). In the isoflurane group, angiotensin II at a mean dosage of 0.15 µg/kg b.w. min was given to support the blood pressure. Arterial and venous catheters were placed in femoral vessels for monitoring (mean arterial blood pressure, blood gases, hematocrit) and for administration of fluids and drugs. After fixation of the head, the left hemisphere was completely exposed by a rectangular trephination. Four platinum needle electrodes (diameter 75 µm) were then placed into the cortical gray matter at the lateral border of the skull window für measurement of rCBF by H_2 clearance. The electrodes were placed at different distances

* Supported by the Deutsche Forschungsgemeinschaft grant Ba 452/6–7

1 Anästhesiologisches Institut, Klinikum Großhadern, Ludwig-Maximilians-Universität, Marchionistr. 15, W-8000 München 70, FRG

2 Institut für Chirurgische Forschung, Klinikum Großhadern, Ludwig-Maximilians-Universität, Marchionistr. 15, W-8000 München 70, FRG

Advances in Neurosurgery, Vol. 19
W. J. Bock, Ch. Lumenta, M. Brock, M. Klinger (Eds.)

from the lesion, e.g. 5, 9, 13, and 17 mm from the center of trauma. The brain surface was protected by a thick layer of paraffin oil. After control measurements a focal cold lesion according to Klatzko [6] was induced in the occipital region of the brain. Measurements of rCBF were taken at intervals of 15 min in the 1st h, and 20 min during the remaining experimental period until termination of the experiment 6 h after trauma. The brain was then rapidly removed and frozen. For assessment of specific gravity (SG), the brain was sectioned in 7 coronal slices. Small tissue samples taken from standardized areas were immersed in a linear density column (Percoll) for assessment of SG.

Results

PCO_2 and hematocrit remained largely unchanged throughout the experimental course and did not differ between the groups. Arterial pressure was 78, 86, 72, and 88 mmHg in groups I, F, T, and C respectively. Control values of rCBF in the four groups ranged from 40 to 65 ml/100 g min. After induction of the lesion, market hyperemia of 30 60 min duration was observed with fentanyl (increase to 127%) and α-chloralose (increase to 204%) in the vicinity of the focus, while blood flow was only moderately altered with isoflurane (155%), or thiopental anesthesia (86%). In the later course of the experiment, rCBF remained largely unchanged in this area in animals receiving α-chloralose. On the other hand, regional perfusion close to the lesion decreased markedly below control with isoflurane, fentanyl, and thiopental anesthesia (–24%, –23%, –17%) 3–4 h after trauma. Also in areas distant from the lesion, a hyperemic response was observed in all groups subjected to different forms of anesthesia. Later, blood flow remained largely unchanged with thiopental, or increased moderately with α-chloralose. With fentanyl anesthesia, rCBF also decreased in areas distant to the lesion (–11%). Animals with isoflurane anesthesia, however, then had a marked and long-lasting second hyperemic response, with increases of flow to 122%. Further details of the cerebral blood flow response have been published elsewhere [8].

Values of SG averaged from two sections in the region of the lesion and the corresponding contralateral site are given in Table 1. Decreases in SG indicate an increased water content. In the lesioned hemisphere, a marked and significant

Table 1. Specific gravity (g/cm^3) of white matter in the vicinity of a focal lesion and in the corresponding regions of the contralateral hemisphere

Group	Lesion		Contralateral	
Isoflurane	1.0327 ± 0.0004	*n* = 33	1.0347 ± 0.0004	*n* = 24
Fentanyl	1.0321 ± 0.0005	*n* = 28	1.0341 ± 0.0004	*n* = 22
Thiopental	1.0319 ± 0.0005	*n* = 27	1.0341 ± 0.0004	*n* = 18
α-Chloral.	1.0306 ± 0.0006	*n* = 29	1.0332 ± 0.0004	*n* = 18

($p < 0.01$) decrease in SG was found compared to the corresponding region of the contralateral hemisphere. The lowest values for SG were found in α-chloralose anesthesia and were significantly different from the values with isoflurane or fentanyl anesthesia. There were no significant differences in SG between groups I, F, and T.

Discussion

The immediate and pronounced hyperemia after focal cold injury as observed with isoflurane and fentanyl anesthesia in our experiments is in contrast to other studies, where depression of blood flow was found in inverse relationship to distance from the lesion [3, 9]. However, in those studies, rCBF was not measured in the 1st h after trauma. Further, a closed-skull preparation was employed, allowing the intracranial pressure to rise quickly after trauma. This may have blunted the post-traumatic hyperemic response. Recent studies focusing on microcirculatory alterations from cerebral lesions have found brief hyperemia associated with pial vasodilation after fluid percussion injury or cold lesion [2, 11]. Since post-traumatic hyperemia may enhance the formation of brain edema, its extent and duration is of considerable clinical importance. While in our experiments isoflurane led to marked early and late hyperemia, with fentanyl hyperemia was limited to a period of 60–90 min after trauma. This was followed a decrease in flow in all regions later on. Animals receiving thiopental had only a moderate increase in blood flow after induction of the lesion, and the blood flow remained largely unchanged during the later experimental observation period.

In spite of the rather variable flow pattern, measurements of SG revealed no specific influence of anesthesia on the water content in groups C, F, and T. Inhalation anesthetics such as isoflurane are considered less suitable for neurosurgical procedures, since with a traumatized brain the agents may increase intracranial pressure and support the formation of brain edema [4, 10]. Recently, Kaieda et al. [5] have analyzed this question again, but found no differences between inhalation anesthetics and barbiturates in the formation of brain edema from a focal lesion. In addition to a hyperemic blood flow response, an increase of the systemic blood pressure may also contribute to the formation of vasogenic brain edema in the presence of a cerebral lesion. The comparatively high blood pressure observed in animals receiving α-chloralose may be responsible for the somewhat more pronounced extravasation of edema in this group. However, animals receiving fentanyl had an even higher blood pressure than those receiving thiopental, but there was no difference in the effect on brain edema formation in those groups.

In conclusion, despite the marked variety of blood flow response to focal trauma observed in animals subjected to different forms of anesthesia, the development of vasogenic brain edema was obviously not affected by the anesthetic procedures. However, this conclusion is valid only in open-skull conditions, in which brain swelling or increased cerebral blood flow are unlikely to result in an increase in intracranial pressure.

Summary

Anesthetic agents reduce cerebral metabolism and may impair coupling of cerebral blood flow and metabolism. We analyzed the effects of isoflurane (I; 1 MAC), fentanyl (F), thiopental (T; 32.5 mg/kg h) and α-chloralose (C) on regional cerebral blood flow (rCBF) and brain edema formation after a focal cerebral injury (cold lesion) in rabbits ($n = 6$ per group) In the isoflurane group, angiotensin II (0.15 µg/kg min) was given to maintain blood pressure. rCBF of cerebral cortex was measured three times an hour by H_2 clearance with needle electrodes placed at different distances to the lesion for 6 h after induction of trauma. Thereafter, samples of white matter were obtained from near the focal lesion and from corresponding areas of the contralateral hemisphere for measurement of specific gravity (SG) by a linear density column (Percoll). Blood pressure was 78, 86, 72, and 88 mmHg in groups I, F, T, and C, respectively. After induction of the lesion, hyperemia lasting approximately 1 h was observed in all groups. This was most pronounced distant from the lesion. Close to the lesion rCBF remained unchanged in groups C and T, but fell significantly below control in I and F. The blood flow response distant from the trauma was characterized by a moderate increase (C), or no alteration (T), while isoflurane animals had pronounced secondary hyperemia for about 3 h. With fentanyl, however, rCBF was markedly reduced in this area. The SG of white matter close to the lesion decreased significantly to values of 1.032 g/cm^3 (I, F, T) or 1.031 g/cm^3 (C), indicating edema. Specific gravity was 1.034 g/cm^3 in the contralateral hemisphere (control). The differences between groups I, F, and T in SG adjacent to the lesion were not statistically significant. However, significant differences were observed between the SG in group C and in the other groups. It is concluded that in an open-skull preparation, formation of post-traumatic brain edema from a focal cerebral lesion does not seem to be markedly affected by either hyperemia or a reduction of blood flow from various anesthetic agents, at least during the first few hours after trauma.

References

1. Cucchiara RF, Theye RA, Michenfelder JD (1974) The effects of isoflurane on canine cerebral metabolism and blood flow. Anesthesiology 40:571–574
2. DeWitt DW, Jenkins LW, Wei EP, Lutz HJ,. Becker DP, Kontos HA (1986) Effects of fluid percussion brain injury on regional cerebral blood flow and pial arterial diameter. J Neurosurg 64:787–794
3. Frei HJ, Wallenfang W, Pöll H, Reulen HJ, Schubert R, Brock M (1973) Regional cerebral blood flow and regional metabolism in cold induced oedema. Acta Neurochir 29:15–28
4. Grosslight K, Foster R, Colohan AR, Bedford RF (1985) Isoflurane for neuroanesthesia: risk factors for increases in intracranial pressure. Anesthesiology 63:533–536
5. Kaieda R, Todd MM, Weeks JB, Warner DS (1989) A comparison of the effects of halothane, isoflurane, and pentobarbital anesthesia on intracranial pressure and cerebral edema formation following brain injury in rabbits. Anesthesiology 71:571–579
6. Klatzko I, Piraux A. Laskowski EJ (1959) The relationship between edema, bloodbrain barrier and tissue elements in a local brain injury. J Neuropathol Exp Neurol 17:548–564

7. Michenfelder JD (1980) The cerebral circulation. In: Prys-Roberts C (ed) The circulation in anaesthesia. Blackwell, Oxford
8. Murr R, Berger S, Schürer L, Baethmann A (1989) Regional cerebral blood flow and tissue pO_2 after focal trauma: effects of isoflurane and fentanyl. In: Hammersen F, Messmer K (eds) Cerebral microcirculation. Karger, Basel, pp 61–70 (Progress in applied microcirculation)
9. Pappius HM (1981) Local cerebral glucose utilization in thermally traumatized brain. Ann Neurol 9:484–491
10. Smith AL, Marque JJ (1976) Anesthetics and cerebral edema. Anesthesiology 45:64–72
11. Yamamoto L, Soejima T, Meyer E, Feindel W (1976) Early hemodynamic changes at the microcirculatory level following cryogenic injury over the cortex. In: Pappius HM, Feindel W (eds) Dynamics of brain edema. Springer, Berlin Heidelberg New York, pp 59–62

Single-Stage Neuro-rhinosurgical Operation and Management of Malignant Tumors of the Anterior Cranial Skull Base

U. Neubauer[1], R. Fahlbusch[1], M.E. Wigand[2], and M. Weidenbecher[2]

Introduction

The anatomical relationships in malignant tumors of the anterior cranial skull base with additional involvement of both the intracranial space and the paranasal sinuses, the orbit, and the nasal cavity has resulted in different surgical approaches to these tumors. Most authors prefer separate transcranial and transfacial approaches. We present the method and results of a single-stage transcranial–transbasal approach which permits total removal of the tumor without an additional transfacial operation. The authors' experiences with this technique in the treatment of esthesioneuroblastomas have already been reported on elsewhere [5].

Patients and Methods

Twelve patients with malignant tumors of the anterior cranial fossa were treated between 1984 and 1990. The average age of the patients was 43 years; the youngest was 6 and the oldest 76 years old. The sexes were equally affected, with 6 male and 6 female patients. The most frequent symptom was impaired nasal breathing, followed by anosmia and epistaxis (Table 1).

Table 1. Clinical symptoms of 12 patients undergoing the single-stage operation

Symptom	No. of patients
Nasal obstruction	10
Anosmia	9
Epistaxis	6
Proptosis	5
Signs of increased intracranial pressure	2

[1] Neurochirurgische Klinik mit Poliklinik, Universität Erlangen-Nürnberg, Schwabachanlage 6, W-8520 Erlangen, FRG

[2] Hals-Nasen-Ohren-Klinik, Universität Erlangen-Nürnberg, Waldstr. 1, W-8520 Erlangen, FRG

Advances in Neurosurgery, Vol. 19
W. J. Bock, Ch. Lumenta, M. Brock, M. Klinger (Eds.)

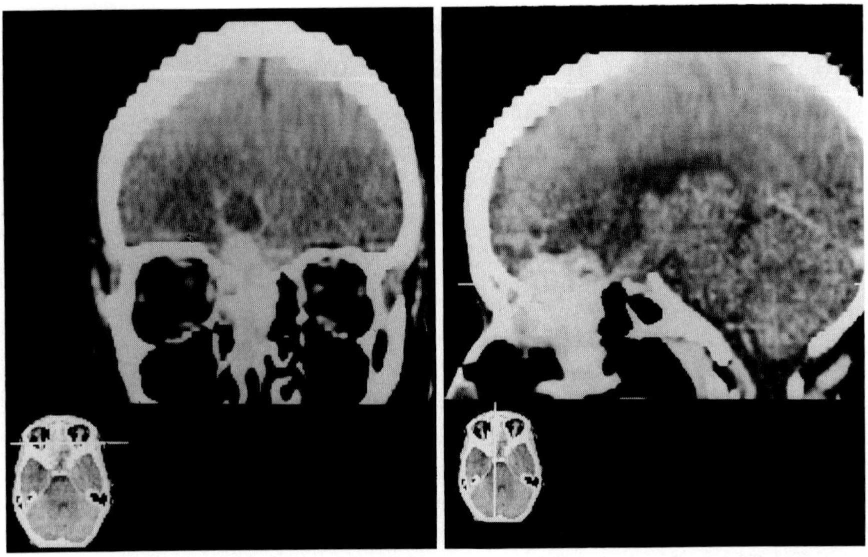

a b

Fig. 1. **a** Frontal and **b** sagittal computed tomograms of adenocystic carcinoma of the anterior skull base with some cystic intracranial growth

Diagnosis

All patients were investigated by plain radiography and computed tomography which clearly revealed the intra- and extracranial extent of tumor growth and the bony destruction of the skull base (Fig. 1). The histological diagnosis was confirmed by endoscopic biopsy.

Operative Treatment

1. The procedure starts with a bifrontal craniotomy with the patient lying supine. A large pedicled pericranial flap is preserved, later to be utilized for the closure of the skull base.
2. The intracranial part of the tumor is removed.
3. The affected basal dura and skull base are resected, giving access to the frontal, ethmoidal and sphenoidal sinuses.
4. The tumor within these sinuses is removed.
5. If the orbit is involved, it is opened from the roof and medial wall and all tumor tissue resected.
6. The tumor in the nasal cavity and maxillary sinuses is resected.
7. The skull base is closed with two layers of autologous material only: fascia lata and a pedicled pericranial flap. No bone grafts or any artificial material is used.

Results

The postoperative follow-up and adjuvant irradiation therapy in our 12 patients has now reached 3–44 months (mean 20.3 months). The long-term survival rate is 83%. Two of our 12 patients died due to local recurrences or distant metastasis between 10 and 13 months after surgery.

Among the survivors with a mean follow-up of 21.9 months, we have five (41%) with tumor recurrence diagnosed 8–30 months postoperatively. These patients have been living with their recurrent tumor for an average of 13.8 months. Five patients (41%) have been free of recurrence for between 3 and 36 months (mean 20.2 months).

Complications of the method are rare: in our series, one infected bone flap and one intracerebral hematoma of uneventful course (Table 2).

Table 2. Management of 12 patients undergoing the single-stage operation

	Age	Sex	Tumor location[a]	Histol. diagnosis	Irradiation	Complications	Follow-up
1.	53	M	1, 2, 4, 6, 7	Adenocystic carcinoma	Postop.	–	Recurrence 30 mo. Alive 43 mo.
2.	52	M	1, 2, 6	Adenocystic carcinoma	Postop.	–	Alive 31 mo.
3.	31	F	1, 2, 4, 7	Adenocystic carcinoma	Postop.	osteo- myelitis	Recurrence 25 mo. Alive 44 mo.
4.	29	M	1, 2, 4, 6	Undiff. carcinoma	Postop.	–	Recurrence 12 mo. Alive 36 mo.
5.	51	M	1, 2, 6	Adenocystic carcinoma	Postop.	–	Recurrence 8 mo. Alive 27 mo.
6.	47	M	1	Adenocystic carcinoma	Preop.	–	Died 10 mo.
7.	53	M	1, 2, 5, 6	Squamous cell carcinoma	Preop.	–	Recurrence 6 mo. Died 13 mo.
8.	76	F	1, 6	Adenocystic carcinoma	Postop.	ICH	Recurrence 22 mo. Alive 28 mo.
9.	51	F	1, 6, 7	Squamous cell carcinoma	Postop.	–	Alive 6 mo.
10.	6	F	1, 2, 4	Rhabdomyosarcoma	Preop.	–	Alive 35 mo.
11.	8	F	1, 2, 4, 6	Rhabdomyosarcoma	Preop.	–	Alive 23 mo.
12.	74	F	1–7	Chondrosarcoma	Postop.	–	Alive 3 mo.

[a] 1, Nasal cavity; 2, Ethmoidal sinus; 3, Frontal sinus; 4, Sphenoidal sinus; 5, Maxillary sinus; 6, Intracranial (subfrontal); 7, Orbit

Conclusion

The transcranial–transbasal approach to malignant tumors of the anterior cranial skull base allows radical removal of these tumors with additional transfacial operation. The use of bone grafts and homologous material for the closure of the skull base, as recommended in the literature [1, 3, 4, 7], is unnecessary. Long-term survival and complication rates are comparable to those associated with the combined approaches [2, 6, 8].

References

1. Arita N, Shintaro M, Sano M, Hayakawa T, Nakao K, Kanai N, Mogami H (1989) Surgical treatment of tumors in the anterior skull base using the transbasal approach. Neurosurgery 24(3):379–384
2. Cheesman A, Lund VJ, Howard DJ (1986) Craniofacial resection for tumors of the nasal cavity and paranasal sinuses. Head Neck Surg 8:429–435
3. Derome PJ (1984) Transbasal approach to tumors invading the base of the skull. In: Schmidek HH, Sweet WH (eds) Operative neurosurgical techniques, 1. Grune and Stratton, New York, pp 357–379
4. Draf W, Samii M (1989) Surgery of malignant space occupying lesions of the anterior skull base. In: Samii M, Draf W (eds) Surgery of the skull base. Springer, Berlin Heidelberg New York Tokyo, pp 224–230
5. Fahlbusch R, Neubauer U, Wigand M, Weidenbecher M, Röckelein G, Thierauf G, Sauer R (1989) Neuro-rhinosurgical treatment of aesthesioneuroblastoma. Acta Neurochir (Wien) 100:93–100
6. Ketcham AS, Chretien PB, Van Buren JM (1973) The ethmoid sinuses: a re-evaluation of surgical resection. Am J Surg 126:469–476
7. Rosen EM, Simeone FA, Bruce DA (1986) Single stage composite resection and reconstruction of malignant anterior skull base tumors. Neurosurgery 18:7–11
8. Van Buren JM, Ommaya AK, Ketcham AS (1968) Ten years experience with radical combined cranio-facial resection of malignant tumors of the paranasal sinuses. J Neurosurg 28:341–350

Vascular Malformations of the Brain

Diagnostic and Interventional Neuroradiology of Brain Arteriovenous Malformations: Implications on Angioarchitecture for Embolization

A. Valavanis[1] and W. Müller-Forell[2]

Introduction

The introduction of high-field, high-resolution magnetic resonance imaging (MRI) and recent advances in the field of superselective neuroangiography have significantly improved the neuroradiologic evaluation of brain arteriovenous malformations (AVMs) and contributed to a more profound understanding of their angioarchitectural and hemodynamic features. In turn, this recently accumulated knowledge has influenced the indications, goals, and techniques of embolization of brain AVMs. This paper summarizes our experience with the use of high-field MRI, superselective angiography, and embolization in assessment and treatment of 108 patients with brain AVMs between 1986 and 1990, and reviews the recent literature on the subject.

Neuroradiologic Assessment

Thorough neuroradiologic assessment of cerebral AVMs is essential before deciding how to proceed with treatment in a given case. The neuroradiologic assessment should include multiplanar T1- and T2-weighted MRI and complete superseletive angiography of the lesion.

MRI has proved superior to computed tomography (CT) in delineating the topography of AVMs and depicting associated changes in the surrounding brain parenchyme [6]. However, for emergency examination of patients with cerebral AVMs, e.g., after acute hemorrhage or stroke, CT still represents the modality of choice, because it is readily accessible and rapidly provides information on the underlying cause of the patient's acute clinical deterioration.

On MRI, AVMs presents a signal-void area consisting of dilated vessels arranged in a coiled, vermiform pattern [2]. In the vicinity of the nidus of the AVM dilated vessels can be recognized, which are the feeding arteries and draining veins. Typically, draining veins are larger and less convoluted than feeding arteries and can be shown to converge towards a superficiall by and/or deeply located sinus, depending on the location of the AVM.

[1] Abteilung für Neuroradiologie, Universitätsspital Zürich, CH-8091 Zürich, Switzerland
[2] Abteilung für Neuroradiologie, Universitätsklinik Mainz, W-6500 Mainz, FRG

Advances in Neurosurgery, Vol. 19
W. J. Bock, Ch. Lumenta, M. Brock, M. Klinger (Eds.)

A complete protocol for MRI examination of any case of cerebral AVM should include a triplanar T1-weighted and an axial T2-weighted series of images. The triplanar T1-weighted series allow precise topographic evaluation of the AVM in respect to gyri, sulci, subcortical white matter, deep nuclei, and the ventricular system. The T2-weighted series is necessary in order to detect new or old parenchymal changes in the brain around the AVM, such as infarction, gliosis, or hemorrhage [6]. The MRI examination is also essential in planning the selective and superselective angiographic evaluation of a cerebral AVM.

The aim of the neuroangiographic assessment is to provide the information on the angioarchitectural features, hemodynamic characteristics, and vascular morphology of the AVM needed in order to plan the treatment strategy.

The neuroangiographic examination should for preference be performed with the patient awake and mildly sedated, using a femoral approach, nonionic contrast material, and the digital subtraction technique. In neonates and children under the age of 12–14 the examination should be performed under general anesthesia.

Angioarchitecturally, an AVM consists of feeding arteries, a nidus, and draining veins. Selective angiography should allow detection of the number and type of arteries participating in supplying the malformation, the size and configuration of the nidus, and the number and type of veins draining it. In addition, associated angioarchitectural features, such as saccular aneurysms located on feeding arteries, direct arteriovenous fistulous connections within the nidus, and stenotic changes and varicose dilatations of draining veins or the absence of expected draining veins, should be detected. Superselective angiography involves catherization of each individual feeding artery identified by selective angiography. It is performed with flow-independent, steerable microcatheters inserted coaxially through the regular catheter used for selective angiography and advanced with the help of a microguidewire towards the target feeding artery.

Topographically, supra- and infratentorial AVMs are classified into two major types: convexial and central [9]. Convexial AVMs are located within sulci and/or gyri. Their dominant supply is from branches of the cortical arteries, i.e., anterior, middle or posterior cerebral arteries, supratentorially, and superior, anterior-inferior or posterior-inferior cerebellar arteries infratentorially. Depending on their size and specific location in respect to vascular territories, one or more cortical arteries may participate into their supply, while depending on their extension towards the subcortical white matter and paraventricular area and/or towards the dural surface of the brain, they are additionally supplied by deep perforating arteries (e.g., lenticulostriate branches of middle cerebral artery) or from meningeal arteries.

Central AVMs involve the deep structures of the brain, such as the striocapsulothalamic area, the caudate nucleus, the corpus callosum, the hippocampus, the mensencephalon, pons, medulla oblongata, choroid plexus of the ventricles, or paraventricular white matter. Their supply is mainly from perforating arteries arising from the circle of Willis or the vertebrobasilar system and from the choroid arteries.

On the basis of superselective angiographic findings and intraoperative observations [9], the feeding arteries of brain AVMs may be classified into two types: terminal and transit. Terminal type feeding arteries end directly in the nidus after giving off normal branches more proximally. A safe microcatheter position for subsequent embolization of terminal type feeding arteries is on the distal segment just proximal to the nidus and beyond normal branches.

Transit type feeding arteries supply the AVM through small branches while the main stem of the artery continues its course to supply normal brain distal to the AVM. Where there are transit feeding arteries, catheterization of each branch feeding artery is necessary for safe embolization, as embolization performed with the microcatheter in the main stem of the transit feeding artery carries a high risk of occluding the normal segment of the artery distal to the AVM causing cerebral infarction.

In approcimately 20% of cases of brain AVMs, superselective angiography discloses saccular aneurysms or microaneurysms located at the branching sites of feeding arteries [3, 8]. Such aneurysms are thought to be caused by the increased flow and altered hemodynamics of the feeding arterial system and are called related aneurysms [9]. Since related aneurysms are flow-induced, embolization of the nidus of the AVM, with subsequent reduction of flow in what was previously a feeding artery, is expected to cause regression of the aneurysm. Related aneurysms represent one of the main risk factors for hemorrhage of an AVM, and their incidence in AVMs which have already bled has been shown to be as high as 41% [8]. If a related aneurysm is present in an AVM classified as inoperable and referred for palliative embolization, a reasonable course appears to be to direct embolization towards that portion of the AVM which is fed by the artery bearing the aneurysm. Regression of such an aneurysm following partial embolization may significantly reduce the risk of future hemorrhage.

Superselective angiography has provided new insights into the instrinsic architecture and vascular composition of the brain AVM nidus. Superselective angiographic studies show the nidus to be composed of a pathologically dilated arteriovenous vascular bundle of plexiform arrangement and variable size and shape. Usually, convexial AVMs have a pyramid-shaped nidus with the base located on the cortical surface of the brain and the tip directed towards the paraventricular area. Central AVMs usually have an oval or round nidus. In up to 4% of cases, superselective angiography reveals direct arteriovenous fistulas within the plexiform nidus [8]. Such high-flow fistulous arteriovenous connections within the nidus may well cause an arterial steal effect and therefore be responsible for ischemic phenomena in the surrounding brain [1]. Selective embolization of such a fistula in an otherwise not totally obliterable plexiform AVM may redistribute flow towards a previously ischemic area and therefore reduce some existing neurologic deficits.

The nidus is usually composed of multiple compartments, the number of which depends on the number of feeding arteries. Each compartment of the nidus represents a vascular hemodynamic unit characterized by a feeding artery and draining vein. The goal of embolization is obliteration of each superselectively identified compartment of the nidus, not merely occlusion of the feeding arteries.

Of special importance in the assessment of brain AVMs is identification of the draining veins and their angioarchitectural and hemodynamic features. The type of veins participating in the drainage of an AVM depends primarily on the specific location of the malformation, its size, and its extension. As a general rule, convexial AVMs are drained by superficial, cortical veins. If such AVMs extend subcortically towards the ventricular system, they are additionally drained by deep, subependymal veins. Central AVMs almost invariably drain towards the deep, subependymal system.

Application of the technique of superselective angiography to the assessment of brain AVMs in the past few years has disclosed a high incidence of anomalies in the draining venous system in brain AVMs. These associated venous anomalies mainly consist of stenosis of draining veins various distances downstream of the AVM, varicose dilatation of the postnidal segment of draining veins, reflux of contrast material into venous systems remote from the AVM, absence of expected draining veins, and recruitment of transcerebral veins [7–9]. Such associated venous anomalies are observed in up to 40% of brain AVMs [8]. From a hemodynamic point of view these associated venous anomalies indicate hyperpressure within the nidus, and, indeed, statistical correlation of the incidence of hemorrhage with such venous anomalies has revealed that high-grade stenosis of the draining vein(s) and varicose dilatation of draining veins are angiographically present in more than 50% of AVMs which have already bled [8].

Embolization

Depending on the complexity of the AVM as assessed angiographically, embolization may be performed either during the same session or at another time. With larger AVMs multiple sessions are usually performed. In children up to the age of 12–14 years, embolization should be performed under general anesthesia. In adults, embolization should be performed with the patient awake and appropriately sedated, so that neurologic testing can be performed throughout the procedure.

Among the various embolic agents currently available for embolization of brain AVMs, including microparticles of polyvinylalcohol (PVA), isobutyl-2-cyanoacrylate, *n*-butyl-cyanoacrylate, silk sutures, microcoils, and avitene, the cyanoacrylates have proved the most efficient material. Cyanoacrylate produces permanent endovascular occlusion and, if properly injected, causes obliteration of the nidus itself. However, this material is rather difficult to handle, may cause gluing of the catheter within the vascular system, and therefore requires considerable experience.

During the past 10 years embolization has constantly gained in acceptance as an important technique in the management of patients with cerebral AVMs. The refinement of technical tools and embolic materials and an improved understanding of the complex angioarchitecture and hemodynamics of cerebral AVMs have contributed to the establishment of embolization as one of the available therapeutic options for cerebral AVMs.

Depending on a variety of factors including the clinical condition and neurologic presentation of the patient, the size and location of the AVM as assessed by multiplanar MRI, and the angioarchitectural and hemodynamic characteristics of the latter as determined by superselective angiography, embolization may be performed as either a preoperative, a palliative, or a curative procedure.

Preoperative embolization is mainly performed in large or medium-sized AVMs that are potentially operable [4]. The goal of embolization is partial obliteration of the lesion and occlusion of surgically inaccessible or less well accessible, mainly deep feeding arteries. These measures contribute to a reduction of operation time and increase the rate of radical removal [4].

Palliative embolization is carried out in AVMs classified as inoperable because of size and/or location and in which partial embolization is expected to improve certain symptoms or neurologic deficits and to reduce the probability of recurrent hemorrhage. The goal of palliative embolization is to occlude arteriovenous fistulous connections within the AVM, thus reducing the steal effect on the surrounding brain, and to obliterate those parts of the AVM that are associated with aneurysms on the feeding arteries or venous ectasias of the draining veins, thus potentially reducing the risk of hemorrhage.

Curative embolization achieved exclusively by endovascular techniques is currently feasible in approximately 8%–20% of cases referred for interventional neuroradiologic treatment [1]. The majority of patients referred for neuroradiologic treatment harbor the more complex types of cerebral AVMs in terms of size, location, number of feeding arteries, and angioarchitectural characteristics, which explains the rather low rate of complete obliteration achieved by embolization. The goal of curative embolization is complete obliteration of the AVM with preservation of the vascular supply to the normal surrounding brain. Technically, this is currently possible in 70%–80% of cases with small and some medium-sized AVMs supplied by a limited number of feeding arteries accessible to superselective catheterization. This group of AVMs includes lesions that are easily and safely resectable by microsurgical techniques, but also deeply located AVMs which are not, or not so easily, accessible to microsurgical techniques.

A further use of embolization of cerebral AVMs is to reduce the size of some medium-sized and small AVMs in which complete endovascular obliteration is technically not possible and surgical removal is thought to be associated with significant risks, so that subsequent radiosurgery may result in complete obliteration of the lesion [5].

The main complications of embolization of brain AVMs include hemorrhage and infarction. Hemorrhage may result from rupture of nidus following early obliteration of a main or single draining vein, or, very rarely, from perforation of a feeding artery during manipulation with the microguidewire. Infarction will result if branches of feeders supplying brain distal to the AVM have been unintentionally occluded. Such complications may lead to recovery, permanent neurologic deficit, or death. Currently, the overall incidence of permanent neurologic deficits following embolization is 5%–7% and the mortality 3%–6% [1].

References

1. Berenstein A (1990) Cerebral arteriovenous malformations. AJNR 11:220 (abstract)
2. Biondi A, Scialfa G (1988) Morphological and blood flow MR findings in cerebral vascular malformations. J Neuroradiol 15:253–265
3. Lasjaunias P, Piske R, Terbrugge K, Willinsky R (1988) Cerebral arteriovenous malformations (C. AVM) and associated arterial aneurysms (AA). Analysis of 101 C AVM cases, with 37 AA in 23 patients. Acta Neurochir (Wien) 91:29–36
4. Pelz DM, Fox AJ, Vinuela F, Drake CC, Ferguson GG (1988) Preoperative embolization of brain AVM's with isobutyl-2 cyanoacrylate. AJNR 9:757–764
5. Steiner L (1984) Treatment of arteriovenous malformations by radiosurgery. In: Wilson CB, Stein BM (eds) Intracranial arteriovenous malformations. Williams and Wilkins, Baltimore, pp 295–314
6. Valavanis A, Schubinger O, Wichmann W (1986) Classification of brain arteriovenous malformation nidus by magnetic resonance imaging. Acta Radiol [Suppl] 369:86–89
7. Vinuela F, Nombela L, Roach MR et al. (1985) Stenotic and occlusive disease of the venous drainage system of deep brain AVM's. J Neurosurg 63:180–184
8. Willinsky R, Lasjaunias P, Terbrugge K, Pruvost P (1988) Brain arteriovenous malformations. Analysis of the angioarchitecture in relationship to hemorrhage. J Neuroradiol 15:225–227
9. Yasargil MB (1988) Microneurosurgery, vol. IIIA. Thieme, New York

Embolization Techniques in the Treatment of Cerebral Arteriovenous Malformations

B. Richling and G. Bavinzski[1]

Cerebral embolization techniques have been modified greatly since Serbinenko first approached the cerebral artery with a microballoon [2]. During the last few years, flow-guided balloon systems with or without calibrated leak have become replaced by microcatheters of so-called "progressive softness". These guidewire-supported catheter systems permit low-flow vessels to be approached independent of flow when the approach is limited more by the small diameter of the vessels than by the sharp angle of the bifurcations [1]. Further reductions in size (e.g. Tracker 10, Target Therapeutic Corporation, California, USA) nowadays allow even the most delicate vessels to be approached effectively, e.g., cerebral vessels in pediatric patients (Fig. 1) or perforating arteries.

There are two disadvantages of the wire-guided catheter as opposed to be ballon-directed system. The first is the considerable resistance encountered as the wire is advanced into the small vessels. The second is the inability to temporarily occlude any small vessel as with the balloon system. This temporary blockage of flow by the calibrated-leak balloons is particularly useful for flushing the distal vasculature with glucose solution, allowing better distribution of the acrylic glue. Notwithstanding, guidewire-supported, flow-independent, progressive-softness microcatheters have revolutionized the possibilities of endovascular neurosurgery.

The choice of embolic material depends on the specific goal of treatment. Traditional calibrated-leak balloon systems only permitted injections of low-viscosity liquids (e.g., acrylates); progressive-softness microcatheters now permit injections of very finely grained particulates [e.g., PVA (Polyvincyl-alcohol) particles]. When the position of the catheter tip is optimum relative to the arteriovenous malformation (AVM; Fig. 1), fine particulates permit stepwise and safe embolization. The slow buildup of the particulates from the level of the AVM fistula to more proximal locations by the controlled slowdown of the flow allows visualization of physicological and pathological vessels that were invisible before the partial occlusion of the shunt.

The use of particulates also has disadvantages. Because particulates mix with blood clots in an angioma, they will not occlude the AVM compartment permanently. Therefore, they can only be used for preoperative embolization. The alcohol present in the mixture of particulates, collagen, and contrast material increases the

[1] Neurochirurgische Universitätsklinik Wien, Währinger Gürtel 18–20, A-1090 Wien, Austria

Advances in Neurosurgery, Vol. 19
W. J. Bock, Ch. Lumenta, M. Brock, M. Klinger (Eds.)

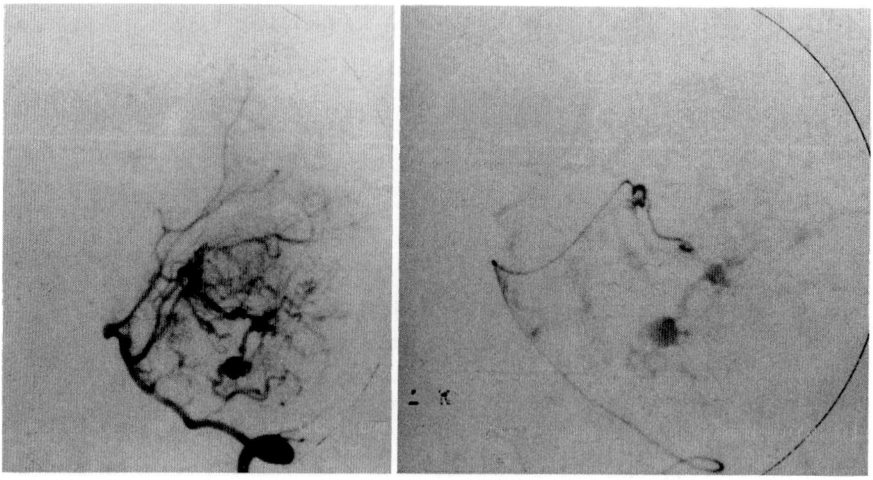

Fig. 1. Child aged 12 years. AVM of the upper vermis with unusual venous drainage. Small microcatheter (Tracker 10) allows endovascular approach close to the nidus via the superior cerebellar artery

formation of fibrotic material but almost never causes permanent occlusion (Fig. 2).

Acrylates are also used to embolize cerebral AVMs. Acrylate, usually as the glue Acryl-Monomer, immediately polymerizes on contact with free H^+ ions. This rapid chemical reaction leads to the typical problems and risks associated with the use of acrylates as embolic material. These problems include a stuck catheter, inadvertent venous occlusion, irreversible occlusion of vital arteries, and animal toxicity. However, the toxic effects observed in animal models have not been seen in patients. The consensus in the literature is that this toxicity does not contraindicate its use [4].

The goal of embolizing cerebral AVMs is to produce a solid cast of the nidus with the acrylate, if possible with no blood inclusions (Fig. 3). Only complete casting of the nidus channels by the embolic material provides optimal assurance against recanalization; otherwise, the angioma will recanalize. The effect of the "drop-by-drop" method (acrylate spots of various size in the angioma) is similar to that of embolization with particulates but lacks the simplicity and assurance of the latter. In multicompartmental AVMs, closure of the feeding arteries by acrylate (like occlusions by detachable balloons, coils, or surgical ligation) does not even produce a temporary effect. Single-vessel occlusion is indicated only for a simple, high-flow fistula; we recommend using detachable balloons or coils rather than the hard-to-control acrylate.

The difficulties associated with controlling the distribution and setting of the acrylate not only contribute to the instability of the embolization, but can also create other complications. For example, the catheter tip can become glued to the vessel wall (usually without further consequences). Worse, the draining vein can become occluded, causing a rupture or venous infarction.

a b

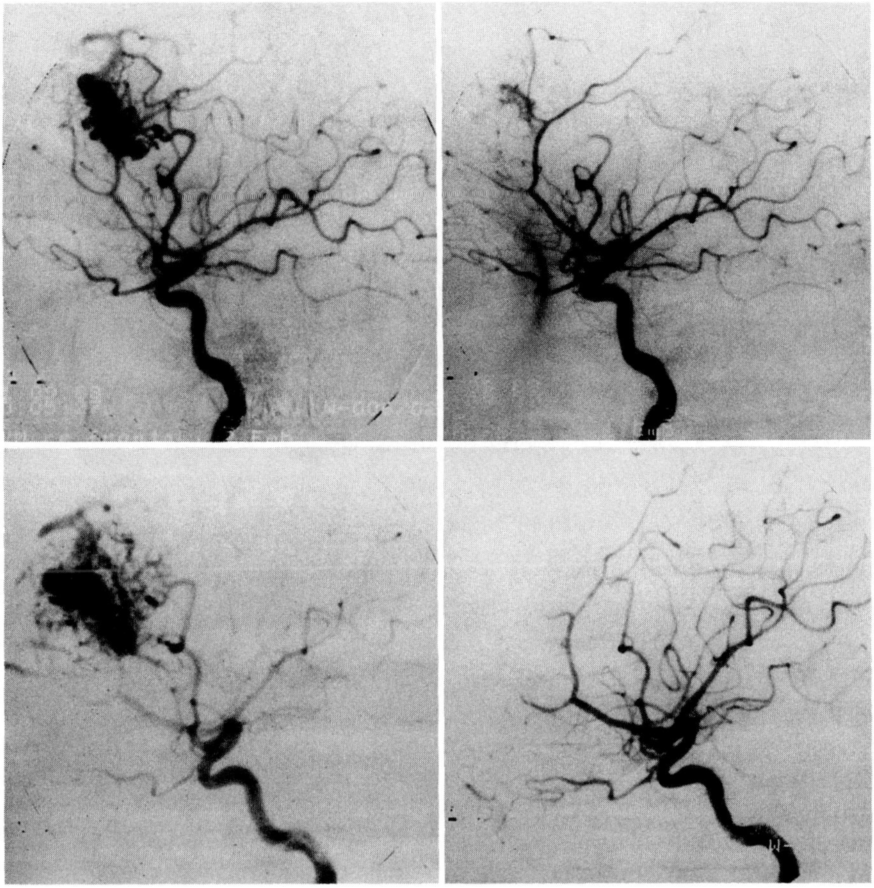

c d

Fig. 2a–d. Left frontal AFM **a** before and **b** after embolization with a mixture of alcohol, collagen, particulates, and contrast media. **c** Angiogram after 6 months showing recanalization of the malformation. **d** After embolization with Histoacryl

Fundamentally, the goal of treatment is total surgical excision or total and permament occlusion. Modern catheter techniques appear to achieve permanent and total occlusion in about 20%–25% of angiomas, although current follow-up periods are no more than 3–5 years (Table 1). However, when the long-term results are evaluated, the outcomes of endovascular and surgical therapy should be compared. The interventional neurosurgeon will also encounter many angiomas considered to be inoperable but amenable to embolization, such as those located in the basal ganglia, large angiomas of the left central area, or diffuse angiomatosis (Table 1). Most surgically "simple" angiomas are likewise easy to embolize; therefore, the rate of total occlusion should also be higher in an identical population of angiomas.

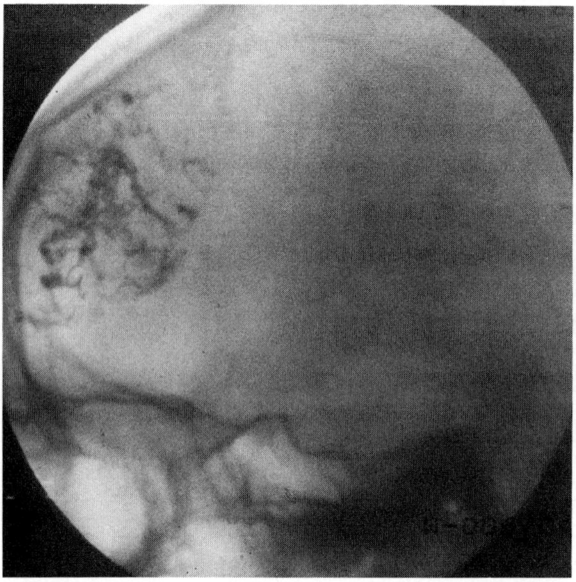

Fig. 3. Plain X-ray showing casting of the frontal AVM (lower left)

The following categories of angiomas are therefore suitable for embolization. First, there are the so-called simple angiomas. These are located in noneloquent regions of the brain and have only one or two feeders (the classification by Spetzler [3] is of limited use from an endovascular point of view). Simple angiomas are not only easily operable but can also be embolized permanently. Secondly, there are nonoperable angiomas or angiomas operable only at high risk, such as those located in the basal ganglia or brain stem. This group of malformations can sometimes be totally, but more often only partially, occluded. From an endovascular point of view, these inoperable or high-risk malformations constitute a primary indication for embolization. In between these two extremes lie a large number of midgrade angiomas that challenge the surgeons's personal skills. In these angiomas, embolization will be used either to achieve a solid casting or, if this is not possible, to make the operation easier through preoperative embolization.

At the University of Vienna, Department of Neurosurgery, embolization is the first step of treatment (even for simple AVMs) when an AVM appears from the angiogram to be endovascularly approachable and if no emergency operation is needed or no space-occupying hemorrhage is present. The embolization (in 1–3 stages) will lead to either a total or a partial occlusion. Again, the stability of the embolization will depend on the solidity of the casting. Partially embolized AVMs are operated on unless the risk associated with the natural history of the lesion is less than the surgical risk, as may be the case with huge AVMs of the basal ganglia.

Table 1. Cerebral AVMs treated from 1985 to July 1990 ($n = 91$): Localization and results

Localization	Emb. only ($n = 68$)	Emb. + op. ($n = 10$)	Op. only ($n = 13$)
Frontal	8	1	1
Temporal	3	1	0
Sylvian	2	1	1
Central	13	2	1
Left angular	4	0	3
Parieto-occip.	1	0	2
Occipital	4	0	1
Corpus call.	3	1	1
Basal ganglia	16 }	0	1
Post fossa	7 } 30 (44%)	2	2
Angiomatosis	7 }	2	0
No. of sessions	135 (1:2)	12+11	17
No. of total occlusions	21 (31%)		
Morbidity	6 (8.8%)	1	1 (7.7%)
Mortality	2 (2.9%)	0	0

The decision to operate will also be determined by the symptoms caused by a vascular steal. These symptoms often disappear after partial embolization. If one or more hemorrhages have occurred, partial embolization will be insufficient. If permanent total occlusion is not achieved in such cases, surgical excision to eliminate the risk of future hemorrhages is the only reasonable goal.

Today's embolization techniques permit more selective approaches to AVMs and more controlled embolization of compartments than was considered possible only a few years ago. This progress should not lead to disputes about therapeutic approaches for the treatment of AVMs. Instead, competently performed embolizations should be considered another option in the armamentarium against these potentially devastating lesions.

References

1. Richling B (1989) The current state in endovascular treatment of cerebral arteriovenous malformations. In: Neuroimaging II, Gustav Fischer Stuttgart New York, 309–315
2. Serbinenko FA (1974) Balloon catheterization and occlusion of major cerebral vessels. J Neurosurg 41:125–145
3. Spetzler RF, Martin NA (1986) A proposed grading system for arteriovenous malformations. J Neurosurg 65:476–483
4. Vinters HV, Galil KA, Lundie MJ, Kaufmann JCE (1985) The histotoxicity of cyanoacrylates. Neuroradiology 27:279–291

Results of Combined Endovascular and Surgical Treatment of Intracranial Arteriovenous Malformations

D. Wijnalda[1] and T.G. Tjan[2]

Introduction

For assessment of treatment of intracranial arteriovenous malformations (AVMs) it is important to know the natural history. The incidence of intracranial AVMs in the population is 0.5%. The risk of bleeding is 3% per year. The mortality with bleeding is 10% and the morbidity is 30% [2, 3, 4]. Since the introduction of microsurgical techniques there has been a tremendous improvement in treatment. In spite of this there are still many large AVMs in vulnerable areas of the brain which are hardly or not at all accessible to surgical treatment. The development of endovascular superselective techniques has given us a powerful alternative [1, 5, 7]. The aim of treatment is radical occlusion of the AVM for prevention of bleeding.

Patients, Methods, and Results

Since 1983, 96 patients have been treated by superselective embolization with bucrylate or histoacryl in 283 sessions. Indications were: previous bleeding, seizures, progressive neurological deterioration, severe headache.

Table 1. Results of superselective embolization completed in 209 sessions in 72 patients with AVMs

	No. of patients
100% Obliteration	5
50%–95% Obliteration	24
Surgical excision	23
Failure	12
Death due to embolization	6
Death after recurrent bleeding	2
Total	72

[1] Department of Neurosurgery, St. Elisabeth Hospital, 5000 LC Tilburg, The Netherlands
[2] Department of Neuroradiology, St. Elisabeth Hospital, 5000 LC Tilburg, The Netherlands

Advances in Neurosurgery, Vol. 19
W. J. Bock, Ch. Lumenta, M. Brock, M. Klinger (Eds.)

In the almost 300 embolization sessions the mortality was 2% per session and morbidity 8%. There has been a clear decline in these figures in more recent series because of the learning effect.

The treatment has been completed in 72 patients and is still continuing in 24. Table 1 shows the results.

In five cases obliteration was complete and lasting. A partial occlusion was obtained in 24 cases (80%–95% in seven, 60%–80% in eight, and < 60% in nine). Surgical excision was performed in 23 patients after partial embolization. In a further 12 cases embolization was technically impossible or the patient refused further treatment.

Six patients died because of bleeding during embolization and two patients died after recurrent bleeding due to the nature of the AVM.

In the same period, 64 patients were treated by microsurgery and the AVM was radically removed in 63. In this series mortality was 0%. This result is of course biased by a very strict preoperative evaluation of the risks. In 14 cases preoperative partial embolization was performed to facilitate the surgical procedure (Fig. 1–3). Nine patients presented after incomplete endovascular obliteration, having been previously considered inoperable. The AVM could be removed completely in eight of them and partially in one.

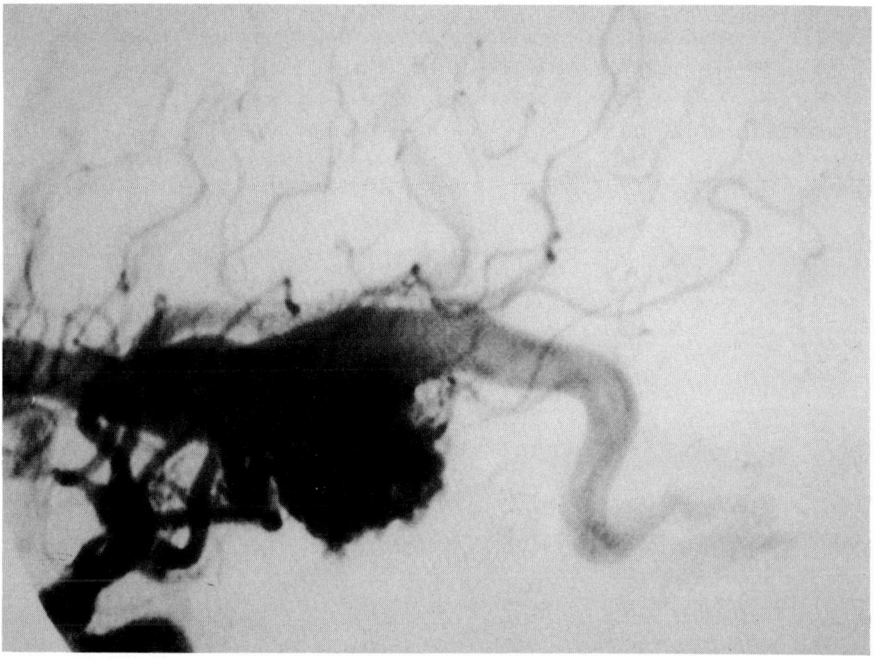

Fig. 1. Woman, 38 years old: transient ischemic attacks in the right hemisphere due to a high-flow AVM on the left side

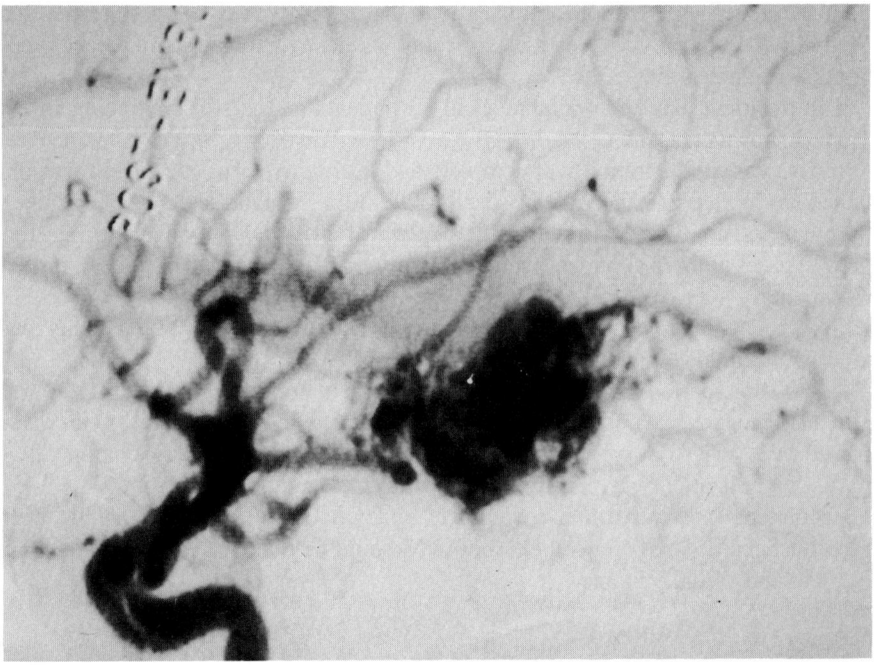

Fig. 2. After embolization there is a strong reduction in flow, an improvement in the filling of normal vessels, and a reduction in the size of the AVM

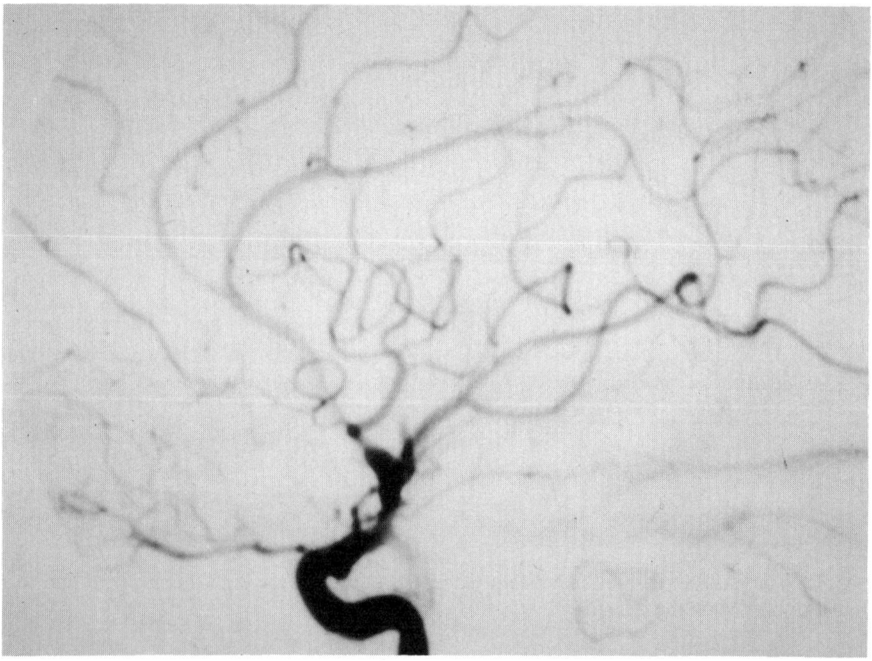

Fig. 3. The picture after surgical excision

All AMVs removed were examined for their pathology. There was a strong lymphocytic reaction in the surrounding tissue and many foreign-body giant cells in the embolized cases only. The long-term effects of these reactions to bucrylate are unknown [6].

Discussion

Close cooperation between neuroradiologist and neurosurgeon are essential because of the timing of the operation after embolization. In partially embolized AVMs we saw strong leptomeningeal recanalization within half a year and it became extremely difficult to coagulate these very thin-walled vessels. We now plan the operation to take place within a few days to weeks after the last embolization session.

In only a small percentage of cases was there complete obliteration of the AVM by endovascular treatment alone. We became aware of the possibilities, the impossibilities, and the risks of endovascular treatment. The most important thing we learned, however, was that invasive neuroradiology and neurosurgery are strong allies in the struggle against the devastating effects of AVM. We would like to stress the importance of a combined approach to this difficult disorder.

References

1. Debrun G, Vinuela F, Fox A, Drake CG (1982) Embolization of cerebral arteriovenous malformations with bucrylate. J Neurosurg 56:615–627
2. Fults D, Kelly DL Jr (1984) Natural history of arteriovenous malformations of the brain: a clinical study. Neurosurgery 16:658–662
3. Graf CJ, Perret GE, Torner JC (1983) Bleeding from cerebral arteriovenous malformations as part of their natural history. J Neurosurg 58:331–337
4. Jane JA, Kassell NF, Torner JC, Winn HR (1985) The natural history of aneurysms and arteriovenous malformations. J Neurosurg 62:321–323
5. Picard L, Moret J, Lepoire (1984) Traitement endovasculaire des angiomes artérioveineux intracérébrauc. Technique-Indication-Résults. J Neuroradiol 11:9–28
6. Vinters HV, Lundie MJ, Kaufmann JCE (1986) Long-term pathological follow-up of cerebral arteriovenous malformations treated by embolization with bucrylate. N Engl J Med 314:477–483
7. Vinuela F (1985) Interventional therapy of intracerebal angiomas. In: Poeck K, Freund HJ, Gänshirt H (eds) Proceedings of the XIIIth world congress of neurology. Springer, Berlin Heidelberg New York

Indications, Technique, and Results of Microsurgical Treatment of Intracranial Arteriovenous Malformations

Ch. Lumenta, M. Bettag, A. Bertels, and W.J. Bock[1]

Introduction

In the past few years treatment of intracranial arteriovenous malformations (AVMs) has become the subject of various clinical specialities. Endovascular therapy using embolic agents, sterotactic radiosurgery, and "conventional" microsurgery are sometimes supplementary and sometimes competitive methods in the treatment of brain AVMs. Especially in ruptured AVMs, we prefer microsurgical treatment, because with microsurgery the malformation can in the vast majority of cases be completely excised in one session [2, 9, 10, 11, 14, 15, 16], which markedly reduces the risk of recurrent hemorrhage. The results of microsurgical excision have steadily improved [7], as we can demonstrate in our follow-up study of 57 patients with a brain AVM.

Patients and Methods

From January 1986 to March 1990, 57 patients with brain AVMs were referred to our neurosurgical unit: 41 (72%) male and 16 (28%) female. The age of the patients ranged from 15 to 68 years, with a peak incidence at 20–30 years. The commonest mode of presentation in this series was intracranial hemorrhage which had occurred in 31 (54%) patients. In 17 (30%) patients the initial symptom was epilepsy without any bleeding. Six (11%) patients complained of recurrent headache and 3 (5%) presented with deteriorating neurological signs. The time interval between initial symptom and admittance to surgery ranged from a few hours to 24 years, with an average of 2.4 years.

Thirty-five (61%) patients were treated by microsurgical excision, 9 (16%) patients had radiosurgery and in 3 (5%) patients an endovascular approach was taken. In 8 (15%) cases no therapy was performed because of infaust prognosis. Two (4%) patients refused any treatment.

The surgical technique was always similar: AVM was directly dissected from the adjacent brain tissue as described by several authors in previous works [2, 17].

In the 35 surgically treated patients, 33 (94%) AVMs were located supratentorially, with only 2 (6%) angiomas in the infratentorial region. The most frequent lo-

---

[1] Neurochirurgische Klinik, Medizinische Einrichtungen der Heinrich-Heine-Universität Düsseldorf, Moorenstr. 5, W-4000 Düsseldorf 1, FRG

Advances in Neurosurgery, Vol. 19
W. J. Bock, Ch. Lumenta, M. Brock, M. Klinger (Eds.)

cation was the parietal lobe, followed by the temporal and occipital lobe. Nineteen (54%) AVMs were located in the left hemisphere, 13 (37%) in the right hemisphere and 3 (9%) had a median location. In 10 (29%) patients the AVMs were smaller than 2 cm, in 18 (51%) they were between 2 and 4 cm, and in 7 (20%) they were larger than 4 cm. According to the Spetzler–Martin grading system [12] there were 3 (9%) grade I lesions, 6 (17%) grade II lesions, 11 (31%) grade III lesions, 13 (47%) grade IV lesions, and 2 (6%) grade V lesions.

For pre- and postoperative investigations we used angiography and contrast enhanced computed tomography or magnetic resonance imaging. All patients have been followed up for a minimum of 3 months and a maximum of 4 years, with an average of 1.4 years.

Results

To compare the patient's state on admission and at follow-up we used the criteria proposed by Forster et al. [3] and Jennett and Bond [8] (Table 1). Of 35 surgically treated patients there were 9 (25.5%) at grade 0 or I on admission; that means they had no neurological deficit. Nine (25.5%) had minor neurological deficits or recurrent epileptic fits, 10 (29%) had severe neurological deficits with a depressed level of consciousness or coma I or II, and 7 (20%) were deeply comatose (Fig. 1).

From the results at last follow-up, 15 (43%) patients were clinically grade 0 or I, 8 (23%) had moderate disability and reduced working capacity, 8 (23%) patients were suffering severe disability and were not able to work regularly, and 4 (11%) patients had died (Fig. 1).

Table 1. Classification of patient's state on admission and follow-up (after Forster et al. [3] and Jennett and Bond [8])

Grade	State on admission	Follow-up
0	Fully responsive, no symptoms and signs	Good recovery, full working capacity
I	Fully responsive, headache only, seizures less than 1/month	Good recovery, full working capacity
II	Fully responsive, neurological deficit, seizures more than 1/month	Moderate disability, reduced working capacity
III	Depressed level of consciousness, coma I–II, major neurological deficit	Severe disability, unfit for regular employment
IV	Unconscious, coma III–IV	Persistent vegetative state, death

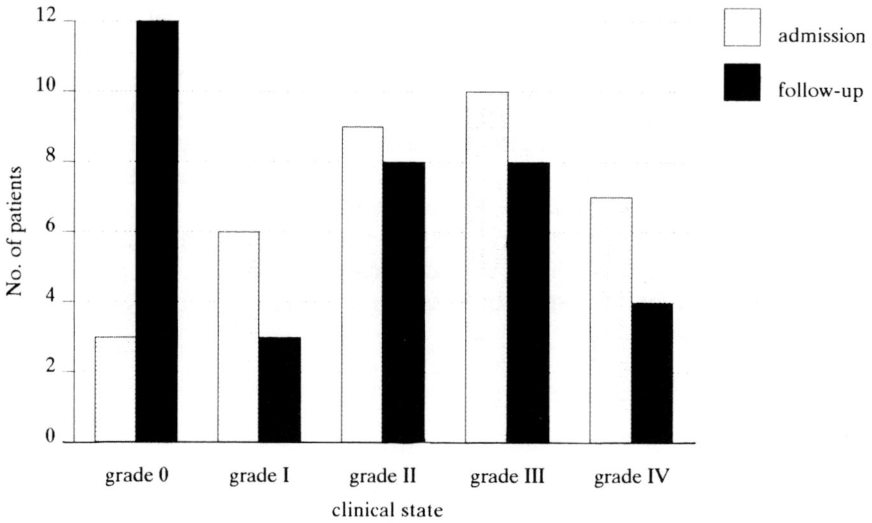

Fig. 1. Clinical state on admission and at follow-up in 35 surgically treated patients with brain AVMs

Comparing the clinical state on admission with the outcome at last follow-up, 19 (54%) patients were improved, 11 (32%) unchanged, and 5 (14%) patients deteriorated (Table 2). There was no deterioration in patients with small AVMs and no deterioration in patients admitted without symptoms of hemorrhage. Five out of 24 patients presenting with intracranial hemorrhage on admission deteriorated after complete surgical excision of the AVM (Table 2).

Table 2. Clinical outcome compared with state on admission, in relation to size of AVM and occurrence of intracranial hemorrhage (*n* = 35)

	Improved	Unchanged	Deteriorated	Total
Small AVM (< 2 cm)	7	4	–	11
Medium AVM (2–4 cm)	10	6	3	19
Large AVM (> 4 cm)	2	1	2	5
With hemorrhage	12	7	5	24
Without hemorrhage	7	4	–	11
Total	19 (54%)	11 (32%)	5 (15%)	

The late morbidity due to surgical treatment was 8.5% (three patients). Two of these three patients had medium-sized AVMs and one had a large AVM. All of these AVMs were Spetzler–Martin grade IV, i.e. they were located in an eloquent region and had a deep venous drainage. On admission these patients had only headaches or focal seizures; postoperatively two had hemiparesis and one hemianopia.

The mortality due to surgical treatment was 11.4% (four patients). Three of the four patients had medium-sized AVMs and one a large AVM. All of these AVMs were Spetzler–Martin grade IV [12]. On admission, one patient had a minor neurological deficit, one had a severe neurological deficit and was mildly comatose, and two were deeply comatose with abnormal flexor or extensor response.

In 31 (89%) of 35 patients it was possible to completely excise the AVM in one session. Four (11%) patients were brought to theater again because of angiographically confirmed remaining malformation.

At the last follow-up, only 1 of 11 patients with epileptic fits in their preoperative history had presistent seizures after surgical excision of the AVM. There was no case of postoperative epilepsy in patients without a history of seizures and admission.

Discussion

An intracranial AVM may manifest with intracranial hemorrhage or seizures. In our series hemorrhage occurred in more than 50% of patients, and in about one third seizures were the first symptom. This is similar to other series by Drake [2], Heros [7], and Yasargil [17].

Our data demonstrate that early postoperative deficits (7/35 = 20%) resulting from excision of an intracranial AVM may improve in a certain number of cases (3/35 = 8.5%) after approximately 4–8 months. Steinmeier et al. [13] reported an early neurological morbidity of 44% in a series of 48 patients, but 6 months after surgery only three patients had residual major morbidity. In a study of 153 patients, Heros et al. reported an immediate major neurological deficit of 24% which decreased to 8% after a mean follow-up period of 3.8 years.

Four (11.4%) patients died in our series due to surgical treatment. All of them had a grade IV intracranial AVM according to the classification of Spetzler and Martin. Late mortality in the studies of Heros et al. was 1.3% (three patients).

In reference to epilepsy, we were able to establish that no patients without a history of seizures ever suffered from an epileptic fit after excision of the AVM. On the other hand, only one out of 11 patients with seizures in their preoperative history had fits after surgery, which could be controlled by anticonvulsants. Although there was no increased incidence of epilepsy after surgical excision of a brain AVM in our series, other research groups have reported an average incidence of postoperative epileptic fits of 11.6%–22% [4, 7, 17].

Comparison between the different methods of treating brain AVMs is difficult because of different patient populations and different follow-up periods. It has become increasingly clear that the rate of bleeding of AVMs, whether they have bled in the past or not, is approximately 2%–4% per year [1, 5, 6, 7].

On the other hand late morbidity and mortality resulting from surgical excision of AVMs are low, especially for patients with AVMs grades I–IV. Therefore we are of the opinion that surgery should by undertaken in patients with AVMs of these grades. Caution should be taken in patients with small AVMs in eloquent brain areas and in those with very large AVMs (grade V).

It is advisable to decide for radiation therapy in patients with small AVM, especially if no hemorrhage has yet occurred.

Embolization should be tried in patients with very large AVMs, even if just to reduce the flow so the incidence of seizures and headaches can decrease.

References

1. Brown RD Jr, Wiebers DO, Forbes G, O'Fallon WM, Piepgras DG, Marsh WR, Macinnas RJ (1988) The natural history of unruptured intracranial arteriovenous malformations. J Neurosurg 68:352–357
2. Drake CG (1979) Cerebral arteriovenous malformations: considerations for and experience with surgical treatment in 166 cases. Clin Neurosurg 26:145–208
3. Forster DMC, Steiner L, Hakonson S (1972) Arteriovenous malformations of the brain. A long-term clinical study. J Neurosurg 37:562–570
4. Foy PM, Copeland GM, Shaw MDM (1981) The incidence of postoperative seizures. Acta Neurochir (Wien) 55:253–264
5. Fults D, Kelly DL Jr (1984) Natural history of the brain: a clinical study. Neurosurg 15:658–662
6. Graf CJ, Perret GE, Torner JC (1983) Bleeding from cerebral arteriovenous malformations as part of their natural history. J Neurosurg 58:331–337
7. Heros RC, Korosue K, Diebold PM (1990) Surgical excision of cerebral arteriovenous malformations: late results. Neurosurgery 26:570–578
8. Jennett B, Bond M (1975) Assessment of outcome after severe brain damage. Lancet I:480–484
9. Luessenhop AJ, Rosa L (1984) Cerebral arteriovenous malformations: indications for and results of surgery, and the role of intravascular techniques. J Neurosurg 60:14–22
10. Malis LI (1982) Arteriovenous malformations of the brain. In: Youmans JR (ed) Neurological surgery, vol 3. Saunders, London, pp 1786–1806
11. Nornes H, Lundar T. Wikeby P (1979) Cerebral arteriovenous malformations: results of microsurgical management. Acta Neurochir (Wien) 50:243–257
12. Spetzler RF, Martin NA (1986) A proposed grading system of arteriovenous malformations. J Neusorurg 65:476–483
13. Steinmeier R, Schramm J, Müller HG, Fahlbusch R (1989) Evaluation of prognostic factors in cerebral arteriovenous malformations. Neurosurgery 24:193–200
14. Suzuki J, Onuma T, Kayama T (1982) Surgical treatment of intracranial arteriovenous malformations. Neurol Res 4:191–207
15. Verbiest H (1979) Arteriovenous malformations. Operative surgery/neurosurgery, 3rd edn. Butterworths, London
16. Wilson CB, U HS, Domingue J (1979) Microsurgical treatment of intracranial vascular malformation. J Neurosurg 51:446–454
17. Yasargil MG (1988) Microneurosurgery, vol 3B. Thieme, New York, pp 376–378

Surgical Problems in Partially Embolized Angiomas

J.M. Gilsbach[1] and M. Schumacher[2]

Introduction

Five years ago, we changed our policy regarding the treatment of cerebral arteriovenous malformations (AVMs) from a purely surgical technique to a combined procedure with preoperative embolization and operation. Since then, the number of operations on AVMs has decreased. One reason for this is the fact that some AVMs are still under neuroradiological treatment; another may be that in some cases the neuroradiologist was able to completely occlude the malformation. One further reason could be the lack of information on how effectively embolized but still active AVMs can be surgically treated. This article is intended to contribute to some aspects of the problems encountered during surgery on embolized AVMs and to the final result after surgical removal of an incompletely embolized AVM.

Treatment Concept

In Freiburg, and since August 1990, also in Aachen, we operate directly on small AVMs if they can be endovascularly obliterated only at high risk. This we do particularly if the patients have suffered a recent intracerebral bleeding which facilitates the approach. As direct surgical intervention in one session in large AVMs did not always produce convincing results, we changed in 1983 to a stepwise surgical procedure and intraoperative embolization: the dissection and occlusion of the AVM was interrupted when hemostasis became more difficult. The results of this stepwise surgical exclusion were good and the five patients with large AVMs treated in this way adapted uneventfully to the altered hemodynamic conditions (no breakthrough) and suffered no rebleeding during the waiting period of the second operation. As the endovascular procedures became increasingly safe, we changed our strategy again and referred patients for preoperative embolization, hoping that the (stepwise) embolization would work like a staged operation, with the aim of smoothly normalizing the disturbed cerebral hemodynamics and simplifying the final surgical procedure by reducing the flow and the volume of the AVM.

---

[1] Abteilung Neurochirurgie der Medizinischen Fakultät, RWTH Aachen, Pauweselsstr. 30, D-5100 Aachen, FRG

[2] Abteilung Neuroradiologie, Universität Freiburg, Hugstetter Str. 55, D-7800 Freiburg, FRG

Advances in Neurosurgery, Vol. 19
W. J. Bock, Ch. Lumenta, M. Brock, M. Klinger (Eds.)

The operations were performed when no further embolization with idobutyl 2-cyanoacrylate (IBC) seemed possible or reasonable, a decision taken by each neuroradiologist individually. The interval between the last embolization and surgery was not preset and varied from patient to patient. In the beginning we preferred early surgery, but with growing experience the surgical operation was delayed for at least 6 weeks.

The aim of treatment, direct or combined, was total occlusion of the AVM. If this did not seem possible no treatment at all was started, except in the case of AVMs suitable for radiotherapy.

Surgery and Embolizations

All patients were operated upon in the neurosurgical department in Freiburg (of which J.M.G. was a member at that time). The embolizations were performed in Freiburg (Prof. Schumacher), Nancy (Prof. Picard), and Paris (Prof. Merland).

Patients

Our experience is based on only a small number of patients. We operated on 10 patients with partially embolized AVMs (Table 1).

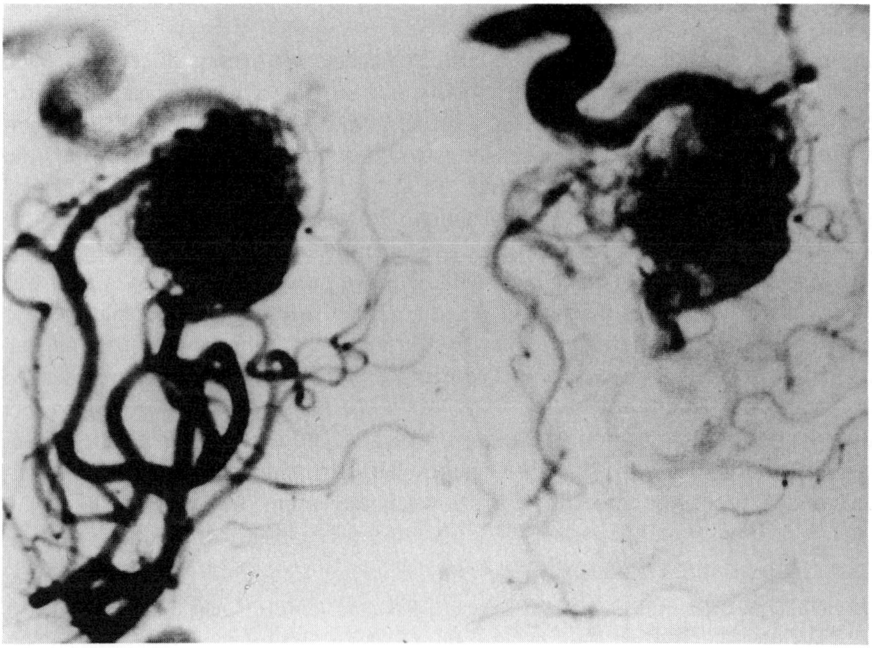

Fig. 1. Parietal AVM before embolization

Table 1. Clinical data and results

Patient	Location	Embolization	Delay[a]	Surgery	Result[b]
E.R. M, 52 yrs	Temporal	Unveventful (30%)[c]	3 mo.	Uneventful, complete removal	Good
P.H. F, 27 yrs	Postcentral	Hemorrhage, latent hemiparesis (50%)	6 mo.	Uneventful, complete removal	Good
F.R. M, 26 yrs	Occipital	Catheter not removable (60%)	2 mo.	Uneventful, complete removal	Good
S.J. M, 46 yrs	Fronto-parietal	Uneventful (80%)	5 mo.	Uneventful, complete removal	Good
R.D. F, 33 yrs	Occipital	Uneventful, internal external territory (50%)	23 days	Difficult hemostasis, complete removal	Good
K.A. M, 32 yrs	Sylvian fissure	Moderate hemi-paresis (60%)	4 mo.	Uneventful, residual, deep AVM	Good
R.B. F, 33 yrs	Corpus callosum, basal ganglia	Uneventful (40%)	5 mo.	Staged op, difficult hemostasis, complete removal	Good
W.R. M, 31 yrs	Parietal	Transient hemi-paresis (60%)	1 mo.	Difficult hemostasis complete removal	Good
K.H. F, 33 yrs	Corpus callosum	Uneventful (50%)	12 days	Difficult hemostasis, complete removal	Good
W.M. F, 33 yrs	Precentral	Uneventful (50%)	9 days	Difficult hemostasis, residual deep AVM	Good

[a] Delay between last embolization and surgery
[b] Acording to Glasgow Outcome Scale
[c] Approximate extent of AVM exclusion by embolization

Intraoperative Findings and Results

One interesting question concerns the surgical problems occurring after endovascular embolization. Theoretically, an AVM partially filled with IBC could be hard and difficult to handle. This problem was in practice not encountered in any case: the embolized parts were more or less soft and could be manipulated with instruments or cut (Figs. 2, 3). Another as yet unresolved question involves the local and hemodynamic reactions after embolization: an early operation could be complicated by an inflammatory reaction and a disturbed autoregulation, while late surgery would increase the risk of rebleeding and the recruitment of new feeders. In recently embolized AVMs hemostasis proved difficult from the beginning; especially in AVMs with a low degree of occlusion, the small penetrating vessels were under high pressure, while the larger ones, often partially or completely occluded, posed no problems. No bleeding occurred during waiting for the final surgical procedure, but did occur once immediately after embolization.

Discussion and Preliminary Conclusion

Due to the individual decisions on how to treat an AVM and due to the lack of prospective studies on the overall morbidity and mortality associated with embolization plus surgery in an unselected series, a comparison of surgery alone with preoperative embolization plus surgery is difficult [1–5]. Moreover, no large study exists which proves that partially embolized AVMs can be operated on safely and easily. For this reason, only preliminary impressions can be described here.

The intraoperative findings show why complete embolization of AVMs is difficult to achieve. Deep parts of the AVM remained open, and even in some arteries which were filled with IBC a residual flow could be observed.

The IBC was often located very distally in veins and normal arteries, and in one early-operated case the embolization was accompanied by a hyperemic and inflammatory reaction. These findings and long-lasting circulatory disturbances after total or partial occlusion [6–8] suggest that very early surgical intervention is not

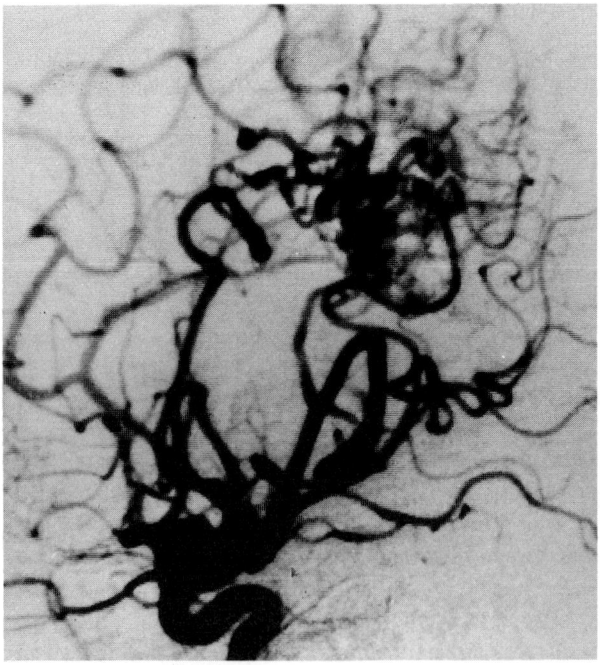

Fig. 2. AVM after partial embolization

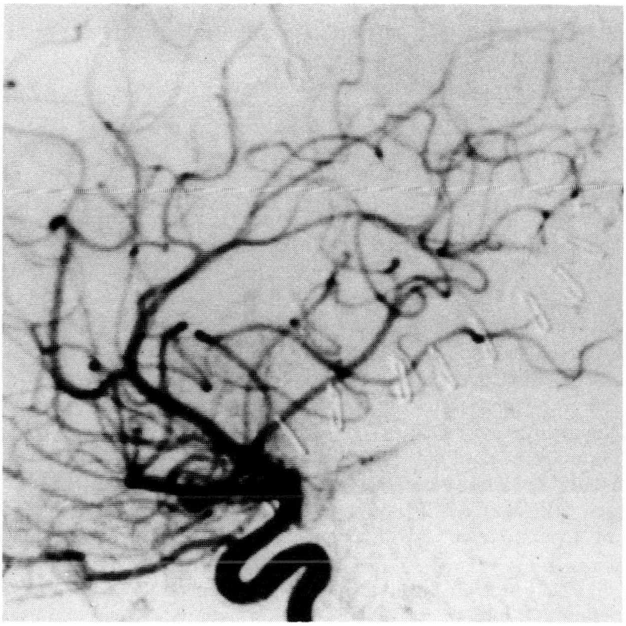

Fig. 3. Control angiogram after surgical exclusion

advisable. On the basis of these observations, we decided to wait at least 6–8 weeks after the last embolization, until the inflammatory and circulatory disturbances had subsided. The advantages of this policy, which includes a control angiogram on the day before the planned operation, are that further new pedicles can be detected and perhaps embolized again, instead of being operatively occluded, and that further spontaneous thrombosis can occur in the waiting period. Six to eight weeks should not be too long to allow the recruitment and enlargement of new feeders.

From the surgical point of view, preoperative embolization reduced the active parts of the AVMs and the surgical difficulties with large feeding arteries and also normalized circulation without problems for the patient in the adaptation period. Theoretically, the stone-like IBC may hinder dissection or provoke hemorrhage, and the disturbed circulation may complicate hemostasis by an increased pressure in perforating vessels [1, 4, 9–11]. In practice the first problem did not occur, but the second one did: in comparison to nonembolized AVMs, embolization did not substantially reduce the problems with small penetrating, feeding, and draining vessels, so that one of the main problems in AVM surgery still remained. These problems may be due to incomplete exclusion (30%–60%) or too early surgical intervention when the pressure in arteries origiating from large "stagnating" arteries is still too high. The incomplete removal of two AVMs was due to these problems with hemostasis of deep penetrating vessels.

In the future, prospective studies will be needed to evaluate whether combined treatment of preoperative embolization and operation is superior to staged operation with or without intraoperative embolization.

References

1. Cromwell LD, Harris AB (1980) Treatment of cerebral arteriovenous malformations. A combined neurosurgical and neuroradiological approach. J Neurosurg 52:705–708
2. Cromwell LD, Harris AB (1983) Treatment of cerebral arteriovenous malformations: combined neurosurgical and neuroradiological approach. AJNR 4:366–368
3. Day AL, Friedman WA, Sypert GW, et al. (1982) Successful treatment of the normal perfusion pressure break-through syndrome. Neurosorgery 11:625–630
4. Debrun G, Fox A, Drake C (1981) Comments on Samson D, Ditmore QM, Beyer CW Jr Intravascular use of isobutyl 2-cyanoacrylate: Part 1: Treatment of intracranial arteriovenous malformations. Neurosurgery 8:51
5. George B, Riche MC, Gaston A, et al. (1983) Embolisation peropératoire des malformations arterio-veineuses à partir de l'artère vertébrale. Neurochirurgie 30:269–272
6. Harders A, Bien S, Eggert HR, et al. (1988) Haemodynamic changes in arteriovenous malformations induced by superselective embolization: transcranial Doppler evaluation. Neurol Res 10:239–245
7. Hassler W, Gilsbach J, Gaitzsch J (1983) Results and value of immediate postoperative angiography after operations for arteriovenous malformations. Neurochirurgia 26:146–148
8. Hassler W, Gilsbach J (1984) Intra- and perioperative aspects of the hemodynamics of supratentorial AVmalformations. Acta Neurochir 73:35–44
9. Peerless SJ (1982) Comments on Day AL, Friedmann WA, Sypert GW, et al. Successful treatment of the normal perfusion breakthrough syndrome. Neurosurgery 11:629–630
10. Samson D, Ditmore QM, Beyer CW Jr (1981) Intravascular use of isobutyl 2-cyanoacrylate: Part 1. Treatment of intracranial arteriovenous malformations. Neurosurgery 8:43–51
11. Spetzler RF, Martin NA, Carter LP, et al. (1987) Surgical management of large AVMs by staged embolization and operative excision. J Neurosurg 67:17–28

Arteriovenous Malformations of the Brain: What is the Best Way to Treat Them?

J. Brotchi[1], O. Dewitte[1], A. Vandesteene[2], G. Rodesch[3], D. Baleriaux[3], and J. Noterman[1]

Introduction

Many modes of treament are proposed for curing arteriovenous malformations of the brain (AVMs): surgery, embolization, radiosurgery. Usually, every specialist presents arguments in favor of the superiority of his or her particular choice. Some try to convince us that embolization is less risky than surgery, that it gives better results. Others think radiosurgery is better, forgetting that this treatment takes many months to become effective and that during this delay the AVM may rebleed. Unconditional supporters of surgery prefer multistaged operations to embolization in huge AVMs. Where does the truth lie?

Patients and Method

In our department, 48 AVMs have been treated the last 5 years (Table 1). Having access to superselective endovascular neuroradiology, we decided to discuss case by case the choice of treatment according to the size, the location, the accessibility, and the grade of the AVM. Patients were sent abroad for radiosurgery, which is not available in Belgium at the moment.

Table 1. Modes of treatment of 48 AVMs

Surgery	40	Alone 38
		After embolization 2
Embolization	10	Without surgery 8
		Before surgery 2
Postembolization radiosurgery 3		

[1] Department of Neurosurgery, Erasme Hospital, Free University of Brussels, 808 Route de Lennik, B-1070 Brussels, Belgium
[2] Department of Anesthesiology, Erasme Hospital, Free University of Brussels, 808 Route de Lennik, B-1070 Brussels, Belgium
[3] Department of Neuroradiology, Erasme Hospital, Free University of Brussels, 808 Route de Lennik, B-1070 Brussels, Belgium

Advances in Neurosurgery, Vol. 19
W. J. Bock, Ch. Lumenta, M. Brock, M. Klinger (Eds.)

Results

Postoperative mortality was 4% (two cases). Postoperative morbidity was 8% (four cases). There was no mortality or morbidity due to embolization or radiosurgery, but two patients rebled while awaiting the next step in multistaged embolization. The first of these was a 40-year-old woman with a rolandic AVM causing epilepsy only. Surgery was considered too dangerous and she sustained an uneventful first stage of embolization. The second stage was scheduled for 6 weeks later. However, 1 month after the first stage she had a massive hemorrhage and died 2 days later.

The second rebleeding was in a 55-year-old woman. After a first moderate bleeding, she underwent angiography which showed a huge right sylvian AVM (Fig. 1). Embolization was decided upon and performed. The postembolization angiogram (Fig. 2) showed a pleasing but incomplete result. Two weeks later the patient bled again (Fig. 3). She is still alive, but her neurological status is poor.

Discussion

In our department, every AVM is approached in a multidisciplinary fashion by neurosurgeons and neuroradiologists together. A common strategy is decided with the aim of offering patients the best treatment with the lowest risk, according to the grade of the malformation [3]. In our opinion, embolization, surgery, and

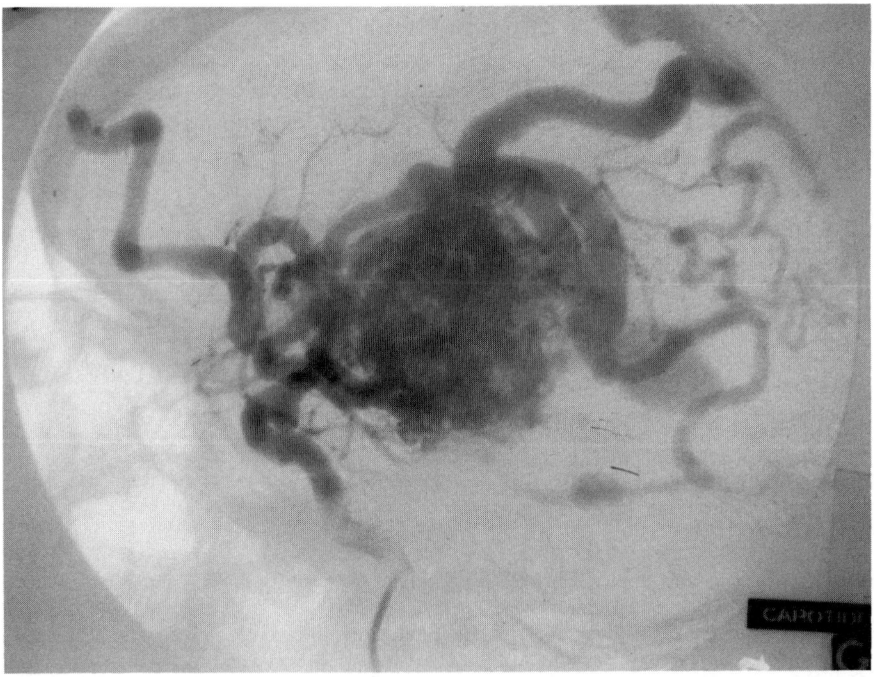

Fig. 1. Huge right sylvian AVM. Right internal carotid angiogram

radiosurgery are not in competition but are complementary. One must never forget that the only way to cure an AVM is to induce its total disappearance, by whatever technique. As we have reported, an AVM may rebleed while waiting complete eradication, so incomplete obliteration of the AVM by embolization also fails to provide protection from subsequent hemorrhage [1].

The most important area of application for endovascular techniques alone is in patients with large AVMs [2]. Embolization may also be used to prepare for surgery, either by reducing the degree of shunting, which lessens the risk of normal perfusion pressure breakthrough, or by occlusion of major feeding arteries difficult of access, in order to reduce the size of the AVM. Stereotactic radiosurgery has proven its efficacy in small AVMs [5], but it must be borne in mind that delayed radiation necrosis may not occur until about 6 months later, and during that time patients are not protected against rebleeding! However, this technique is useful for little nidi impossible to cure either by embolization or by surgery [4].

All these techniques have their advantages and inconveniences. We must take the best they can offer us and if necessary combine them.

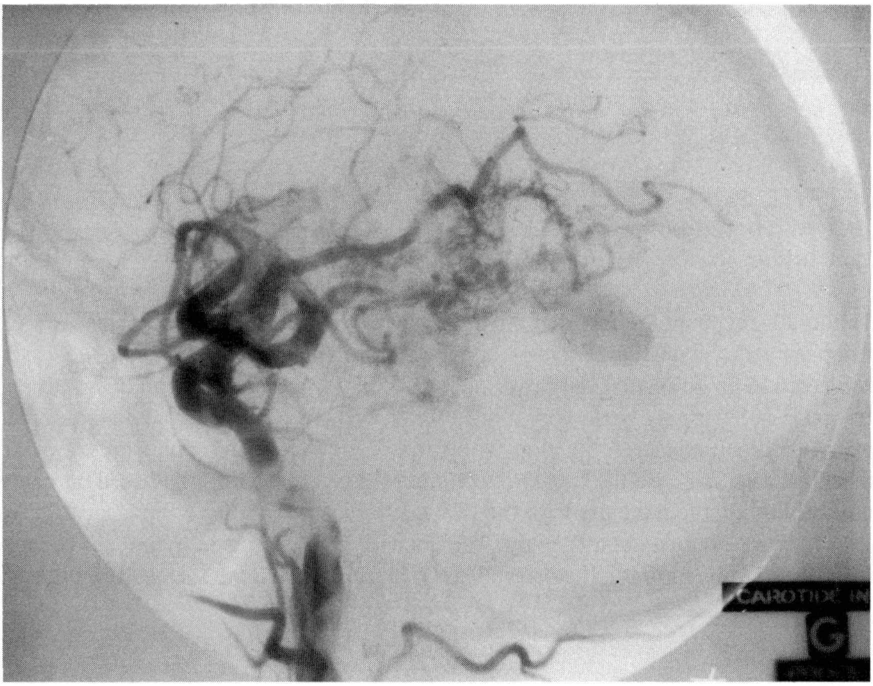

Fig. 2. Postembolization angiogram: More than 80% of the AVM thrombosed

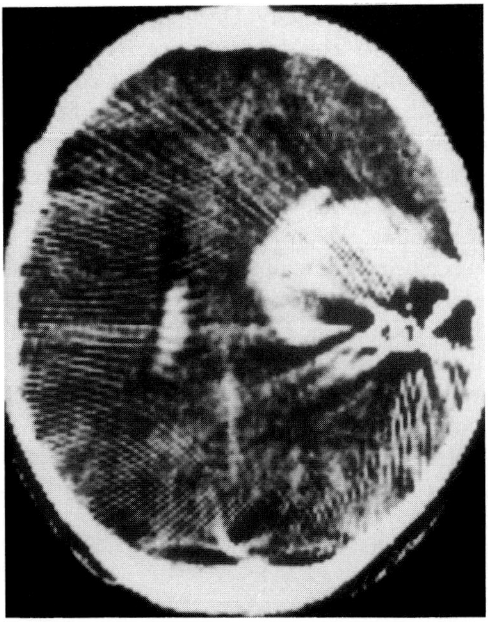

Fig. 3. Computed tomogram showing intracerebral hemorrhage 2 weeks later

Conclusion

Taking into account the fact that the only way to cure an AVM is to induce its total disappearance, even if we do not know what will happen in the future to cases subjected to embolization only, we must offer patients the best technique with the lowest risk. That may be surgery alone, which is the most radical, an endovascular approach alone or in combination with surgery, or stereotactic radiosurgery alone or in combination with the first two techniques. The choice must be based on many criteria, among them the grade of the lesion and its accessibility or nonaccessibility to surgery or endovascular therapy. The decision must be made by a team of neurosurgeons and neuroradiologists wellexperienced in managing this malformation.

References

1. Luessenhop AJ, Presper JH (1975) Surgical embolization of cerebral arteriovenous malformations through internal carotid and vertebral arteries. Long-term results. J Neurosurg 42:443–451
2. Luessenhop AJ, Rosa L (1989) Cerebral arteriovenous malformations. Contemp Neurosurg 11 (15):6
3. Spetzler RF, Martin NA (1986) A proposed grading system for arteriovenous malformations. J Neurosurg 65:476–483

4. Steiner L (1984) Treatment of arteriovenous malformations by radiosurgery. In: Wilson CB, Stein BM (eds) Intracranial arteriovenous malformations. Williams and Wilkins, Baltimore, pp 295–314
5. Steiner L, Lindquist C (1987) Radiosurgery in cerebral arteriovenous malformation. In: Tasker RR (ed) Neurosurgery: state of the art reviews, vol 2, No 1. Hanley and Belfus, Philadelphia, pp 329–336

Arteriovenous Malformations of the Medial Surface of the Parieto-occipital Region and the Basal Ganglia

G.H. Spincemaille[1]

Introduction

Arteriovenous malformations (AVMs) of the medial surface of the hemisphere around the posterior part of the corpus callosum and of the medial side of the trigone of the lateral ventricle are operable lesions [1, 9, 13, 14]. There are various reports in the literature of successful removal of these malformations without major neurological deficit [8, 11, 13, 14]. According to the classification system proposed by Spetzler and Martin [10], these lesions are grade III AVMs. If the interhemispheric approach is used as described by Kempe and Blaylock [4], then no special precautions regarding circulatory and cardiac complications need be taken by the anesthesiologist.

Intravascular techniques (embolization) are helpful in reducing the size of these malformations but rarely exclude them from the circulation because of the multiple vascular territories involved [2, 7]

Patients and Method

We treated six patients with trigonal AVMs during the period 1984–1987. The mean age was 30.6 years (18–46); the sex ratio was 3:3. All AVMs were symptomatic, the patients presenting with intracranial bleeding and additional problems such as seizures and neurological deficits. We operated on four; the two remaining patients (5 and 6) underwent endovascular embolization (Table 1).

The interhemispheric approach was used with the patient in the prone position. The surgical procedure following the descriptions of Kempe and Yasargil proved to be quite easy. By changing the patient's position slightly, it was possible to reach the malformation almost at right angles to the surgeon's visual axis. The only difficulty resided in the distance from the outside of the skull to the malformation. Proggressive elimination of the malformation was performed in the usual way by partial coagulation of the malformation and the main feeding vessels. Complete removal required exploration of the lateral ventricle via a cortical incision of the gyrus cinguli, or dissection in the splenium of the corpus callosum. Postoperative angiograms and follow-up angiograms 1 year later were taken in all cases.

---

[1] Department of Neurosurgery, De Wever Hospital, H. Dunantstr. 5, 6419 PC Heerleen, The Netherlands

Advances in Neurosurgery, Vol. 19
W. J. Bock, Ch. Lumenta, M. Brock, M. Klinger (Eds.)

Table 1. Patient characteristics, clinical data, and postoperative status and angiography

Patient no.	Sex	Age (years)	Preop. status	Treatment	Postop. status	Postop. angio-graphy
1	F	20	Bleeding, coma, hemiparesis (pregnant)	Surgery	Normal	Complete obliteration
2	M	45	Bleeding, epilepsy previous surgery	Surgery	Controlled seizures	Complete obliteration
3	F	18	Two previous bleedings	Surgery (two-stage)	Seizures difficult to control	Complete obliteration
4	M	30	Bleeding, R hemi-paresis, recovery after 1 week, major cortical disturbances	Surgery	Progressive recovery	Complete obliteration
5	M	25	Bleeding, no neorological deficit	Open embolization	Hemiplegia	Partial obliteration
6	F	46	Several bleedings, no neurological deficit	Several sessions of endovascular embolization	Transient neuro-logical deficit, then died after recurrent bleeding	Remaining nidus

Results

In three patients (nos. 1, 2, and 4) the AVM was removed without problems. The postoperative course was uneventful; in those cases where the neurological situation had been disturbed preoperatively, it showed significant improvement. Some cortical deficits remained, as in patient 4, and were responsible for the morbidity due to bleeding. In patient 3 the postoperative angiogram revealed a remnant of the AVM in the roof of the third ventricle. At reexploration the corpus callosum was exposed and the vessels still present coagulated. The postoperative angiogram this time showed complete obliteration of the malformation.

Patient 5 was referred to another neurosurgical department for open embolization. The major feeding vessel being the posterior cerebral artery, the option of embolization with butylacrylate by catheterization of the branch feeding the AVM was undertaken, the artery being exposed surgically. Postoperatively dense hemiplegia was present, probably due to extensive retraction of the temporal lobe. The postoperative angiogram showed revascularization of the malformation through other vessels not previously visualized. No further steps were planned because the patient refused further surgery.

The last patient was referred for endovascular embolization using the floating catheter technique. A well-defined nidus still remained after four sessions of embolization. Eight months after the last session the patient suddenly developed hemiplegia. Computed tomography (CT) showed a huge intracerebral and intraventricular hematoma, and the patient died 1 week after admission to our department.

Discussion

Intracranial bleeding is the most frequent clinical sign leading to detection of AVMs of the trigonal area. CT reveals unilateral intraventricular bleeding extending to the nearby white matter [11].

The feeding arteries of these AVMs originate in the three major vascular territories and sometimes come from both hemispheres. The most frequent feeding arteries are the pericallosal artery, the anterior and posterior choroid arteries, and the posterior cerebral artery and its tributaries such as the posterior temporal artery. The more central the location of the AVM, the more complex the vascular supply.

Different treatment modalities exist, including radiosurgery, endovascular techniques, and surgery. Radiosurgery may be a good choice for the smaller malformations in this region [12], but the technique is not widely available, so the discussion whether to use endovascular embolization or surgery remains.

Both techniques carry morbidity and mortality. If the main feeders are large vessels, endovascular embolization seems a reasonable choice [2, 7]. If a nidus still remains after several sessions of embolization, however, surgery should be scheduled. The operation can be done via the transtemporal or the interhemispheric approach [3, 6, 9]. The transtemporal route described by Heros [3] has the disadvantage of a transcortical and transcerebral route: good exposure is limited. The approach may be well suited for medial temporal lesions, but for lesions of the trigonal area the real interhemispheric approach is preferable. The technique can be carried out with the patient in semi-sitting or prone position; with the latter positioning, it is easy to reach the lesion. The approach has been described by several authors with small variations [4, 8, 11].

Although the location of the AVM is quite a distance from the outside of the skull, the terminology "deep" AVM is not correct in relation to the brain surface. It is important to be aware of some general points in order to reach the malformation without damaging the brain and its vascular supply. The venous phase of the angiogram is important as it allows localization of the large cortical veins. The surgeon should proceed along the falx between the large bridging veins. Drilling should be generous on the side of the malformation in order to avoid problems with retracting the hemisphere.

An important advantage of paramedian approach resides in the fact that the feeding arteries can be approached earlier than when using the transtemporal approach [8].

The aim of surgery should be total removal of the malformation. Due to the compartmental organization of AVMs, some parts of the malformation may be overlooked through being hidden in the corpus callosum [11, 13]. As in the case of patient 3, postoperative angiography may reveal a remnant of the AVM. If there is any doubt about the completeness of the removal, postoperative angiography should be performed.

Conclusion

1. In young patients with a symptomatic AVM surgical treatment is superior to conservative treatment [5].
2. Endovascular techniques are of great help in obliterating the major feeders; however, in this particular localization of the medial parieto-occipital region, they seldom eliminate the angioma completely. Embolization is the treatment of choice when the malformation has a dominant feeder like the posterior cerebral artery. Its advantage resides in its making surgery much easier [2, 7].
3. Radiosurgery (proton beam, gamma knife) is a reasonable alternative for the treatment of small, medially located angiomas [12].

References

1. Batjer HH, Samson D (1986) Surgical approaches in trigonal AVM. J Neurosurg 67:511-517
2. Harders A et al. (1988) Haemodynamic changes in arteriovenous malformations induced by superselective embolization: transcranial Doppler evaluation. Neurol Res 10:239–245
3. Heros RC (1982) AVM of the medial temporal lobe: surgical approach and neuroradiological characterization. J Neurosurg 56: 44–52
4. Kempe LG, Blaylock R (1976) Lateral trigonal intraventricular tumors. A new operative approach. Acta Neurochir (Wien) 35:233–242
5. Luessenhop AJ (1984) Cerebral AVM: indications for and results of surgery. J Neurosurg 60:14–22
6. Martin NA, Wilson CB (1982) Medial occipital AVM. Surgical treatment. J Neurosurg 56: 798–802
7. Riche MC et al. (1986) Embolization of arteriovenous malformations using compression. A propos of 11 cases. J Mal Vasc 11:162–167
8. Solomon RA, Stein BM (1986) Surgical management of AVM that follow the tentorial ring. Neurosurgery 18:708–715
9. Solomon RA, Stein BM (1987) Interhemispheric approach for the surgical removal of thalamocaudate AVM. J Neurosurg 66: 345–351
10. Spetzler RF, Martin NA (1986) A proposed grading system for AVM. J Neurosurg 65: 476–483
11. Stein BM (1984) AVM of the medial hemisphere and the limbic system. J Neurosurg 60:23–31
12. Steiner L (1984) Treatment of arteriovenous malformations by radiosurgery. In: Wilson CB, Stein BM (eds) Intracranial arteriovenous malformations. Williams and Wilkins, Baltimore, pp 295–313
13. Yasargil MG, Jain KK, Antic J (1976) AVM of the splenium of the corpus callosum. Microsurgical treatment. Surg Neurol 5:5–14
14. Yasargil MG, Jain KK, Antic J (1976) AVM of the anterior and middle portion of the corpus callosum. Surgical treatment. Surg Neurol 5:67–80

Considerations on the Coexistence of Intracranial Arteriovenous Malformations and Aneurysms

J.A. Grotenhuis and J.A.N. van der Spek[1]

Treatment of intracranial arteriovenous malformations (AVMs) is still one of the great challenges in neurosurgery. In a considerable number of cases a special dimension is added to the problem by the simultaneous detection of one or sometimes more than one intracranial aneurysm.

Three hypothesis have been propounded to explain the nature of this coexistence: (1) the association of AVM and aneurysms is coincidental; (2) both lesions are congenital vascular malformations that tend to occur simultaneously; (3) aneurysms are caused by the hemodynamic stress resulting from the augmented blood flow to the AVM.

The first hypothesis is considered unlikely, though possible. The incidence of aneurysms occuring simultaneously with AVMs is, according to recent clinical studies covering a large number of AVMs, 6%–9% [5, 7, 9, 12, 14], higher than that of aneurysms alone in a general population, which definitely suggests a special relationship between these two lesions. The second hypothesis cannot be accepted because intracranial aneurysms are not purely congenital. Although the congenital medial defect of the arterial wall is an important factor in the development of an aneurysm, it is also found in many parts of arterial bifurcations, where aneurysms do not develop. Furthermore, in an autopsy study on 215 subjects with intracranial aneurysms, the prevalence of AVMs was not higher than in a control group of 849 subjects without intracranial aneurysms [11].

Our study suggests, together with most other recent studies, that the hemodynamic stress due to the increased blood flow to the AVM plays a decisive role in the development of aneurysms located on the arterial route supplying the AVM. This hypothesis is supported by the following observations: aneurysms frequently occur at sites remote from the circle of Willis and are to a very high percentage located on arteries contributing to the AVM [1, 2, 4, 6, 8, 10]; there have been several observations of shrinking of the aneurysm after surgical treatment of the AVM as well as of an increase in size of the aneurysm on angiographic follow-up of conservatively treated AVMs [5, 7, 13]; in a postmortem study of a patient with an AVM and an aneurysm, it was found that the media of the dilated artery varied in thickness and the elastic lamina was interrupted in some places [3]. That the increased blood flow can cause distension and degeneration of arterial walls has also been shown experimentally [11].

---

[1] Neurosurgical Center Nijmegen, Canisius-Wilhelmina Hospital and St. Radboud University Hospital, Postbus 9015, 6500 GS Nijmegen, The Netherlands

Advances in Neurosurgery, Vol. 19
W. J. Bock, Ch. Lumenta, M. Brock, M. Klinger (Eds.)

In the present study we report six of our owns cases and a review of the literature on the coexistence of intracranial AVMs and aneurysms. The following data are based upon 158 AVMs associated with 196 aneurysms; 121 were associated with one aneurysm, 37 AVMs with more than one.

The first group consisted of 98 supratentorial and 23 infratentorial AVMs. In 91 out of the 98 supratentorial and in all 23 cases of infratentorial AVM, the aneurysm was located on an artery related to the AVM.

The second group consisted of 32 supratentorial and 5 infratentorial AVMs, associated with altogether 75 aneurysms. In 16 out of the 32 supratentorial and in 3 out of the 5 infratentorial AVMs all aneurysms were on arteries supplying the AVM, while in the other 16 supratentorial and 2 infratentorial AVMs, at least one aneurysm was related to the AVM.

It is not always obvious which of the two lesions is the symptomatic one, and in the case of spontaneous intracranial hemorrhage it can be impossible to determine unequivocally which of the lesions has bled. In many cases the primary CT scan will provide the decisive evidence, but in doubtful cases one should recall the following indications compiled from the literature: there was no correlation between probability and kind of hemorrhage on the one hand and size of the AVM, number of associated aneurysms, and localization of AVM and aneurysms on the other.

From the 158 AVMs associated with 196 aneurysms, we found unequivocal data concerning kind of hemorrhage and source of the bleeding in 82 cases. In 50 cases a subarachnoid hemorrhage and in 32 cases an intracerebral hemorrhage occurred. In 43 out of the 50 cases with subarachnoid hemorrhaging the aneurysm was the source of the bleeding (86%), the remaining 7 cases being caused by the AVM. Out of the 32 cases with intracerebral hemorrhage, 25 were due to rupture of the AVM (78%), the other 7 were caused by rupture of the aneurysms (22%). Finally, the age of the patient appeared to be important. Below 30 years of age there was a higher probability of bleeding from the AVM. With increasing age, there was a higher probability of aneurysm rupture.

From 1980 to 1989 76 patients harboring 77 AVMs were diagnosed in the neurosurgical center Nijmegen. In 6 cases we found associated aneurysms (7.8%). The mean age of the 70 patients with AVM was 30.2 years (range 1–59 years), where that of the 6 patients with associated aneurysms was 42.0 years (range 33–52 years). This marked difference in mean age has also been reported in the literature. The data of the 6 patients with AVM and aneurysm can be gathered from Table 1.

Regarding the treatment of patients harboring an AVM and aneurysm, one should concentrate first on the symptomatic lesion. If the AVM is the source of the hemorrhage and surgery is considered as the best option, all aneurysms related to the AVM should be treated in the same session. Although aneurysms may shrink and even angiographically disappear after excision of the AVM, it is very doubtful that this disappearence can be regarded as actual healing. There will always be a change, however remote, of hemorrhage, from the permanently damaged arterial wall.

Even more important is the simultaneous treatment of aneurysms located on adjacent normal arteries or adjunctive feeding arteries, because these vessels often

Table 1.

Pat. age	Pat. sex	AVM Localization	AVM Feeders	Aneurysm Localization	Initial symptom	Source of hemorrhage	Operation (1st stage) Aneurysm	Operation (1st stage) AVM	Follow-up
33	M	Frontal L	ACA L	AcoA/A1A R oaICA L	SAH	Aneurysm (ACoA/AlA)	++	–	Symptom-free
51	F	Parietal L	ACA L MCA L	ACA L	Seizure (1972) SAH (1984)	Aneurysm	+	+	Right hemi-paresis (post-operative rebleeding)
42	M	Cerebellar L	SCA L PICA L	PICA L	SAH	Aneurysm	+	+	Symptom-free
45	F	Parietal R	ACA R MCA R	pcaICA R	Seizure (1969) SAH (1981)	Aneurysm	+	–	Symptom-free (with antiepilep-tics)
42	M	C. callosum	ACA R	AcoA	SAH + ICH	AVM	+	+	Memory defect, decreased activity
39	M	Parietal R	ACA R MCA R	AcoA	SAH	Aneurysm	+	–	Symptom-free, surgery of AVM scheduled

ACA, anterior cerebral artery; *ACoA*, anterior communicating artery; *A1A*, A1-segment of ACA; *ICA*, internal carotid artery; *ICH*, intracerebral hemorrhage; *MCA*, middle cerebral artery; *oaICA*, offspring of ophthalmic artery from ICA; *pcaICA*, offspring of posterior communicating artery from *ICA*; PICA, posterior inferior cerebellar artery; SAH, subarachnoid hemorrhage; *SCA*, superior cerebellar artery

increase in size after excision of the AVM and the concomitant decrease in size of the AVM's feeding arteries and their main branches, leading to a higher probability of aneurysm rupture. Surgical treatment of these aneurysms is also strongly advisable directly before nonsurgical treatment e.g., embolization of the AVM.

If the aneurysm is the source of bleeding, then it should be surgically treated. The AVM should then be regarded as an incidental, unruptured AVM. Treatment of this lesion should depend on individual considerations, including the age of the patient and size and localization of the AVM, the latter also in relation to the aneurysm to be approached surgically. In these cases, decision analysis, a mathematical aid to clinical reasoning, may be useful where judgment is difficult.

References

1. Anderson RM, Blackwood W (1959) The association of arteriovenous angioma and saccular aneurysm of the arteries of the brain. J Pathol Bacteriol 77:101–110
2. Boyd-Wilson JS (1959) The association of cerebral angiomas with intracranial aneurysms. J Neurol Neurosurg Psychiat 22:218–223
3. Brihaye J, Blackwood W (1957) Arterio-venous aneurysm of the cerebral hemispheres. J Pathol Bacteriol 73:25–31
4. Gacs G, Vinuela F, Foy AJ, Drake CG (1985) Peripheral aneurysms of the cerebral arteries. J Neurosurg 58:63–68
5. Hayashi S, Arimoto T, Itakura T, Fujii T, Nishiguchi T, Komai N (1981) The association of intracranial aneurysms and arteriovenous malformation of the brain. J Neurosurg 55:971–975
6. Hudgins RJ, Day AL, Quisling RG, Rhoton AL, Sypert GW, Carcia-Bengochea F (1983) Aneurysms of the posterior inferior cerebellar artery. J Neurosurg 58:381–387
7. Miyasaka K, Wolpert SM, Prager RJ (1982) The association of cerebral aneurysms, infundibula and intracranial arteriovenous malformations. Stroke 13:196–203
8. Patterson JM, McKissock W (1956) A clinical survey of intracranial angiomas with special reference to their mode of progression and surgical treatment; A report of 110 cases. Brain 79:233–266
9. Perret G, Nishioka H (1966) Report on the cooperative study of intracranial aneurysms and subarachnoid hemorrhage. Section VI. Arteriovenous malformations. An analysis of 545 cases of cranio-cerebral arteriovenous malformations and fistulas reported to the cooperative study. J Neurosurg 25: 467–490
10. Reigh EE, Lemmen LJ (1960) Cerebral aneurysms with other intracranial pathology. J Neurosurg 17:469–476
11. Stehbens WE (1968) Blood vessel changes in chronic experimental arteriovenous fistulas. Surg Gynec Obstet 127:327–337
12. Suzuki J, Onuma T (1979) Intracranial aneurysms associated with arteriovenous malformations. J Neurosurg 50:742–746
13. Tognetti F, Limoni P, Testa C (1983) Aneurysm growth and hemodynamic stress. Surg Neurol 20:74–78
14. Waga S, Itoh H, Kojima T (1985) Posterior inferior cerebellar artery aneurysm associated with arteriovenous malformation fed by the same artery. Surg Neurol 23:617–620

Follow-up After Treatment for Intracranial Arteriovenous Malformations

H.M. Mehdorn[1], S.P. Müller[2], D. Koch[1], and W. Grote[1]

Introduction

Despite refinement of surgical techniques, intracranial arteriovenous malformations (AVMs) continue to challenge neurosurgeons in the way of selecting the best treatment for any particular patient with regard to the medical history, clinical findings, location and size of the AVM, and in the light of their personal experience. In order to clarify the long-term results of various forms of treatment, a follow-up analysis was performed on outcome in 300 consecutive patients treated at the Department of Neurosurgery of University of Essen Medical Center between 1970 and 1989 for symptoms due to an angiographically demonstrated intracranial AVM.

Patients and Methods

The 300 consecutive patients treated for clinical symptoms attributable to an AVM came from a total of 319 patients treated for intracranial angiomas between 1970 and 1989 in our department. Charts were reviewed and clinical follow-up was carried out where possible. If no long-term clinical follow-up was available, information about long-term results of treatment was sought from relatives or referring physicians. Particular care was directed toward the social outcome. The follow-up interval ranged between 0 and 291 months after the first event which had led to the diagnosis of an AVM, with an average follow-up interval of 60 months.

In the patients who had undergone proton beam therapy (PBT), in addition to clinical follow-up, computed tomography (CD) scans every year and control angiography 2 years after therapy were performed. This led to 41 control angiographies and 104 CT scans in 54 patients.

Transcranial Doppler sonography (TCDS) was used for frequent monitoring of flow velocities in intracranial arteries supplying angiomas, in order to better understand changes in intracranial hemodynamics following this kind of treatment. Technical details have been published previously [7, 8]. A total of 210 TCDs examinations were performed in 64 patients. Finally, in 11 patients, single photon emission computed tomography (SPECT) studies were performed using techne-

---

[1] Neurochirurgische Universitätsklinik, Hufelandstr. 55, W-4300 Essen 1, FRG
[2] Abteilung für Nuklearmedizin, Neurochirurgische Universitätsklinik, Hufelandstr. 55, W-4300 Essen 1, FRG

Advances in Neurosurgery, Vol. 19
W. J. Bock, Ch. Lumenta, M. Brock, M. Klinger (Eds.)

tium-labelled erythrocytes to determine the size and intensity of the blood pool in the AVM itself.

Results

One hundred and fifty-three patients presented with intracranial hemorrhage, and their age distribution showed a peak in the second decade of life, while patients with seizures as initial symptoms (85 patients) had their highest incidence in the third decade, and other initial symptoms such as neurological deficit or headaches (58 patients) mostly occurred even later in life.

Primary treatment consisted of surgical excision of the AVM in 108 patients, radiation therapy using the stereotactic proton beam technique (PBT) (4–7) in 68 patients, and ligation of the feeding artery in 30 patients; interventional neuroradiology was employed in 11 patients, followed by excision of the lesion or by radiation therapy, or performed as the only procedure (upon patient request); a conservative approach was chosen in 6–7 patients. (Of the remaining 16 patients, 5 died within 24 h of admission and 11 were treated by a variety of other methods.) Figure 1 shows the treatments employed in relation to the primary symptoms.

Because this was a retrospective analysis covering a period of 20 years, the size and location of the AVMs could not be determined with sufficient accuracy to grade the AVMs according to one of the recently published grading systems [11, 12]. For historical reasons, several patients harboring large AVMs which had been considered elsewhere as inoperable were referred to our department specifically to be further referred for PBT by Dr. Kjellberg in Boston. Most of these patients decided against surgery or neuroradiological interventions when the therapeutic risks and benefits were discussed with them again and preferred the lower-risk therapies even with the residual risk of later hemorrhages.

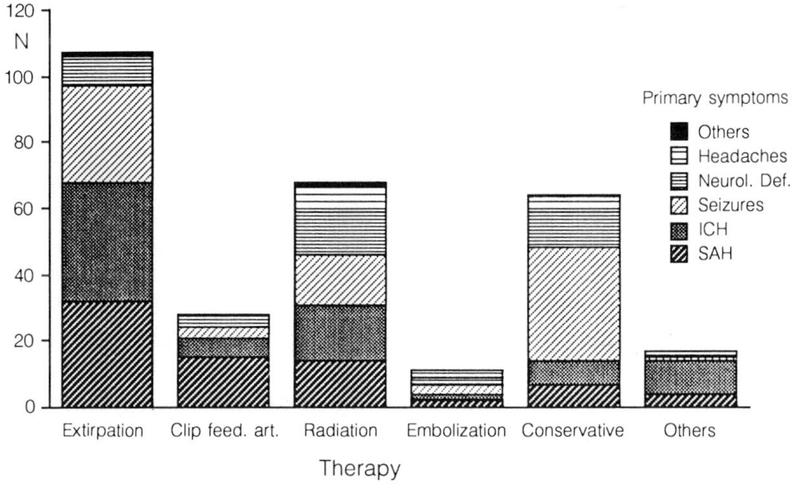

Fig. 1. Treatment in relation to primary symptoms

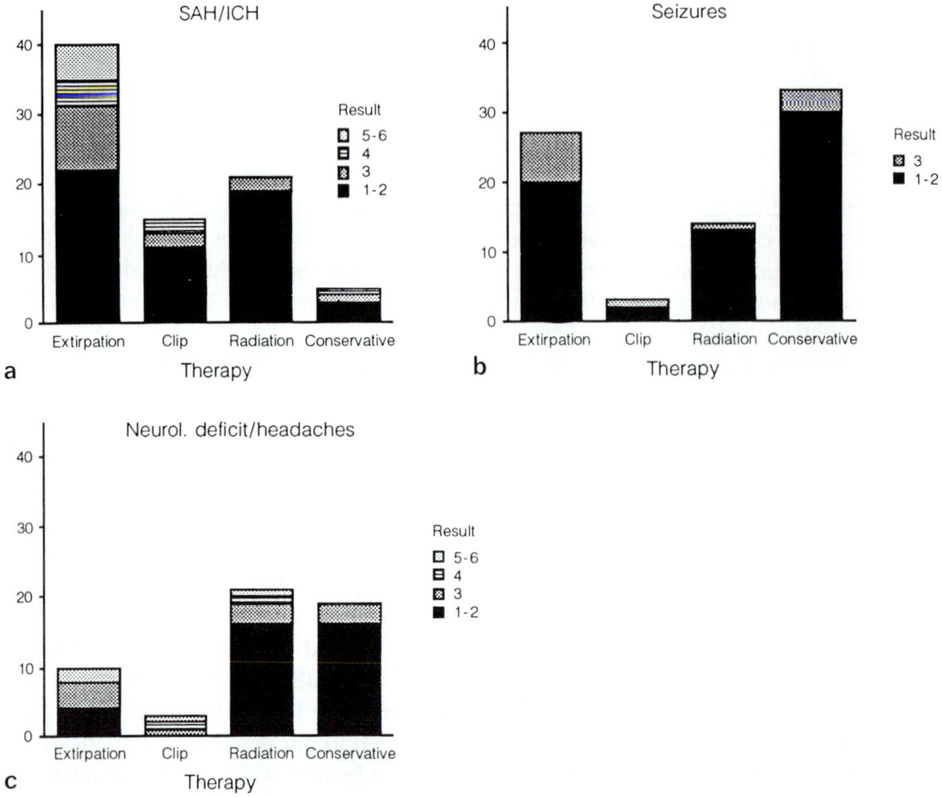

Fig. 2a–c. Long-term results following different treatment forms for different primary symptoms. SAH, subarachnoid hemorrhage; ICH, intracerebral hemorrhage. Results: 1–2, working; 3, independent; 4, needs help; 5, requires daily care or dead

Clinical Follow-up

In order to compare the results of different treatment modalities (Fig. 2) in relation to initial clinical symptoms, we first looked at patients presenting with intracranial hemorrhage and whose clinical condition was classified as Hunt and Hess grades I–III upon admission to our department. In the surgically treated group, combined long-term mortality and invalidity (defined as requiring intense daily care) was 12% (including two deaths due to cancer and suicide). Fifty-five percent of the patients had returned to their previous work. In the group of patients undergoing PBT, 90% of the patients had gone back to their previous occupation. Among the patients operated upon because of seizures, one patient died, and 69% returned to their previous work. Among 15 patients who had undergone radiation therapy after seizures had led to the diagnosis of an AVM, one died of a massive hemorrhage while the others led a useful life. Finally, in the group of patients who were diagnosed because of a neurological deficit and/or headaches, only 1/3 were able to return to

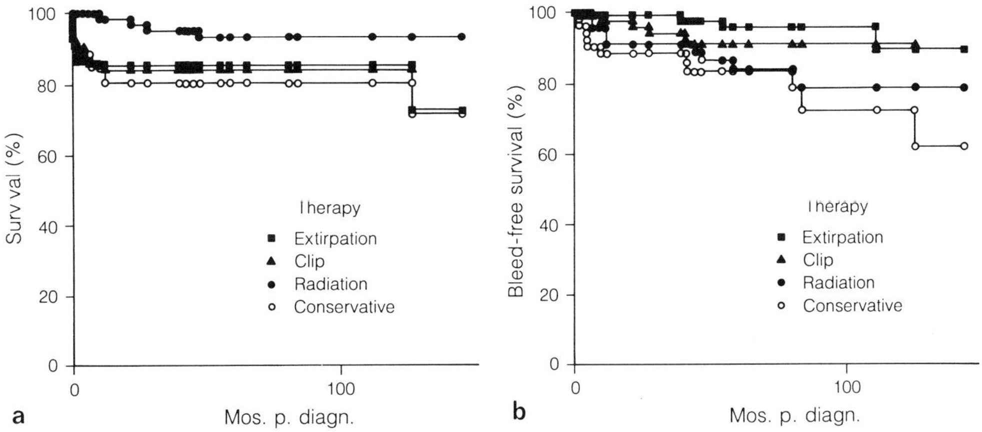

Fig. 3a, b. Life table analysis of the effect of different treatment forms: **a** survival; **b** bleed-free survival

their previous occupation; their percentage was higher among the irradiated or conservatively managed patients.

Long-term results for each treatment modality were obtained by using the Kaplan-Meyer method of life-time analysis. Figure 3 clearly shows that surgical removal of an AVM provides the lowest risk of a recurrent hemorrhage – the recurrent hemorrhages are due to incomplete AVM removal or additional AVMs at other locations. Also, patients with radiated AVMs run a risk of recurrent hemorrhage only slightly lower than that in the natural history – at least in the follow-up time of up to 153 months (average 86 months). On the other hand, patients who have undergone PBT have the best course as far as AVM-related mortality and invalidism is concerned, when compared to surgically treated, and conservatively managed patients, although it should be said that particularly the surgical group contains patients who arrived at our institution in Hunt and Hess grades IV and V condition.

Additional Investigations

Control CT scans were reviewed for a total of 54 patients who had undergone PBT; 20 showed a reduction of contrast enhancement, and the AVM was no longer visible in five. Contrast enhancement diminished, in rare instances, even over several years. No signs of parenchymal brain damage were detected in a single instance. Control angiography was performed in 41 patients of the same cohort, 2 years after PBT; it showed disappearance of the AVM in four patients and reduction of size and/or flow through the AVM in ten. While only small AVMs (less than 2 cm in diameter) actually disappeared some larger AVMs showed a reduction in size.

TCDs showed in most instances a reduction in mean flow velocity within the first 6 months following radiotherapy; however, over the ensuing time, a return to

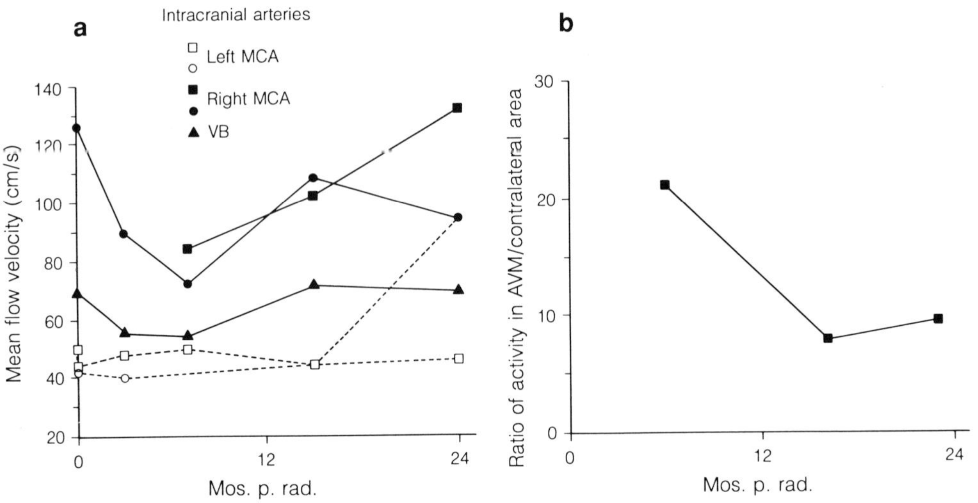

Fig. 4a, b. Patient with a right parieto-occipital AVM who has undergone proton beam therapy. **a** Development of blood flow velocities in the arteries feeding the AVM and normal brain; MCA, middle cerebral arteries. **b** Development of the blood volume as determined by SPECT, calculated as the ratio between the AVM and the contralateral areal

flow velocities close to the preradiation levels was noted. A typical example of the changes in the angioma-feeding arteries over time is given in Fig. 4a, indicating a reduction in flow velocity in the angioma-feeding arteries while the velocities in the arteries of the contralateral (left) hemisphere did not change.

SPECT investigations using technetium-labelled erythrocytes showed a reduction of blood volume in the AVM in only 6 of 11 patients within the 12 months following proton beam therapy. In the other patients, the time course varied remarkably. In addition to TCDs findings, Fig. 4b also shows the course over time of blood pool for the same patient. It is obvious that the reduction of blood volume occurs later than reduction of flow velocities and again is only temporary.

Discussion

Since the natural history of symptomatic AVMs carries a 2.23%–3%/year risk of recurrent hemorrhage [1, 9, 15], any kind of treatment should reduce this long-term risk as long as the immediate risk remains acceptable. Although different grading systems have been proposed in order to evaluate the surgical risks [11–13], mortality and morbidity still vary remarkably in different series [2, 3, 12, 14], depending on patient referral and management. Therefore, the term "inoperable lesion" should also be regarded as an expression of personal experience and judgment.

In the series of 300 patients with a clinically symptomatic intracranial AVM referred to our department between 1970 and 1989, the yearly risk of hemorrhage in untreated patients was approximately 3%, with a higher risk during the early follow-up time. This risk could best be reduced by surgery, with three late recurrent hemorrhages due to contralateral or residual AVMs. On the other hand, surgery resulted, as calculated by the life table analysis, in a mortality of approximately 12% at 1 year, with no further deaths during the average follow-up of 5 years. This, however, includes all patients treated over a 20-year period for AVM-related intracerebral hemorrhage of any severity and all causes of death. These figures, of course, are to a certain degree historical figures and therefore cannot be unconditionally used for comparison of surgical risks against the risks of other forms of modern treatment (Fig. 3).

Still, from what appears in Figs. 2 and 3, the other preferred method of treatment was referral for PBT ([4–6], R.N. Kjellberg 1989, personal communication), and these patients had the best course as far as mortality and invalidism are concerned. The follow-up results in these patients make evident the risk of recurrent hemorrhage, which, in agreement with the literature, was not reduced in the first years after therapy. For the patients presented here, who represent only a small subgroup of Dr. Kjellberg's overall series of more than 800 patients with AVMs, it is too early to give any long-term results; in the overall experience, a significant reduction of mortality from recurrent hemorrhage has been observed to occur after a latency period of 8 years.

The clinically obvious benefit of PBT is at odds with its results as shown by other investigations: the "wipe-out" rate [3] following PBT as evidenced by control angiography and CT is very low, but on the other hand, the risks with PBT seem to compare effectively with those of any kind of treatment, bringing no early complications and a late complication rate of 1.8% ([4]; R.N. Kjellberg 1989, personal communication). In our patients, no complications related to PBT have been observed yet; they will continue to be followed in the future.

Because the clinical effects of PBT are so difficult to measure in the early phase, it was thought interesting regularly to follow these patients with additional noninvasive investigations. Previously, our early experience with TCDs has been reported [7], and it was suggested that the initial reduction of flow velocities in intracranial arteries subsequent to PBT may be related to a reduction of arteriovenous shunt in the AVM and therefore might correlate with the protection against hemorrhage. The additional data gained since then regarding flow velocities further support the idea that the flow reduction is only temporary and may be related to an early postradiation swelling in the nidal vasculature. So far, however, the flow reduction cannot be directly related to the long-term benefit of PBT, as is shown by the fact that the patient whose TCDs data were previously presented [8] has since died from massive intracerebellar hemorrhage 20 months after PBT. Autopsy examination in this particular patient [10] did not show any of the alterations in the vasculature which have been proposed to occur after radiation therapy [5, 6].

The later re-rise of flow velocities is also difficult to explain; it may be related to a reduction in diameter of feeding arteries, although no sufficiently comparable control angiographies have been performed in these patients to study this assumption.

It had been hoped that the additional data obtained from SPECT relating to the blood pool in the AVM would help in understanding the TCDs findings. Although in some patients a reduction of blood pool has been observed, a later re-rise in blood pool also occurred. So far, these data are controversial and further experience and correlation with patients' clinical development will be needed to make them helpful.

To conclude, surgical excision of an intracranial AVM remains the best choice of treatment provided it can be performed safely. Close cooperation with interventional neuroradiologists may be one way of further reducing surgical risks. Radiation therapy should be reserved for patients harboring truly inoperable lesions, because of the long delay until it really provides protection against future hemorrhages.

References

1. Crawford PM, West CR, Chadwick DM (1986) Arteriovenous malformations of the brain. Natural history in inoperable patients. J Neurol Neurosurg Psychiatry 49:1–10
2. Drake CG (1979) Cerebral arteriovenous malformations of the brain: considerations for and experience with surgical treatment in 166 cases. Clin Neurosurg 26:145–208
3. Drake CG (1983) Arteriovenous malformations of the brain. The options for management. N Engl J Med 309:308–331
4. Kjellberg RN (1987) Proton beam therapy for inoperable arteriovenous malformations. Neurosurgery Update Course, Boston, November 1978 (cited from [9])
5. Kjellberg, RN, Hanamura T, Davis KR, Lyons S, Adams RD (1983) Bragg peak proton beam therapy for arteriovenous malformations of the brain. N Engl J Med 309:269–274
6. Kjellberg RN, Davis KR, Lyons S, Butler W, Adams RD (1984) Bragg peak proton beam therapy for arteriovenous malformations of the brain. Clin Neurosurg 31:248–290
7. Mehdorn HM, Grote W (1988) Non-invasive follow-up of patients undergoing proton beam therapy for intracranial arteriovenous malformations. Acta Neurochir [Suppl] (Wien) 42:98-102
8. Mehdorn HM, Hense J, Hoffman B (1988) Applications for transcranial Doppler sonography in neurosurgery. Adv Neurosurg 16:62–66
9. Ogilvy CS (1990) Radiation therapy for arteriovenous malformations: review. Neurosurgery 26:775–735
10. Reinhardt R, Mehdorn HM, Gerhard L, Grote W (1989) Neuropathologische Studien zum Therapieeffekt der Protonenbestrahlung bei arteriovenösen Angiomen. Das intrakranielle Gefäßsystem, 10th Mainzer Herbsttagung, 14–16 Sept 1989
11. Shi YQ, Chen XC (1986) A proposed scheme for grading intracranial arteriovenous malformations. J Neurosurg 65:484–489
12. Spetzler RF, Martin N (1986) A proposed grading system for arteriovenous malformations. J Neurosurg 65:476–483
13. Steinmeier R, Schramm J, Müller HG, Fahlbusch R (1989) Evaluation of prognostic factors in cerebral arteriovenous malformations. Neurosurg 24:193–200
14. Svien HJ, McRae JA (1965) Arteriovenous anomalies of the brain. Fate of patients not having definite surgery. J Neurosurg 23:23–28
15. Wilinks RH (1985) Natural history of intracranial arteriovenous malformations: review. Neurosurg 16:421–430

Posterior Fossa Arteriovenous Malformations: Angioarchitecture in Relation to Hemorrhagic Episodes

G. Rodesch[1, 2], R. Garcia Monaco[1], H. Alvarez[1], A. Goulao[1], and P. Lasjaunias[1]

Introduction

Posterior fossa arteriovenous malformations (AVMs) are rare in comparison with supratentorial lesions: they represent about 10%–15% of all intracranial AVMs [1, 2]. Their presenting symptoms are mainly hemorrhages [3], but the question whether there is an increased risk of bleeding in this infratentorial localization is still unanswered. In order to try to analyze the relationship between hemorrhagic episodes and posterior fossa localization, we have reviewed the files of 32 patients referred to one of us (P.L.) and analyzed the angioarchitecture of the AVMs involved.

Results

Seventy-eight percent of all AVMs in our series (foramen magnum lesions, dural fistulas, cavernomas, and venous anomalies were excluded from our series) presented with hemorrhage; 9.5% were revealed by progressive neurological symptoms; 6.5% were incidental findings. In the pediatric population (five patients in our series), cardiac failure developed in one newborn (3%) and in another baby a cranial bruit was heard (3%) which led secondarily to the diagnosis.

In the population with cerebellar AVMs, 24 of the 28 patients (86%) presented with hemorrhage and only one with neurological symptoms. On the other hand, of the four brain stem lesions, two presented with progressive deficit, one with intracranial bruit (see above) and one with hemorrhage.

Discussion

We have tried to penetrate the angioarchitectural data of the AVMs and compare them with those obtained previously by analysis of supratentorial lesions [2, 4] Twenty (62.5%) were nidus-type lesions and 5 (15.5%) belonged to the group of micro-AVMs [5]. Four (12.5%) were associated with dilatation of the vein of Galen (false vein of Galen aneurysm malformations). Multiple AVMs were seen in three patients (10%).

---

[1] Hôpital Bicêtre, Neuroradiologie Diagnostique et Thérapeutique, 78 rue du Général Leclerc, 94275 Le Kremlin Bicêtre, France
[2] Hôpital Erasme, Neuroradiologie, 808 Route de Lennick, B-1070 Brussels, Belgium

Advances in Neurosurgery, Vol. 19
W. J. Bock, Ch. Lumenta, M. Brock, M. Klinger (Eds.)

Table 1. Angioarchitecture of posterior fossa AVMs in 32 patients[a]

Angioarchitecture	Patients overall		Patients who bled ($n = 25$)	
	n	%	n	%
Venous ectasia	24	75	18	72
Venous stenosis or thrombosis	22	68	18	72
Aneurysms	7	22	6	24
Transdural supply	6	19	6	24
Transmesencephalic supply	6	19	4	16

[a] The difference between the overall population and the group that bled is minimal since 78% of them are the same patients.

The following aspects of angioarchitecture were particularly looked for: venous thrombosis, stenosis, or ectasia, associated flow-related aneurysms (pre- or intranidal), transdural supply, and transmesencephalic supply. The analysis is summarized in Table 1 and shows that bleeding is mainly due to rupture of venous ectasias subsequent to venous stenosis or thrombosis and to associated aneurysms. Since these elements represent high risk factors, they should be treated first by endovascular therapy in order to decongest the venous system and disconnect the arterial pouches. The angioarchitectural analysis of posterior fossa AVMs shows no major further differences to supratentorial lesions. The risk factors have equal incidences in both locations [3]. On the other hand, according to Crawford et al. [2], infratentorial location is not synonymous with higher risk of hemorrhage, as temporal lobe location is, for example. The same conclusions can be drawn from a comparison of clinical and autopsy data [3].

Though apparently supporting the "classical" concept that posterior fossa AVMs have a high tendency to bleed, our series suggests that hemorrhagic accidents are rather the dominant expression of cerebellar AVMs, as in micro-AVMs [5]. We speculate that clinical tolerance of these lesions is guaranteed by the functional anatomy of the cerebellum [3]: this could mean that the "best way" for these AVMs to reveal their presence is the hemorrhagic episode. By contrast, brain stem lesions would reveal themselves primarily by neurological deficits, because of the eloquence of this structure and its great concentration of nervous pathways, so that any pathological condition will rapidly produce symptoms.

Conclusion

Posterior fossa AVMs do not bleed or rebleed more than other AVMs. Hemorrhage is their dominant mode of expression. There are no angioarchitectural differences between supra- and infratentorial lesions. Bleeding is linked to venous hemodynamic changes or associated aneurysms, with the same incidence as in other AVMs.

References

1. Batjer H, Samson D (1986) Arteriovenous malformations of the brain: natural history study. J Neurosurg 64:849–856
2. Crawford P, Pest C, Chadwick D, Shaw M (1986) Arteriovenous malformations of the brain: natural history in unoperated patients. J Neurol Neurosurg Psychiatry 49:1–10
3. Garcia Monaco R, Alvarez H, Goulao A, Pruvost P, Lasjaunias P (1990) Posterior fossa arteriovenous malformations. Angioarchitecture in relation to their hemorrhagic episodes. Neuroradiology 31:471–475
4. Willinsky R, Lasjaunias P, Terbrugge K, Pruvost P (1988) Brain arteriovenous malformation. Analysis of the angioarchitecture in relationship to hemorrhage. J Neuroradiol 15:225–237
5. Willinsky R, Lasjaunias P, Terbrugge K, Pruvost P (1988) Cerebral micro-arteriovenous malformations (mAVMs). Review of 13 cases. Acta Neurochir (Wien) 91:37–41

Clinical and Radiological Prognostic Factors in Cerebral Arteriovenous Malformations

H.-G. Höllerhage, K.-M. Dewenter, and H. Dietz[1]

Introduction

Progress in microsurgery has meant that operative treatment of arteriovenous malformations (AVMs) has nowadays become to a high degree safe. In consequence there is a clear indication for surgery in the majority of these lesions, whereas some 25 years ago conservative treatment was recommended in 85% of all cases [10]. Thus, progress in surgical techniques has abrogated a lot of restrictions to surgery of AVMs. However, this new surgical freedom is increasingly offset by the progress made in endovascular techniques, which are not limited to lesions not amenable to surgery but are becoming established as an alternative form of treatment or even the treatment of choice in malformations well accessible to the surgeon. These developments require careful consideration during decision making, which should be based on empirical data allowing the best assessment of the prognosis in each individual case. Since the term AVM designates relatively heterogeneous lesion, mere comparison of different series of surgically treated or surgically vs. endovascularly treated cases provides only more or less anecdotal information. This is the reason why grading systems have been published. In a previous paper [3] we discussed the value and practicability of the systems of Luessenhop and Genarelli [5], Spetzler and Martin [9], and Shi and Chen [8]. We arrived at the conclusion that, although the system of Spetzler and Martin has some advantages, strictly speaking all these grading systems are rather arbitrary and have a low accuracy in predicting the outcome of surgery of AVMs. In the present paper we present a method of evaluating prognosis by multivariate analysis of radiological and clinical data.

Methods

From 1972 to 1987 107 patients underwent surgery for histologically verified AVMs. We obtained the relevant clinical data such as age, sex, grade of clinical condition on admission, history of bleeding or seizures, clinical course, and early and late outcome from the patients' records. The clinical grade on admission and the outcome grading were assessed according to a 5-point scale as published else-

[1] Neurochirurgische Klinik, Medizinische Hochschule Hannover, Konstanty-Gutschow-Str. 8, W-3000 Hannover 61, FRG

Advances in Neurosurgery, Vol. 19
W. J. Bock, Ch. Lumenta, M. Brock, M. Klinger (Eds.)

where [2]. This admission scale was graduated as follows: no deficit, grade I; slight deficit, grade II; distinct deficit, such as palsy or disturbance of consciousness, grade III; severe deficits, grade IV, comatous moribund state, grade V. The outcome scale is very similar to the Glasgow outcome scale, with grade I signifying an excellent result and grade V death. Late outcome was according to the last follow up, which was never less than 3 months postoperatively. Only patients who were in a good clinical state (grade I, II) on discharge were lost to follow up. In these cases we took it for granted that the late follow up was the same. Out of all 107 patients, six had no angiographic signs of the lesion preoperatively. The angiograms of eight more had not been performed at the Medizinische Hochschule Hannover and were no longer available at the admitting hospitals. This left 93 sets of angiograms for analysis, which was carried out as follows. All feeding arteries and draining veins as well as the exact location and size of the malformations were listed, and the statistical analysis was based on these data. The correlation between grading and the outcome was calculated by means of Spearman's rank correlation coefficient ϱ corrected for ties [7]. For multivariate analysis we used a software implementation of a generalized linear model [4] developed at the University of Linz, Austria (ALMO Statistik-System, Prof. Dr. Kurt Holm, University of Linz, Austria). We used a submodel for multiple dichotomous independent and one dichotomous dependent variable. The dependent (target) variable was the late outcome. The independent (predictor) variables were entered into the multiple regression model in a stepwise procedure. In this procedure variables are entered in succession and only those which contribute significantly to the regression are retained; others are eliminated. Many variables were naturally dichotomous (e.g., venous drainage: superficial/deep; feeders from a particular artery: yes/no) and the rest were dichotomized as follows. Clinical grade on admission and outcome were dichotomized into good (grades I and II) and poor (grades III–V). Age and size were divided into young/old and small/large, depending on whether they were above or below the respective median value. The influence of the significant predictors is represented in terms of effects which are given with standard deviation and significance level.

Results

The significant variables are shown in Table 1. The strongest adverse effect seen on the prognosis was from lenticulostriate feeding arteries. Feeders from the rolandic branches of the middle cerebral artery had a similar effect to feeders from the A1 segment of the anterior cerebral artery. Interestingly, feeding of the AVM from the contralateral side through the anterior communicating artery had an adverse effect on prognosis, too, even when the lesion was remote from the anterior cerebral territory.

Compared to the effects of these radiological data, the effect of clinical grade on admission was not so strong. All other variables had no effect at all or only weak

Table 1. Significant prognostic factors confirmed by multivariate analysis

	Effect[a]	Standard deviation	Partial correlation coefficient	Significance ($p <$)
Feeders from M1 segment (lenticulostr.)	0.6852	0.1875	0.3649	0.0005
Feeders from rolandic branches	0.3737	0.1075	0.3492	0.001
Shunt through anterior commun. artery	0.3160	0.1565	02116	0.05
Feeders from A1 segment	0.3060	0.1440	0.2221	0.05
Poor clinical grade	0.1338	0.0524	0.2642	0.02

[a] Effects can be understood as quantification of the adverse influence of the factors on outcome.

Multiple correlation: 0.5747; $p < 0.0001$

Table 2. Grading of AVMs on the basis of our analysis

Feature		Points assigned
Clinical grade on admission		
	good (I, II)	1
	poor (III–V)	2
Feeding vessels from A1 segment		
	no	0
	yes	1
M1 segment		
	no	0
	yes	1
P1 segment		
	no	0
	yes	1
Rolandic branches		
	no	0
	yes	1
Shunt through anterior communicating artery		
	no	0
	yes	1

Table 3. Results of surgery in relation to our grading

		Grading I	II	III	IV	Total
Outcome	I	26	11	1	0	38
	II	13	17	0	0	30
	III	4	7	4	1	16
	IV	0	3	3	1	7
	V	0	1	1	0	2
Total		43	39	9	2	93

$\varrho = 0.55$

effects that were not statistically significant. In particular, there was not even the slightest support for the hypothesis that the type of venous drainage was of any prognostic significance. The number of feeders and the size of the lesion each had only a slight but not significant effect on the outcome. In general, feeders from the posterior cerebral artery tended to be prognostically favorable, although in one case with a feeding artery from the P1 segment, a poor outcome (grade IV) due to thalamic infarction was seen. With regard to the clinical data, age had only a slight effect. Whether bleeding had occurred or not only affected the clinical grade on admission; it had no direct effect on outcome. The history of seizures did not influence the result of surgery.

On the basis of these findings we graded our cases as shown in Table 2. The inclusion of feeders from the P1 segment among relevant prognostic factors may seem unreasonable, but its importance is supported by our findings even though with only one case it could not be statistically confirmed. A theoretical maximum of 7 points could be given if all unfavorable prognostic criteria were met. However, the maximum score in our patients was 4.

Table 3 shows our results on the basis of this grading. The rank correlation coefficient ϱ of 0.55 shows that this grading correlates quite well with outcome. Exclusion of the P1 feeders from the scoring does not change the rank correlation coefficient except for the rounded third place behind the decimal point.

Discussion

One of the points we made in our previous paper [2] was that present grading systems of AVMs provide only weak prognostic tools because they are based on rather arbitrary categories. Consequently the correlations between gradings and outcomes are not very clear: the correlation coefficient ϱ between the Spetzler and Martin's classification and outcome in our patients was 0.22, for Luessenhop and Generalli's scheme it was 0.14, and for Shi and Chen it was 0.12. All correlations coefficients were thus closer to zero (which is equivalent to no correlation at all) than to 1 (which is equivalent to perfect correlation). We were able to show that clinical grade on admission is a better predictor than all three grading systems ($\varrho = 0.34$), but this is not a particularly satisfying correlation either. By contrast, much higher correlations exist between the grading system of Hunt and Hess and outcome after aneurysmal subarachnoid hemorrhage. For example, calculation using the data given by Chyatte et al. [1] yields $\varrho = 0.52$ and calculation of the placebo group of Petruk et al. [6] yields $\varrho = 0.58$. It is obvious from this that the grading scale of Hunt and Hess has important implications in finding the best treatment of subarachnoid hemorrhage and the best timing of aneurysm surgery. A similarly effective prognostic system for AVMs would certainly be worthwhile, especially if it were as easy to use as the Hunt and Hess scale. The problem with the three grading systems mentioned is that they are based not on an analysis of clinical and radiological data but on the opinion of the authors. For example, a deep venous drainage leads to a more unfavorable classification in both Spetzler and Martin's and Shi and Chen's system; our results make it unlikely that the type of venous drainage is of great prognostic importance. Similarly, feeders from the posterior cerebral artery lead to a higher (less favorable) score in Shi and Chan's system; our results even show a tendency to better outcomes in this group.

An advantage of Spetzler and Martin's system is that it is easy to apply. However, this does not compensate for low prognostic accuracy. Our grading system is quite easy, too, and is based on statistical analysis of clinical and radiological factors. We are aware of the objection that these factors only showed their significance in a retrospective study in our patients and cannot readily be generalized, and that therefore it would be desirable to verify the value of the predictors in a prospective series. On the other hand, our results do not only make sense because they were extracted from our patients' data by a computer program: they are plausible, too. If we look at the factors that influence the prognosis unfavorably we have "poor grade on admission," which is obvious without further comment. The others are "feeding vessels from the A1 and M1 segments and rolandic branches." These are vessels that supply eloquent regions of the brain, especially the basal ganglia and the central region. Although it could not be confirmed statistically, it is obvious that feeders from the P1 segment have probably the same adverse effect on the prognosis of surgery. That is why our proposed grading scheme takes feeders from the P1 segment of the posterior cerebral artery into account. The adverse effect of a shunt through the anterior communicating artery even in remote lesions is less straightforward but may be explained by the fact that excision of such lesions must induce a considerable change in hemodynamics because of the abolishment of the shunt volume.

Our proposed grading scheme is generally applicable in supratentorial AVMs. The rank correlation coefficient between grading and outcome of 0.55 achieved by our scheme is high, comparable to the correlation of the Hunt and Hess scale, with outcome in aneurysmal subarachnoid hemorrhage. It could therefore be a most valuable prognostic tool in the treatment of AVMs.

References

1. Chyatte D, Fode NC, Sundt TM (1988) Early versus late intracranial aneurysm surgery in subarachnoid hemorrhage. J Neurosurg 69:326–331
2. Höllerhage HG (1988) Zur neurochirurgischen Behandlung von zerebralen arteriovenösen Mißbildungen. Neurochirurgia 31:139–143
3. Höllerhage HG, Zumkeller M, Dewenter KM (1990) Zum prognostischen Wert von Graduierungssystemen bei zerebralen arteriovenösen Mißbildungen. Neurochirurgia 33:59–64
4. Holm K (1979) Das allgemeine lineare Modell. In: Holm K (ed) Die Befragung, vol 6. UTB Francke, Munich, pp 11–213
5. Luessenhop AJ, Genarelli TA (1977) Anatomical grading of supratentorial arteriovenous malformations for determining operability. Neurosurgery 1:30–35
6. Petruk KC, West M, Mohr G et al. (1988) Nimodipine treatment in poor-grade aneurysm patients. Results of a multicenter double-blind placebo-controlled trial. J Neurosurg 68:505–517
7. Raatz U (1971) Die Berechnung des Spearmanschen Rangkorrelationskoeffizienten in einer bivariaten Häufigkeitstabelle. Biomed Z 13:208–214
8. Shi YQ, Chen XC (1986) A proposed scheme for grading intracranial arteriovenous malformations. J Neurosurg 65:484–489
9. Spetzler RF, Martin NA (1986) A proposed grading system for arteriovenous malformations. J Neurosurg 65:576–483
10. Svien HJ, McRae JA (1965) Arteriovenous anomalies of the brain. Fate of patients not having definite surgery. J Neurosurg 23:23–28

Venous Angiomas: Experience with Surgical and Nonsurgical Management

J.C. Tonn[1], U. Schuchard[2], C.R. Hornig[3], A.L. Agnoli[2], and K. Roosen[1]

Introduction

Venous angiomas have until now been considered a rare vascular malformation. Especially before the era of computerized tomography (CT) they were infrequently diagnosed by clinicians. Nevertheless, they are a relatively common incidental finding at autopsy, representing 16%–59% of all cerebral angiomas and therefore being the second most frequent angiomatous malformations [1]. This indicates that most venous angiomas remain asymptomatic during life. We have performed a retrospective analysis of patients with venous angiomas with the aim of comparing the results and the pitfalls of surgical and nonsurgical management.

Material and Methods

Between 1969 and 1990, 21 patients with 22 venous angiomas were admitted to the Departments of Neurology and Neurosurgery of the University of Giessen; one patient harbored two venous angiomas. Hospital records, angiograms, CT scans and magnetic resonance images (MRI) were reviewed. Only patients with angiographically proven venous angiomas were included into the study. As far as possible, a follow-up and review of the clinical course since the time of diagnosis was carried out.

Results

The mean age of patients was 31.0 ± 16.1 years (range 5–74 years), with a predominance of males ($n = 16$). In nine patients the lesion was located in the frontal lobe. In four of these cases, a cutaneous manifestation was visible in the periorbital ($n = 2$) or frontotemporal ($n = 2$) region. In our series, venous angiomas within the posterior fossa were most commonly found in the brainstem (Table 1). The lesions

[1] Abteilung Neurochirurgie, Justus-Liebig-Universität Gießen, Klinikstr. 29, W-6300 Gießen, FRG
[2] Abteilung Neuroradiologie, Justus-Liebig-Universität Gießen, Klinikstr. 29, W-6300 Gießen, FRG
[3] Abteilung Neurologie, Justus-Liebig-Universität Gießen, Klinikstr. 29, W-6300 Gießen, FRG

Advances in Neurosurgery, Vol. 19
W. J. Bock, Ch. Lumenta, M. Brock, M. Klinger (Eds.)

Table 1. Localization of venous angiomas

Site	n
Frontal lobe	9
Temporal lobe	4
Parietal lobe	2
Occipital lobe	1
Cerebellum	2
Brainstem	4
	22

Table 2. Initial symptoms

	All patients n	Patients operated upon n
Seizures	7	3
Incidental finding	6	
Cutaneous manifest.	4	4
Subarachnoid hemorr.	2	2
Intracerebral hemorr.	2	1
Dysarthria/ataxia	1	

showed a definite propensity for the left side ($n = 12$) in comparison to the right side ($n = 5$) and the midline ($n = 5$). Most of the malformations ($n = 7$) were diagnosed during investigations following seizures, usually of the grand mal type. In six cases, a venous angioma was found incidentally during examination for minimal or vague complaints not related to the angioma. In two cases a subarachnoid hemorrhage had been the initial symptom, in another two patients a minor intracerebral hemorrhage with cranial nerve palsies (Table 2).

Ten out of 22 angiomas were operated upon (for the initial symptoms of these patients see Table 2). The diagnosis was confirmed histologically in nine cases – in the missing one the biopsy specimen unfortunately got lost. We observed postoperative complications in eight patients (Fig. 1). The most frequent was a hemiparesis with or without aphasia, due to hemorrhagic infarction of the area in which the venous angioma had been located. There were no deaths in either treatment group. A significant difference was evident in the functional outcome of the patients: although the neurological deficits were comparable in both groups at the beginning of the treatment, morbidity was far lower in patients without surgical treatment. Whereas 9 out of 11 patients without surgery had no neurological deficits during follow-up this outcome was only achieved in 3 out of 10 patients operated upon

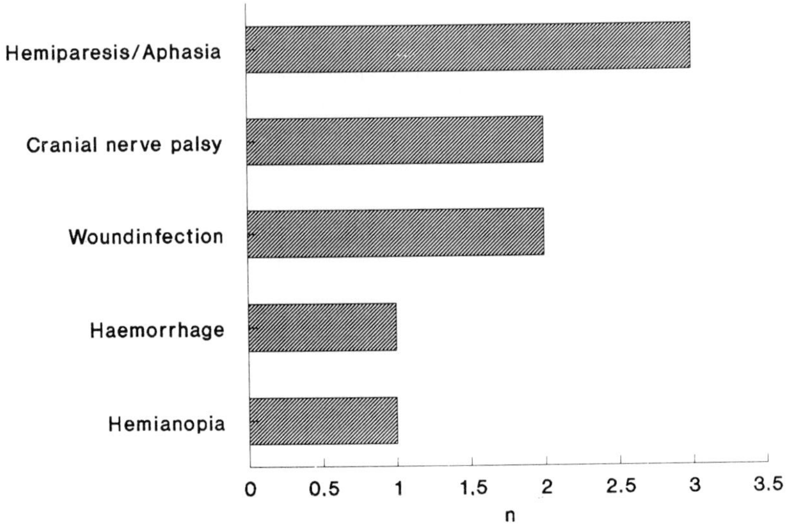

Fig. 1. Postoperative complications

(Fig. 2). During the follow-up period no hemorrhage occurred in those patients who had not undergone surgery.

Discussion

According to Jellinger, venous angiomas consist of anomalous veins within intact neural parenchyma [1]. Neither the number nor the size of the arterial feeders is increased. Lasjaunias stresses the fact that venous angiomas drain a territory of regular arterial vasculature and intact neural tissue; there is no alternative system of drainage. These anomalous veins run into a normal extraparenchymatous venous system. He calls the small deep veins converging towards a transhemispheric collector a "developmental venous anomaly" [2]. This description implies that removal of this drainage might be hazardous for that region of the brain [5] and would explain the high incidence of postoperative hemorrhagic infarction of the brain. Such experiences have already been described in other publications [4]. The low incidence of symptomatic hemorrhage in our series of venous angiomas diagnosed during life might be due to the fact that these lesions are "low flow" vascular malformations. In this respect one might doubt whether a venous angioma is responsible for subarachnoid hemorrhage (SAH) at all. One could speculate that these patients suffered from an SAH of unknown origin and in addition harbored a venous angioma. The high incidence of asymptomatic venous angiomas in postmortem studies supports this hypothesis. Minor hemorrhages in the brainstem associated with venous angiomas have turned out to have a good clinical course without any invasive therapy.

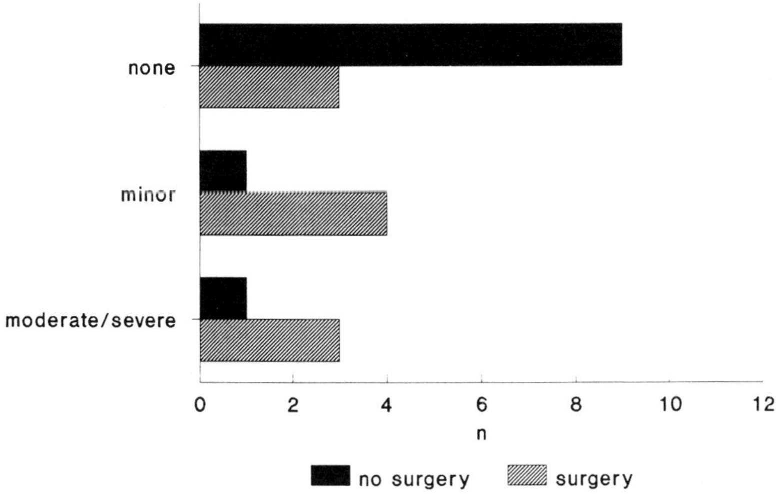

Fig. 2. Functional deficits of 21 patients with a venous angioma after either surgical or nonsurgical treatment

Grand mal seizures are not necessarily caused by a venous malformation and may really be considered a separate disease. In our experience, appropriate anticonvulsive medication is superior to surgery for venous angioma in controlling epileptic fits.

In agreement with other authors [3, 4, 5] we conclude that the only indication for operation upon a venous angioma is when it is associated with a large space-occupying hematoma which has to be evacuated. Merely because the apparent incidence has gone up due to an increasing frequency of CT and MRI investigations is no reason to carry out surgery more often.

References

1. Jellinger K (1986) Vascular malformations of the central nervous system: a morphological overview. Neurosurg Rev 9:177–216
2. Lasjaunias P, Burrows P, Planet C (1986) Developmental venous anomalies (DVA): the so-called venous angiomas. Neurosurg Rev 9:233–244
3. Moritake K, Handa H, Mori K, Ishikawa M, Morimoto M, Takebe Y (1980) Venous angiomas of the brain. Surg Neurol 14:95–105
4. Senegor M, Dohrmann GJ, Wollmann RL (1983) Venous angiomas of the posterior fossa should be considered as anomalous venous drainage. Surg Neurol 19:26–32
5. Yasargil MG (1988) Microneurosurgery, vol III B. Thieme, Stuttgart, pp 405–438

Intracranial Venous Angiomas

C. Plets[1], G. Wilms[2], J. Goffin[1], and Y.S. Ho[1]

Introduction

Venous angiomas are defined as consisting of venous structures only, without arterial or capillary components. According to Fierstein et al. [2], venous angiomas are devoided of large quantities of smooth muscle and elastic tissue; hyalinization and thickening of the walls are common. The first report on a venous angioma demonstrated by angiography came in 1967 [7] and described a structure consisting of a collection of fine dilated medullary veins converging into a central vein draining into a superficial or deep venous system. In 1981, Saito and Kobayashi [4] were the first to propose that venous angiomas are formed as a result of maldevelopment of the medullary veins and their tributaries during embryogenesis. The actual incidence of venous angiomas is unknown but current consensus is that with the availability of gadolinium the detection rate of venous angiomas will undoubtly increase.

Materials and Methods

Our study is a retrospective analysis of 18 cases of venous angiomas seen from 1984 to 1989 inclusive. There were 18 patients: 10 male and 8 female. The average age was 31.4 years with range of 10–84 years. There were 10 supratentorial angiomas which drained into the superior sagittal sinus and 8 infratentorial venous angiomas draining into the superior petrosal sinus or the confluence of sinuses. Computed tomographic (CT) scans were performed in all patients on third-generation scan equipment. Fifteen patients underwent magnetic resonance (MRI; Magnetom R, 1.5 Tesla-Siemens Erlangen). Transfemoral selective angiography was performed in 12 patients.

---

[1] Department of Neurosurgery, University Hospital Gasthuisberg, Catholic University of Leuven, B-3000 Leuven, Belgium
[2] Department of Radiology, University Hospital Gasthuisberg, Catholic University of Leuven, B-3000 Leuven, Belgium

Advances in Neurosurgery, Vol. 19
W. J. Bock, Ch. Lumenta, M. Brock, M. Klinger (Eds.)

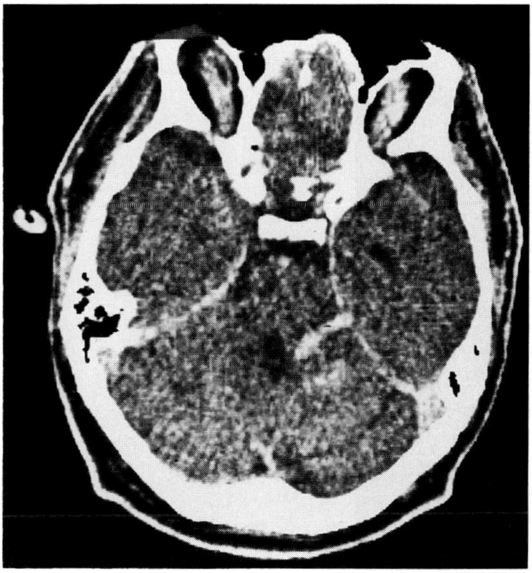

Fig. 1. Contrast-enhanced CT scan. Very typical picture of a venous angioma, showing linear and nodular enhancement in the right middle cerebellar peduncle

Results

The most common symptom was headache (44.4%), followed by sensorimotor disturbance (22.2%). The incidence of hemorrhage was 20% in the patients with supratentorial angiomas and 12.5% in those with infratentorial angiomas.

Contrast-enhanced CT showed an abnormality in 16 patients. Of these, the scans of only two patients, with linear and nodular enhancement, were considered diagnostic of a venous angioma (Fig. 1).

On T2-weighted MRI the draining vein was seen in all instances. It appeared hypointense in 67% of cases, which is consistent with the flow-void appearance of fast-flowing blood. Definitive diagnosis of a venous angioma depends on visualization of the medullary veins. This was seen in only 20% of cases using T2-weighted imaging (Fig. 2). With gadolinium enhancement and T1-weighted imaging, the medullary veins could be seen clearly in all cases in addition to the draining vein (Fig. 3).

We wish to emphasize that gadolinium-enhanced MRI gives a very similar picture of venous angiomas to angiography (Fig. 4). Angiography confirmed a venous angioma in all instances; the typical pattern of medullary veins and draining veins was well seen.

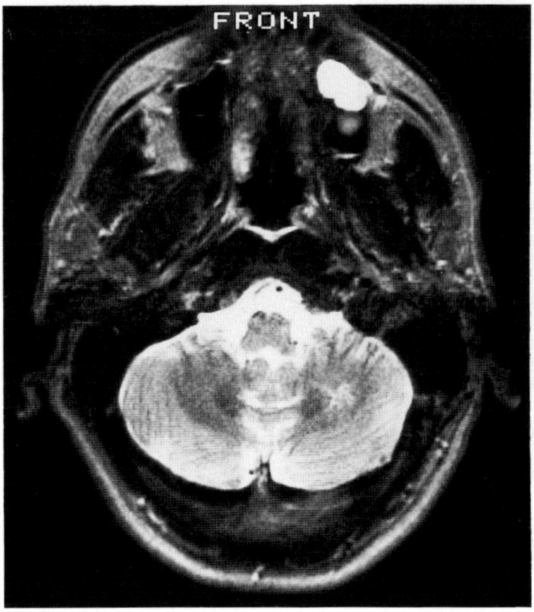

Fig. 2. T2-weighted MRI. A group of medullary veins is seen in the left cerebellar hemisphere. This image is diagnostic for a venous angioma but was found in T2-weighted images in only 20% of our cases

Although all our patients presented with symptoms, only three were operated upon: two of them had bled, and the third case had an intracerebellar angioma causing severe vertigo. One patient with a venous angioma in the deep white matter of the left parietal lobe underwent radiosurgery with the gamma knife in Stockholm. His condition remained good at 3-year follow-up.

Discussion

Intracranial venous angiomas are largely silent lesions, being detected with increasing frequency since the advent of CT and MRI. Nevertheless, both the natural history of these lesions and the absolute indications for operative treatment remain unknown. We compared the patterns of contrast enhancement on CT in our series to those reported by Valavanis et al. [5]. According to these authors a round, enhancing, non-space-occupying lesion in the white matter associated with transcerebral or transcerebellar linear enhancement is a highly specific CT pattern for a venous angioma. Assuming this to be so, CT was diagnostic in 12.5% of the cases in our series and in 18.6% of the cases of Valavanis et al.

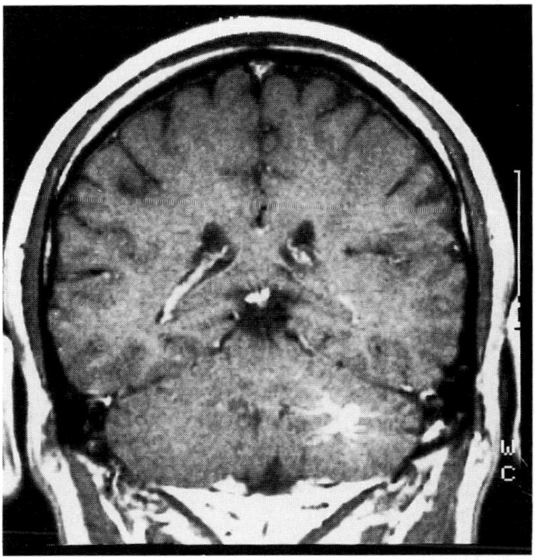

Fig. 3. Gadolinium-enhanced T1-weighted image (same case as Fig. 2). The medullary veins and a small part of the draining vein are clearly visible and look very similar to the way they are seen in venous angioma (see Fig. 4)

It is now widely accepted that MRI is a useful method in detecting venous angiomas. According to Augustyn et al. [1], T2-weighted imaging is more successful in demonstrating venous angiomas than T1-weighted imaging. In their opinion, the transcerebral draining veins were detected in 86% of cases and appeared as hypointense structures. In contrast to this, the body of the venous angioma, corresponding to the medullary veins, was visible in 57% of cases as hyperintense areas. The increased signal could be accounted for by the increased blood pool in the body of the angioma. Our noncontrasted T2-weighted imaging showed the transcerebral draining vein as hypointense in 67% of cases and as hyperintense in 33%. The increased signal can be explained by even echo rephasing as a result of slow laminar flow [6]. The medullary veins were seen in only 20% of the cases in our series.

To date, the use of paramagnetic contrast media in the detection of venous angiomas has not been widely studied. We have performed gadolinium-enhanced T1-weighted MRI studies in 8 patients. In all cases the venous angioma could be visualized and the images strongly resemble the angiographic pictures. On the basis of our experience, we would propose that in patients who are not being considered for operative treatment, the diagnosis of a venous angioma can be provided by a gadolinium-enhanced MR examination, thus obviating the need for angiography.

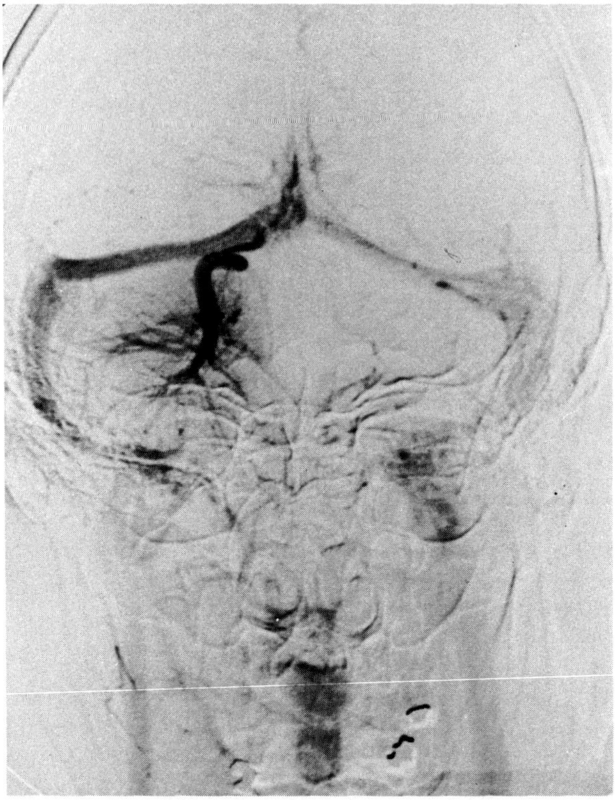

Fig. 4. Frontal vertebral angiogram of a venous angioma draining into the confluence of sinuses (same case as Fig. 2)

The absolute indications of surgery of venous angiomas remain unclear. This is largely due to the poor correlation between the symptomatology and the venous angioma itself. Moreover, these angiomas are frequently asymptomatic. Evidence from the literature suggests large hemorrhage as the primary indication of surgery. Cerebellar venous angiomas have a higher propensity to bleed than supratentorial lesions [3]. We would like to stress that the main danger of the operative procedure is the interruption of the transcerebral or transcerebellar draining vein too close to the venous sinus, which would result in venous infarction, e.g., of the brain stem in a case of cerebellar venous angioma. The aim of the operation must be to interrupt the medullary veins and the proximal part of the draining vein within the white matter, well away from the entrance into the venous sinus or the deep vein. With this approach we had no significant morbidity and no mortality.

Conclusions

1. Venous angiomas are more frequent than was previously thought.
2. They can easily be diagnosed on contrast-enhanced T1-weighted images. Angiography is not necessary.
3. Operative indications are limited to large hemorrhages and perhaps to operable infratentorial angiomas.
4. During operation, the medullary veins and the proximal part of the draining vein should be interrupted, but far away from the sinus.

References

1. Augustyn GT, Scott JA, Olson E, Gilmor RL, Edward MK (1985) Cerebral venous angiomas: MR imaging. Radiology 156:391–395
2. Fierstein SB, Pribram HW, Hieshima G (1979) Angiography and computed tomography in the evaluation of cerebral venous malformations. Neuroradiology 17:137–148
3. Rothfus WE, Albright AL, Casey KF, Latchaw RE, Roppolo HMN (1984) Cerebellar venous angioma: "Benign" entity? AJNR 5:61–66
4. Saito Y, Kobayashi N (1981) Cerebral venous angiomas. Clinical evaluation and possible etiology. Radiology 139:87–94
5. Valavanis A, Wellenauer J, Yasargil MG (1983) The radiological diagnosis of cerebral venous angioma: cerebral angiography and computed tomography. Neuroradiology 24:193–199
6. Waluch V, Bradley WG (1989) NMR even echo rephasing in slow laminar flow. J Comput Assist Tomogr 8 (4):594–598
7. Wolf PA, Rosmans NP, New PFJ (1967) Multiple small cryptic venous angiomas of the brain mimicking cerebral metastases. A clinical, pathological and angiographic study. Neurology 17:491–501

Congestive Cardiac Manifestations from Cerebrocranial Arteriovenous Shunts

G. Rodesch[1,2], R. Garcia Monaco[1], D. Devictor[1], C. Mann[1], A. Hannedouche[1], K. Terbrugge[1], and P. Lasjaunias[1]

Introduction

Cerebral arteriovenous shunts (CAVS) are an infrequent cause of congestive cardiac failure (CCF; 15%–19%). These systemic phenomena are of variable intensity, going from mild cardiac overload to acute heart distress. In newborns, the natural history of severe heart failure due to CAVS has always been considered very poor, with almost 100% mortality. It is the purpose of this presentation to demonstrate that arterial embolization allows dramatic improvement of cardiac function and satisfactory growth in children affected [1].

Material and Methods

Our series consists of 30 children (18 male, 12 female), all less than 15 years old: 19 were less than 1 month, 7 were between 1 and 12 months, and 4 were more than 1 year old. For 23 of them (77%), early CCF was the main complaint; in 7 patients (23%) it was macrocephaly and/or hydrocephaly that was the main problem.

The vascular lesions involved were of different types: 22 vein of Galen aneurysm malformations (VGAM), two cerebral arteriovenous (AV) malformations, two dural AV fistulas, one cerebral AV fistula, two facial capillary hemangiomas, and one facial AV fistula.

The goal of treatment aimed for at that moment was to reduce the flow of the AV shunts by embolization, this leading to a decrease in volume and pressure overload to the right atrium and secondary stabilization of cardiac function.

Arterial embolization was indicated in 24 patients and has so far been performed in 22: five newborns, 11 infants, and six children. Nine patients weighed less than 5 kg, nine between 5 and 10 kg, and four over 10 kg. These embolizations treated 57 occluded cerebral arteries in 42 sessions. Ten were performed as emergency procedures.

All procedures were done under general anesthesia after direct femoral puncture. No cut down has ever been made in our series. Therapeutic endovascular approach was through microcatheters (Tracker from Target Therapeutics or Minitorquer

---

[1] Hôpital Bicêtre, Neuroradiologie Diagnostique et Thérapeutique, 78 rue du Général Leclerc, F-94275 Le Kremlin Bicêtre Cédex, France

[2] Hôpital Erasme, Neuroradiologie, 808 route de Lennik, B-1070 Brussels, Belgium

Advances in Neurosurgery, Vol. 19
W. J. Bock, Ch. Lumenta, M. Brock, M. Klinger (Eds.)

from Ingenor Company) placed through a 4F introducer sheath. We always used low-osmolarity contrast medium (Hexabrix 320, Lab. Guerbet) at a dose of 4–6 ml/kg. Embolization was performed with fluids iso-butyl-cyanoacrylate or *N*-butyl-cyanoacrylate in cases of true vascular lesions or with particles (polyvinyl alcohol foam) in capillary hemangiomas. Systemic hypotension was never used because it would have a deleterious effect on myocardial and cerebral perfusion.

Careful selection of patients and correct choosing of the moment of appropriate treatment are in our eyes essential for satisfactory results. We therefore subdivided our pediatric population into three groups.

Group 1 (four patients). We decided to abstain from treatment because of severe brain damage (demonstrated by either ultrasonography (US), computed tomography (CT), and/or magnetic resonance imaging (MRI) or technical limitations (size of the feeding pedicles).

Group 2 (seven patients). In these patients CCF developed early and was rapidly stabilized by medical treatment. In such cases embolization can be postponed until the age of 6–8 months if cardiac function remains stable. The children are submitted every month to pediatric examination and every 2 months to CT or MRI. If the systemic situation no longer responds to treatment or if neurological deterioration occurs, "emergency" embolization is performed more rapidly than initially decided. Complete cure is not mandatory at that stage: control of about 30% of the shunt is in our experience sufficient to stabilize the systemic situation and allow the child to grow further in a satisfactory way. Medical treatment can then even be rapidly reduced. If anatomical cure can be achieved in one session (in case of brain AVMs or VGAMs) the child is kept asleep for 36–48 h in the pediatric intensive care unit in order to allow an uneventful return to equilibrium of the cerebral hemodynamics. We have performed this in three babies so far, who are now neurologically normal and free of cardiac symptoms. Delayed endovascular therapy was proposed in four other patients: two have been safely embolized and are now cured; two others are awaiting treatment.

Group 3 (19 patients). For these patients embolization was chosen as direct adjuvant therapy to medical treatment after careful analysis of the brain parenchyma (US, MRI, CT). These children are resistant to medical treatment: 10 procedures were performed as an emergency for stabilization of CCF. Of the remaining nine patients, two had treatment refused by their family and are now lost to follow-up. In the seven remaining, nonsystemic symptoms were the main complaint: minor neurological signs, seizures, hydrocephaly, failure to thrive, etc.

Results

To date, 22 patients have been embolized. In 16 of them (73%), CCF resolved completely and digitalis and diuretic treatment could be stopped. Four patients

(18%) improved clinically after endovascular treatment and the medical treatment could be satisfactorily reduced.

The mortality in our embolized patients is 9%: one baby born with VGAM died of massive gastrointestinal bleeding and acute hepatic failure and another of intracranial hemorrhages during management of brainstem AVM. This brings the overall mortality (embolized and nonembolized patients) in our series to 20%. The neurological morbidity was nil; skin necrosis occurred as the only complication after embolization of facial capillary hemangioma.

Conclusion

We believe that the classical bad prognosis of CCF due to cerebrocranial AVS has to be revised. Embolization may control, improve, or cure the shunts and give babies chances of normal development. The endovascular procedures can be associated with low mortality and morbidity if they are performed according to a precise protocol subject to appropriate multidisciplinary management.

References

1. Garcia Monaco R, Devictor D, Mann C, Hannedouche A, Lasjaunias P (1990) Congestive cardiac manifestations from cerebrocranial arteriovenous shunts. Endovascular management in 30 children. Childs Nerv Syst (in press)

Neuropsychological Abnormalities in Patients with Cerebral Arteriovenous Malformations: A Pilot Study

N. Muik[1], U. Zoworka[1], B. Kimmig[2], E. Irle[3], and B. Wowra[4]

Introduction

Stereotactic irradiation is the treatment of choice for inoperable cerebral arteriovenous malformations. At the University of Heidelberg a device for stereotactic radiotherapy using a modified linear accelerator has been developed and used for therapy of nearly 100 patients since 1984 [6, 11, 16].

The clinical experience of dealing with those patients gave rise to the following study, since we found a considerable number of patients suffering from organic psychosyndromes which might have been due to the vascular lesion and which could not be sufficiently covered by description in clinical terminology. The aim of this pilot study was to evaluate neuropsychological testing for detailed analysis of those "psychosyndromes" and to identify probable causative factors associated with those lesions, e.g., bleeding episodes, epilepsy, and vascular steal syndromes.

Patients and Methods

Patients

Twenty-six patients with cerebral vascular lesions treated in 1989 entered the study. Of these patients 24 had arteriovenous malformations (AVM), one patient suffered from a cavernous angioma, and one patient had a hemangioblastoma. Apart from the patient with the cavernoma, who underwent microsurgery, all patients were treated by stereotactic single-dose irradiation [6, 11, 16]. The clinical data of these patients are summarized in Table 1.

The angioma patients were tested using various neuropsychological tests; the results were compared to the results obtained from 20 patients treated for lumbar disk herniation (clinical control group) and 30 normal volunteers (normal control group). Both control groups were matched for age and education to the angioma group.

---

[1] Abteilung Psychologie, Universität Heidelberg, W-6900 Heidelberg, FRG
[2] Abteilung Radiologie, Radiotherapie, Universität Heidelberg, W-6900 Heidelberg, FRG
[3] Abteilung Psychiatrie, Universität Göttingen, W-3400 Göttingen, FRG
[4] Neurochirurgische Klinik, Universität Heidelberg, Im Neuenheimer Feld 400, W-6900 Heidelberg, FRG

Advances in Neurosurgery, Vol. 19
W. J. Bock, Ch. Lumenta, M. Brock, M. Klinger (Eds.)

Table 1. Clinical data of angioma patients

Lesion type	24 AVMs, 1 cavernoma, 1 hemangioblastoma	
Sex	17 Male, 9 female	
Age	Mean: 44 years (range: 22–65 years)	
Location of lesion	Frontal	2
	Frontotemporal	1
	Temporal	5
	Temporoparietal	3
	Parietal	6
	Basal ganglia	6
	Midbrain/pons	2
	Midline	1
Symptoms	Hemorrhage	11
	Recurrent hemorrhage	4
	Epilepsy	11
	Vascular steal	4

Neuropsychological Tests

Intellectual Functions. General intellectual abilities were tested with a shortened version of the Wechsler Adult Intelligence Scale (WAIS) [4] using the four subtests "Information," "Similarities," "Picture completion," and "Block design." Concentration and psychomotor speed were tested with a German version of the Stroop Test [1] and the Trailmaking Test [15]. Possible receptive language disturbances were examined with the Token Test [5, 14]. Memory functions were tested with a paired associate paradigm [12], the selective reminding procedure [3], the Benton Visual Retention Test [2], a visual form of the selective reminding procedure [13], and the Gollin's Incomplete Figures Test [17].

Personality and Mood. The German version of the MMPI (Minnesota Multiple Choice Personality Inventory) [8] was presented with the dimensions depression, hypomania, schizophrenia, psychasthenia, and psychopathic deviation. Furthermore, the FPI (Freiburg Personality Inventory) [7] was used with the subsets depression, sociability, dominance, extraversion, neuroticism, and inhibition. The current mood state was assessed by a short version of the EWL (Eigenschaftswörterliste) [10] including the dimensions vigor, fatigue, depression, anger-hostility, extraversion, anxiety, and irritability.

Results

Intellectual Functions

Comparisons (U tests) of the AVM patients with each of the two control groups revealed strong impairments in all intellectual tests applied ($p < 0.05$ in both cases). The clinical control group was slightly but insignificantly impaired compared to the normal control group. The impairments of the angioma patients were most prominent in the verbal memory designs. The results for the verbal selective reminding paradigm in the angioma and the clinical control group are presented in Fig. 1.

Within the group of angioma patients strong performance differences were revealed in patients who had had more than one episode of intracranial hemorrhage. These patients were strongly impaired in all cognitive variables compared to patients who had had none or not more than one. However, patients with just one hemorrhage still did worse than those in both control groups. Epilepsy, on the other hand, was apparently unrelated to substantially impaired test scores. The performances of patients with recurrent hemorrhage in the verbal selective reminding paradigm are described in Fig. 2. The Benton Test results of patients who had had at least one hemorrhage are shown in Fig. 3.

Personality and Mood

Compared to the clinical control group, the group of AVM patients had significantly elevated scores on the depression scales of all three tests. Furthermore,

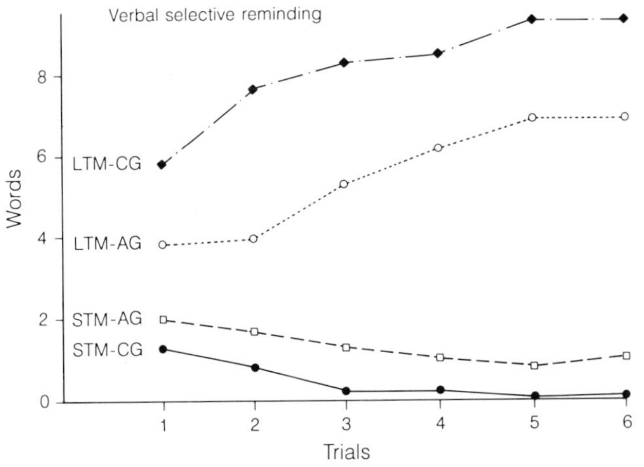

Fig. 1. Results for the verbal selective reminding paradigm. The amount of words recollected from short-term (*STM*) and long-term (*LTM*) memory are shown for the six trials of the task. *AG*, angioma group; *CG*, clinical control group

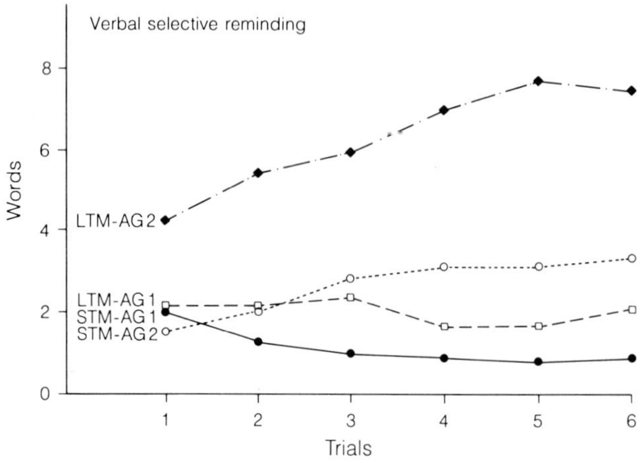

Fig. 2. Results for the verbal selective reminding paradigm. The amount of words recollected from short-term (*STM*) and long-term (*LTM*) memory are shown for the six trials of the task. *AG1*, patients with recurrent hemorrhages; *AG2*, patients with one or no hemorrhagic episode

AVM patients obtained significantly higher scores on the neuroticism scale of the FPI, and on the scales for hypomania, schizophrenia, and psychopathic deviation of the MMPI. The same results were obtained when the angioma patients were compared to the normal control group, except for the schizophrenia scale ($p > 0.05$). The results of all three groups in the MMPI are shown in Fig. 4.

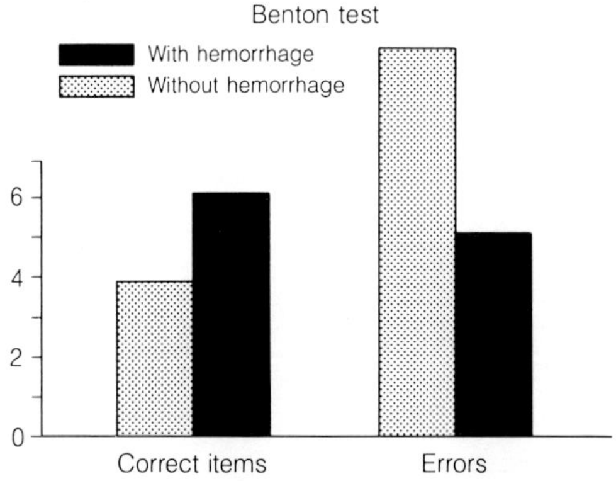

Fig. 3. Results in the Benton Test. The amount of correct items (out of 10) and the amount of errors performed in all items are shown. Patients with one or more episodes of hemorrhage are compared to those without a history of hemorrhage. The performances differ significantly for both kinds of measure ($p < 0.001$ in both cases)

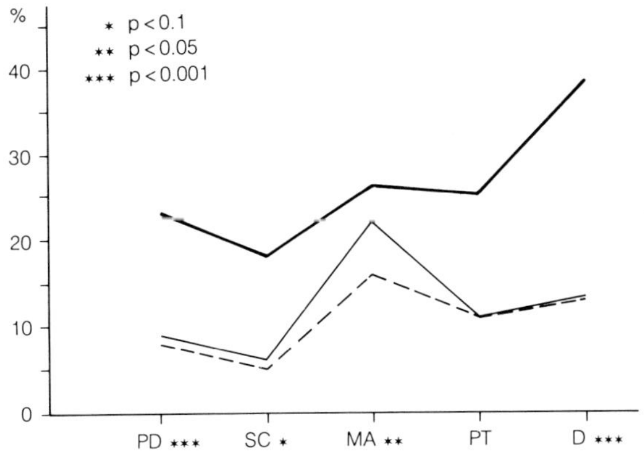

Fig. 4. Results in the MMPI. The percentages of confirmed items are shown for the scales psychopathic deviation (*PD*), schizophrenia (*SC*), hypomania (*MA*), psychasthenia (*PT*), and depression (D). The *thick solid line* indicates the angioma group, the *thin solid line* the normal control group, and the *broken line* the clinical control group. The values relate to comparisons between angioma group and the clinical control group

Within the AVM group, individuals with lesions in the frontal lobe or in close connection to limbic structures showed the most striking deviations in the test score of the MMPI. The scores of these patients, especially on the scales for depression and hypomania, were significantly higher than those obtained by the other AVM patients.

Discussion

The results of neuropsychological testing in cerebral angioma patients confirm the initial clinical impression that these patients are considerably impaired with respect to their intellectual abilities. Furthermore, all patients reported considerable depression and also showed deteriorations in their emotional behavior.

The most important finding may be the considerable intellectual, especially mnemonic deficits of patients who had experienced recurrent intracranial hemorrhages. This finding supports a strong indication for stereotactic irradiation of angioma patients thought to be inoperable, after their first bleeding episode.

In general, patients are believed to have a good chance of full recovery after a first intracranial hemorrhage from an AVM. Our data, however, clearly show that these patients, too, suffer from substantial intellectual deterioration (see Fig. 3). This indicates that these patients also require appropriate therapy, e.g., stereotactic irradiation.

In contrast to the pronounced cognitive effects of hemorrhage, neither the possibility of an influence of epilepsy nor steal-related effects could be generally substantiated.

As regards personality and emotion, severe deteriorations were found in all AVM patients. Here, the location of the angioma seemed to have considerable influence on the specific mood regulation.

While all angioma patients confirmed more statements than controls in relation to depression, schizophrenia, hypomania, psychopathic deviation, and neuroticism, the changes, at least in the scales for hypomania and depression, were most pronounced in patients with frontal or limbic AVMs. Similar observations were made in patients with frontal lesions due to cerebral trauma [9]. Thus, unlike in the intellectual domain, the AVM seems in itself to be the most important predictor of mood disturbance, rather than sequelae of hemorrhages. However, at present we are not able to differentiate between direct effects mediated for example by vascular steal, and reactive behavioral changes in the course of a long-term illness. We hope that follow-up investigations of these patients, including more specific questionnaires, will help to clarify these questions. The latter, too will hopefully provide information about the effects of stereotactic therapy on intellectual and emotional disturbances.

References

1. Bäumler G (1985) Farb-Wort-Interferenztest (FWIT) nach J.R. Stroop. Hogrefe, Göttingen
2. Benton AL (1986) Der Benton-Test. Huber, Bern
3. Buschke H, Fuld PA (1974) Evaluating storage, retention, and retrieval in disordered memory and learning. Neurology 24:1019–1025
4. Dahl G (1972) WIP – Reduzierter Wechsler Intelligenztest. Anwendung, Auswertung, statistische Analysen, Normwerte. Hain, Meisenheim am Glan
5. DeRenzi E, Vignolo AL (1962) The Token test: a sensitive test to detect receptive disturbances in aphasics. Brain 85:665–678
6. Engenhart R, Kimmig B, Wowra B, Sturm V, Höver KH, Schneider S, Wannenmacher M (1989) Stereotaktische Einzeitbestrahlung cerebraler Angiome. Radiologie 29:219–223
7. Fahrenberg J, Selg H, Hampel R (1973) Das Freiburger Persönlichkeitsinventar. Hogrefe, Göttingen
8. Gehring A, Blaser A (1982) MMPI Minnesota Multiphasic Personality Inventory. Deutsche Kurzfassung für Handauswertung. Huber, Bern
9. Grafman J, Vance SC, Weingartner H, Salazar AM, Amin D (1986) The effects of lateralized frontal lesions on mood regulation. Brain 109:1127–1148
10. Janke W, Debus G (1978) Die Eigenschaftswörterliste (EWL). Hogrefe, Göttingen
11. Kimmig B, Engenhart R, Wowra B, Höver KH, Marin-Grez M, Sturm V (1989) Stereotaktisch gezielte Strahlentherapie zerebraler arteriovenöser Gefäßmißbildungen. Strahlenther Onkol 165 (9):652–656
12. Kinsbourne M, Winocur G (1980) Response competition and interference effects in paired associate learning by Korsakoff amnesics. Neuropsychologia 18:541–548
13. Muramoto O (1984) Selective reminding in normal and demented aged people: auditory verbal versus visual spatial task. Cortex 20:461–478
14. Orgass B (1976) Eine Revision des Token Tests. II. Validitätsnachweis, Normierung und Standardisierung. Diagnostica 22:141–156
15. Reitan RM (1958) The validity of the Trailmaking Test in organic brain damage. J Consult Psychol 19:393–394

16. Sturm V, Schlegel W, Kimmig B, Worwa B, Schabbert S, Hartmann G, Pastyr O, Lorenz WJ (1989) Radiosurgery with a linear accelerator: Method, indications and preliminary results. In: Bannasch P (ed): Cancer therapy. Springer, Berlin Heidelberg New York, pp 14–17
17. Warrington EK, Weiskrantz L (1968) New method of testing long-term retention with special reference to amnesic patients. Nature 217:972–974

Cerebral Cavernous Hemangiomas: Treatment and Surgical Decisions

M. Westphal[1], D. Winkler[1], G. Nowak[2], R. Schwachenwald[2], H. Arnold[2], and H.-D. Herrmann[1]

Introduction

Advances in medical diagnostic technology have led to the diagnosis of cavernous hemangioma being made more frequently in recent years than before. Consequently, many of the earlier published series underestimated the incidence of this type of cerebral vascular malformation, otherwise more than 126 cumulated cases should have been reported by 1986 [1]. Knowledge of the clinical course and surgical risk associated with these malformations was thus derived from individual case reports or series compiling surgical results over long periods of time, in which great differences in surgical standards arose [2–5]. Therefore, some of the clinical features and surgical risks of this disease are in need of reassessment in more homogenous series in which a sizable number of patients have been operated upon within a short time period with consistent surgical management.

Cavernous hemangiomas may be located anywhere in the entire central nervous system and the indications for surgery may have to be viewed as being very relative in specially eloquent brain regions. Special emphasis will therefore be given in this report to those criteria in patient's case histories which facilitate decision making, such as the history and risk of hemorrhage, and the relatively low risk of surgery performed with the highest technical standards.

Patients: Clinical and Neuroradiological Data

In the period between October 1985 and April 1990, 27 intracranial cavernous hemangiomas (cavernomas) were treated in our institutions. During the same period we saw six patients with spinal intramedullary caveromas, who will not be reviewed further in this report. The clinical data are summarized in Table 1. Of the four brainstem cavernomas, three were located in the lower brainstem and one in the lamina quadrigemina. Of the supratentorial cavernomas one was located in the optic chiasm and two within the cavernous sinus. The other lesions were located intraparenchymally in different regions within the brain. There was a slight

[1] Neurochirurgische Klinik, Universitätskrankenhaus Eppendorf, Martinistr. 52, W-2000 Hamburg 20, FRG
[2] Neurochirurgische Klinik, Universität zu Lübeck, Ratzeburger Allee 160, W-2400 Lübeck, FRG

Advances in Neurosurgery, Vol. 19
W. J. Bock, Ch. Lumenta, M. Brock, M. Klinger (Eds.)

Table 1. Cerebral cavernous hemangiomas: clinical features

Localization		No. of cases	
Supratentorial,	excluding brainstem	21	
	cavernous sinus		2
	optic chiasm		1
Infratentorial,	excluding brainstem	2	
Brainstem		4	
	upper		1
	lower		3

Females: 16 patients, mean age 30.9 years (range 10–56)
Males: 11 patients, mean age 35.9 years (range 15–68)

prevalence of female patients. Six patients were below 16 years of age, which agrees well with the incidence in children reported by others [6].

Focal or generalized seizures were the leading presenting sign and present in 14 of our 27 patients (Table 1). All patients complained of headaches but only one presented with headaches as the only symptom. Eight patients reported a sudden onset of neurological symptoms. In five patients, this led to immediate hospital admission. Three other patients gave a history of sudden onset of neurological symptoms several years prior to hospital admission. Overall, seven patients presented with residual neurological deficits from presumed previous hemorrhages. The range of the individual case histories was between 29 years and 4 days. The average was 7.9 years, with a tendency to becoming shorter. Seven patients presented with acute hemorrhage and as many with a slowly progressive neurological deficit. In several patients a combination of symptoms was present.

None of our patients reported a family history of cavernoma, which according to some series occurs in up to 50% of patients [7], nor did any patient in our series in whom magnetic resonance imaging (MRI) was performed give evidence of multiple lesions.

All patients underwent computed tomography (CT) scanning. In 52% a calcified lesion was seen as the most characteristic sign. Contrast enhancement was common. In only one case was the lesion hypointense. A CT image suggestive of cavernoma is a hemorrhage without mass effect. This is exemplified in the case of a young girl who had fainted a few hours before admission and underwent CT scanning only because she had hurt her head (Fig. 1).

In addition, MRI was obtained in most patients and was regularly the decisive investigation. In cases presenting with hemorrhage, a discrepancy between size of the clot and neurological deficit, especially in the brainstem, was observed and was judged to be the telltale sign of underlying cavernoma (Fig. 2). Typically, the lesions were inhomogeneous and hemosiderin as an indicator of previous hemorrhages was visible in the T2-weighted images in all cases (Fig. 3).

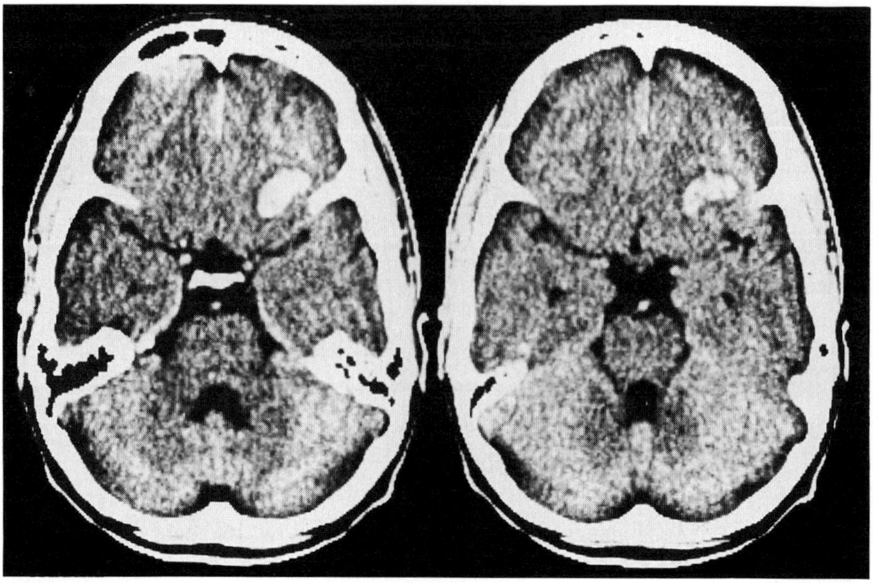

Fig. 1. Unenhanced CT scan of 15-year-old girl who had fainted before admission to the hospital and was neurologically normal at that point except for a slight headache

Angiography was performed in 17 of our patients. It failed to show vascular malformation in 12 cases, in which an avascular space was seen instead. In three patients a vascular lesion was seen in the late venous phase, and in one patient with a cavernous sinus cavernoma, the vascularization was so intense that a meningioma was suspected preoperatively. Indirect signs of a space-occupying lesion were evident in one case. Thus, angiography proved useful in the assessment of the degree of obliteration or vascularization in suspected cavernomas of the cavernous sinus.

Results

All cavernomas were completely resected. The overall outcome was good: 21 out of 27 patients were improved either at the time of discharge or at the first postoperative visit about 4 weeks after leaving the hospital. Four patients were unchanged, either with persistent neurological deficit without further aggravation, or with no deficit before and none after treatment. Two patients were worse. One these two patients, in whom preexistent hemiparesis was aggravated, has improved to better than preoperative level during further follow-up. Only one patient remains ophthalmoplegic 6 months after removal of a cavernous hemangioma within the cavernous sinus.

A CO_2 laser was an essential aid in surgery of cavernomas of the brainstem.

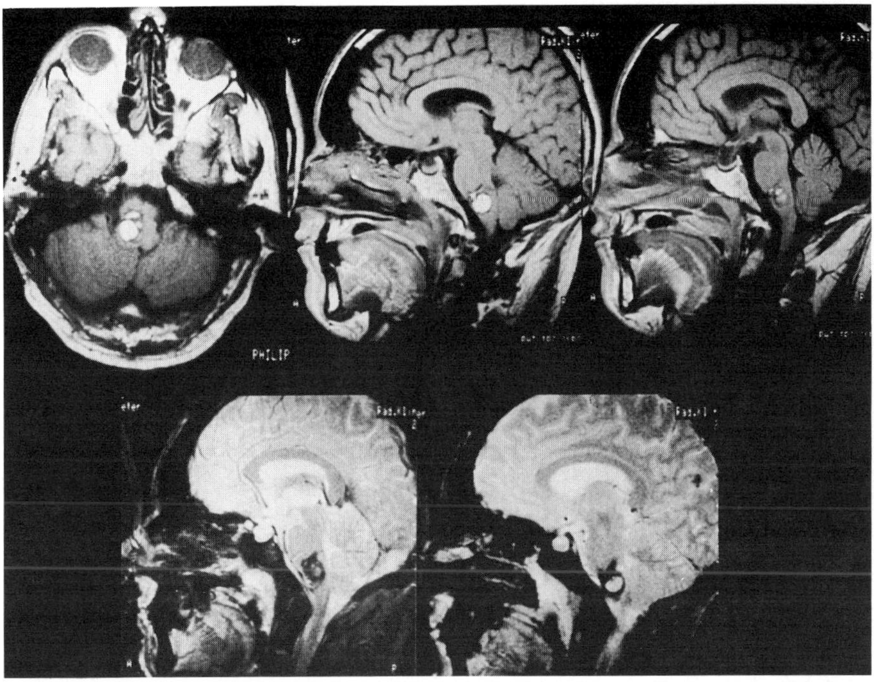

Fig. 2. MR images from a patient who presented with a sudden onset of right-sided dysesthesia and diplopia. On CT scan a fresh pontine hemorrhage was seen. The images demonstrate the discrepancy between the size of the hemorrhage and the neurological symptoms

Discussion

The diagnosis of cavernous hemangiomas has been made more often during the last decade due to the advent of MRI. Thus, patients with only minimal disease and normal neurological status will become eligible for surgery. Our experience shows that these vascular malformations should be managed aggressively in all patients, even those with minimal disease or lesions located in critical regions of the cerebrum or brainstem, provided that certain conditions are met in the latter group.

There is no question that, in addition to the risk of hemorrhage, a persistent seizure disorder associated with a cavernous hemangioma should be an indication for surgical removal, and that these two symptoms are responsible for the majority of referrals for surgical treatment [8].

Hemosiderin around the lesion is an indicator of recurrent microhermorrhages and is present in virtually 100% of cases [7]. Massive hemorrhage, on the other hand, was present in almost 60%, as documented either on admission by CT or MRI or proven indirectly by remnants of old hemorrhages found intraoperatively in patients in whom there was also a history of a past sudden neurological deficit. Thus, a major aspect in deciding for or against surgery is the risk of hemorrhage. We feel that a patient who has had a single hemorrhage with good recovery may be left unoperated upon but needs to be followed and advised about the possibility of a

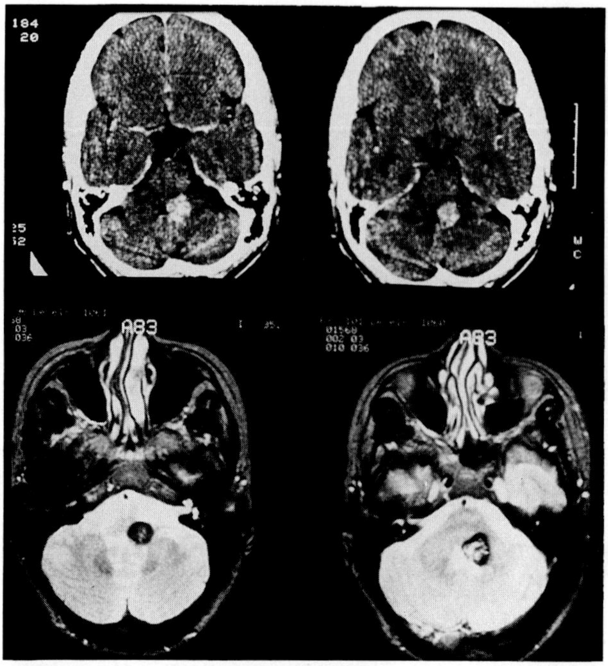

Fig. 3. CT scans and T2-weighted MR images of a lesion in the dorsal pons of 51-year-old woman who presented with a slowly progressive pontine syndrome. The MR images show the hemosiderin around the lesion

recurrence. Patients who present with a hemorrhage and suffer a neurological deficit from the clot should undergo surgery. With other authors, we feel that such operations in eloquent regions like the brainstem are best carried out after clinical stabilization of the patient in the first 4 weeks after the event [9]. That clinical deterioration of the patient invariably follows after removal of eloquent cavernomas [1, 3, 10, 11] has to be disputed [9, 12]. In patients in whom there is a history of recurrent episodic neurological deficit and progressive deterioration, removal of a cavernoma is indicated even in eloquent areas of the brain.

The diagnosis of a cavernoma is most reliably made with MRI [7, 9]. Lack of mass effect or shift is highly suggestive of preformed spaces either from previous small hemorrhages or cystic degeneration. Therefore, hemorrhages originating from cavernomas are frequently less dramatic in their clinical consequences than would be expected from the size or location, especially in eloquent areas such as the brainstem. This phenomenon can also be seen on a CT scan. Such discrepancy is highly suggestive of a cavernous hemangioma. In our series, such presentation was seen in five cases.

The trend towards shorter case histories reflects the improvement of diagnostic tools and at the same time indicates that patients are more readily referred for surgical treatment. Our experience and results with surgical treatment of cavernomas support this trend.

Acknowledgments. We thank Mr. S. Freist for his photographical work.

References

1. Simard JM, Garcia Bengochea F, Ballinger WE, Mickle P, Quisling RG (1986) Cavernous angioma: a review of 126 collected and 12 new clinical cases. Neurosurgery 18:162-172
2. Pozzati E, Giuliani G, Ferracini R, Gaist G (1988) Facial nerve palsy secondary to a dural cavernous angioma of the middle cranial fossa eroding the tegmen tympani. Neurosurgery 23: 245–247
3. Roda JM, Alvarez F, Isla A, Blazques MG (1990) Thalamic cavernous malformations. J Neurosurg 72: 647–649
4. Vaquero J, Salazar J, Martinez R, Martinez P, Bravo G (1987) Cavernomas of the central nervous system: clinical syndromes, CS-scan diagnosis and prognosis after surgical treatment in 25 cases. Acta Neurochir (Wien) 85:29–33
5. Tagle P, Huete I, Mendez J, del Villar S (1986) Intracranial cavernous angioma: presentation and management. J Neurosurg 64: 720–723
6. Herter T, Brandt M, Szuwart U (1988) Besonderheiten der kavernösen Hämangiome im Kindesalter. Neurochirurgia 31:144–149
7. Rigamonti D, Drayer BP, Johnson PC, Hadley MN, Zabramski J, Spetzler RF (1987) The MRI appearance of cavernous malformations (angiomas). J Neurosurg 67:518–524
8. Steiger HJ, Markwalder RV, Reulen H-J (1988) Das zerebrale Kavernom als Ursache von rezidivierenden Hirnblutungen und epileptischen Anfällen. Schweiz Med Wochenschr 118:471–477
9. Fahlbusch R, Strauss C, Huk W, Röcklein G, Kömpf D, Ruprecht KW (1990) Surgical removal of pontomesencephalic cavernous hemangiomas. Neurosurgery 26:449–457
10. Frima-Verhoven PAW, Op de Coul AAW, Tijssen CC, Maat B (1989) Intracranial cavernous angiomas: diagnosis and therapy. Eur Neurol 29:56–60
11. Yamazaki T, Handa H, Yamashita J, Paine J, Tashiro Y, Uno M, Ishikawa M, Asato R (1986) Intracranial and orbital cavernous angiomas. J Neurosurg 64:197–208
12. Yoshimoto T, Suzuki J (1986) Radical surgery on cavernous angioma of the brainstem. Surg Neurol 26:72–78

Microsurgery of Cavernous Angiomas of the Brain with Special Reference to Cerebral Midline Localizations

V. Seifert and D. Stolke[1]

Introduction

Cavernous angiomas or cavernomas of the brain, first described in 1854 by Luschka, comprise between 5% and 16% of all cerebrovascular malformations [6]. However, with the advent and increasing utilization of computerized tomography (CT) and, especially, magnetic resonance imaging (MRI), cavernomas of the central nervous system (CNS) are reported with increasing frequency [11, 12]. Moreover, the superior imaging qualities of MRI have also allowed detection of cavernous angiomas occurring along cerebral midline structures, which were previously missed by angiography or even CT and were therefore summarized under the heading "occult malformations" of the central nervous system [2, 5]. The ability of MRI to provide exact neuroanatomical data on the midline lesion, combined with the routine use of microsurgical techniques, has led to rare attempts at surgical removal of cerebral midline cavernomas [3, 7, 8, 9, 13, 14]. In this paper we report our experiences with 20 cavernous angiomas of the brain, with special reference to five lesions located along the cerebral midline.

Patients and Methods

In a period of 13 years, 20 patients with histologically proven cavernous angiomas were operated on in the Neurosurgical Department of the Hannover Medical School.

Supratentorial Cavernomas

Fifteen patients had cavernous angiomas located in the supratentorial compartment. This group consisted of nine male and six female patients whose ages ranged from 19 to 63 years. Four cavernomas were located in the frontal region, five in the parietal lobe, four in the temporal area, and two occipitally (Fig. 1.). Preoperative neuroimaging procedures consisted of a combination of CT, cerebral angiography, and, more recently, MRI. Although all supratentorial lesions could be detected by

---

[1] Neurochirurgische Klinik, Medizinische Hochschule Hannover, Konstanty-Gutschow-Str. 8, W-3000 Hannover 61, FRG

Advances in Neurosurgery, Vol. 19
W. J. Bock, Ch. Lumenta, M. Brock, M. Klinger (Eds.)

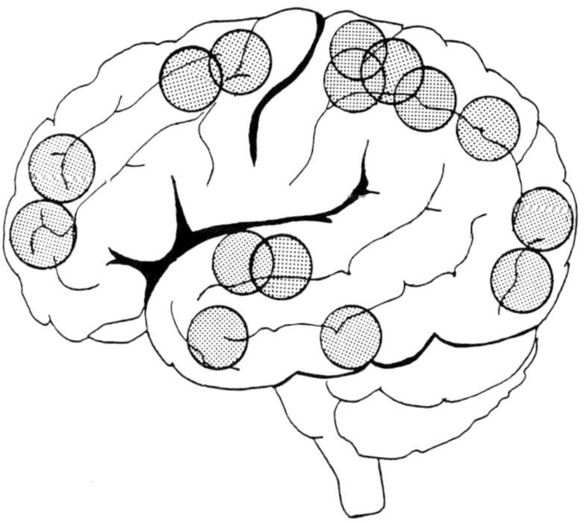

Fig. 1. Distribution of 15 cavernous angiomas within the supratentorial compartment

CT, MRI provided additional excellent information about the extent and localization of the cavernoma. Despite the fact that cerebral angiography was performed on a routine basis, its information in the case of cavernous angiomas was insignificant due to the poor radiological vascularization of these lesions. In ten patients the initial symptoms consisted of either grand mal or focal seizures. Two patients showed focal neurological symptoms, and in three patients an intracerebral hemorrhage had occurred as primary symptom. All patients were operated on using standard microsurgical techniques. There was no postoperative mortality. Postoperative morbidity depended on the location and extent of the lesion. Where cavernomas were located in the motor or speech area, transient postoperative deficits were not uncommon but did resolve almost completely in all patients. In all patients with preoperative intractable generalized or focal seizures, these could be controlled postoperatively using standard anticonvulsive medication.

Cerebral Midline Cavernomas

Five patients had cavernous angiomas located along cerebral midline structures. There were four female patients and one male, their ages from 36 to 66 years. Two cavernomas were located in the cerebellar peduncles, one in the brachium pontis, one in the mesencephalon, and one in the caudate nucleus (Fig. 2). Although CT detected these pathological midline lesions, MRI, performed in all patients, was of absolutely superior imaging quality in terms of pathoanatomical localization, which is of the utmost importance for the planning of the operative procedure. Clinical symptoms consisted of sudden deterioration due to intracerebral bleeding in two patients and of clinical signs of an increasing mass with cranial nerve dysfunction in three patients. Prior to surgery the different options of conservative or operative therapy were extensively discussed with the patients and their relatives.

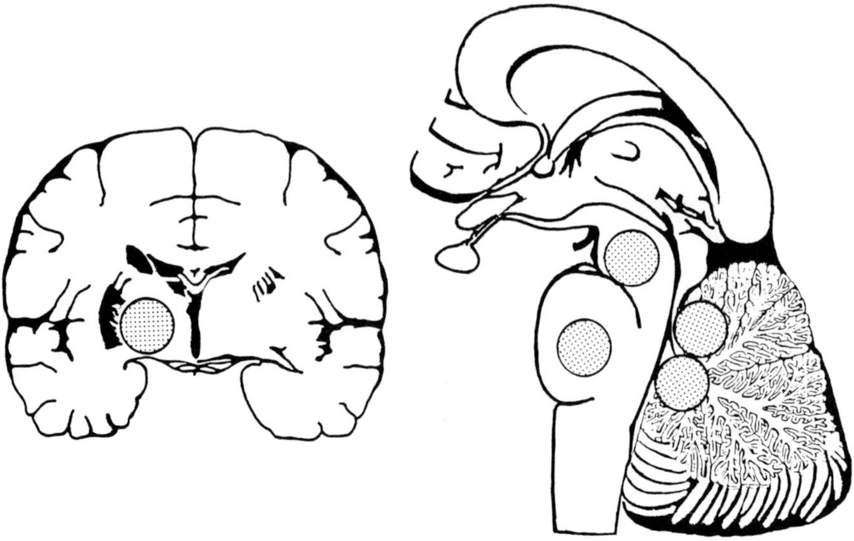

Fig. 2. Distribution of 5 cavernous angiomas located along or close to cerebral midline structures

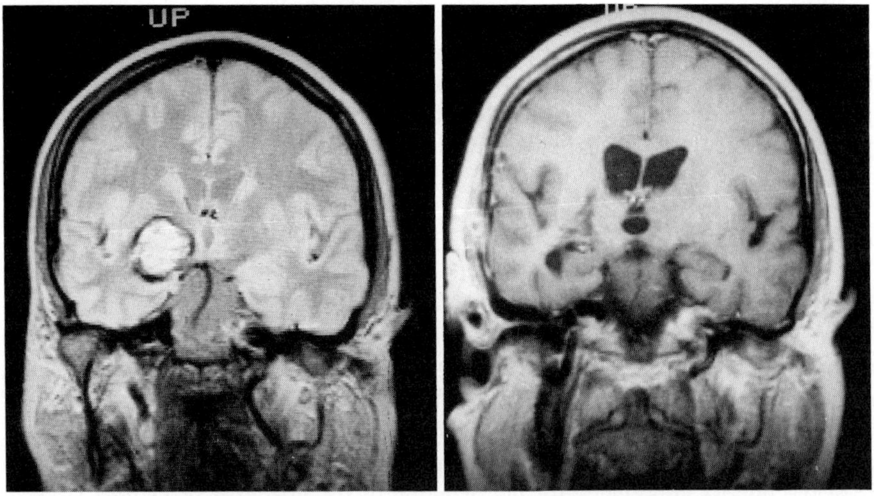

a b

Fig. 3. a Preoperative MRI picture of a cavernous angioma of the right caudate nucleus. **b** Postoperative MRI picture demonstrating complete removal of the cavernoma using a transsylvian microsurgical approach

The operative approaches used were as follows. The cavernoma of the superior cerebellar peduncle was approached using an infratentorial, supracerebellar approach. For the cavernous angioma of the inferior cerebellar peduncle, a sub-/transtonsillar approach through the fourth ventricle was employed. For the cavernoma of the mesencephalon a subtemporal approach was used, while the brachium pontis cavernoma was approached via an infratentorial, retromastoidal approach. Finally, the cavernoma of the caudate nucleus was removed using a transsylvian approach (Fig. 3).

Standard microsurgical techniques were used in all patients. For extirpation of the cavernoma of the pons the additional use of a CO_2 laser was judged to be very helpful.

Four cavernomas were removed completely. In one cavernous angioma recurrence occurred, necessitating a second operation for complete removal.

There was no postoperative mortality. Two patients recovered without any neurological deficit. Two patients with preoperative cranial nerve dysfunction still had cranial nerve defects postoperatively, but with significant improvement in one patient. In the patient harboring the caudate nucleus cavernoma, postoperative hemiparesis occurred, which resolved almost completely within 1 year postoperatively.

Discussion

The predominant location of cavernous angiomas of the brain, as substantiated by our own date, is the subcortical white matter of the hemispheres [4, 15, 16, 18]. Due to their macroscopical pathological appearance, with well-demarcated borders to the surrounding brain parenchyma, these lesions can be removed relatively easily using standard microsurgical techniques. Postoperative results, although depending to some extent on the localization and size of the cavernoma, are usually excellent, especially in terms of reduction of frequency and pharmacological control of focal or generalized seizures.

Computerized tomography and magnetic resonance imaging are the procedures of choice for adequate visualization of cavernous angiomas [11, 16]. MRI especially has proved to be superior to all other neuroimaging techniques, allowing, in addition to precise localization, a preoperative pathological diagnosis with a high degree of reliability [11].

If the diagnosis of a cavernous angioma has been made on MRI, cerebral angiography should be avoided as it is usually unable to show these lesions, owing to the narrowness of the feeding arteries, the slowness of circulation within the cavernoma, and the frequency of intravascular thrombosis [1].

MRI is even more valuable when planning operative intervention in the case of cavernous angiomas located along or close to the cerebral midline. Only recently have scattered reports of surgery of cavernomas of the brain stem, pons or the mesencephalon been published. Our own experience with successful laser-assisted surgery of a pontine cavernous angioma [14] has substantiated our contention that a more aggressive approach in midline cavernomas may be justified. Although little is known about the natural history of cavernous angiomas, the probability of severe and sometimes disastrous bleeding originating from these lesions is well documented in the neurosurgical literature, especially when an initial bleeding had already occurred [4, 15, 16, 18]. Moreover, Pozzatti and coworkers [10] have shown in a recent article that growth of cavernous angiomas within a few months is possible, probably due to multiple intralesional microhemorrhages, or to rapid enlargement of intracavernous cysts [17].

Considering the propensity of cavernous angiomas to bleed or develop significant mass effect due to their growth, once these lesions have become symptomatic an aggressive therapeutic approach in terms of radical resection should be contemplated. Since the introduction of microsurgery, satisfactory approaches to lesions of the brain stem, mesencephalon, and basal ganglia have been developed. From the data extracted from the few reports in the literature dealing with surgery of midline cavernomas, as well as from our own experience, it can be concluded that microsurgical removal of cavernomas of this localization, possibly assisted by CO_2 laser energy, is feasible and may be achieved without mortality and with an acceptable morbidity.

References

1. Bogren H, Svalander CH, Wickbohm I (1970) Angiography in intracranial cavernous hemangioma. Acta Radiol Diagn 10:81–89
2. Chou SN, Erickson DL, Ortiz-Suarez HJ (1975) Surgical treatment of vascular lesions of the brain stem. J Neurosurg 42: 23–31
3. Fahlbusch R, Strauss C, Huk W, Röckelein G, Kömpf D, Ruprecht KW (1990) Surgical removal of ponto-mesencephalic cavernous hemangiomas. Neurosurgery 26:449–457
4. Giombini S, Morella G (1978) Cavernous angiomas of the brain. Account of fourteen personal cases and review of the literature. Acta Neurochir 40:61–82
5. Gomori JM, rossmann RI, Goldberg HI, Hackney DB, Zimmermann RA, Bilaniuk LK (1986) Occult cerebral malformations: high-field MR imaging. Radiology 158:707–713
6. Jellinger K (1986) Vascular malformations of the central nervous system: A morphological overview. Neurosurg Rev 9:177–216
7. Mizutani T, Goldberg HI, Kerson KL (1981) Cavernous hemangioma in the diencephalon. Arch Neurol 38:379–382
8. Ondra SL, Doty JR, Mahla ME, George ED (1988) Surgical excision of a cavernous hemangioma of the rostral brain stem: case report. Neurosurgery 23:490–493
9. Pozzati E, Gaist G, Poppi M, Morrone B, Padovani R (1981) Microsurgical removal of paraventricular cavernous angiomas. J Neurosurg 55: 308–311
10. Pozzati E, Giuliani G, Nuzzo G, Poppi M (1989) The growth of cerebral cavernous angiomas. Neurosurgery 25:92–96
11. Rigamonti D, Drayer BP, Johnson PC (1987) The MRI appearance of cavernous malformation. J Neurosurg 67:518–524
12. Rigamonti D, Hadley MN, Drayer BP, Johnson PC, Hoenig-Rigamonti K, Knight JT, Spetzler RF (1988) Cerebral cavernous malformation. Incidence and familial occurrence. N Engl J Med 319:343–347
13. Seito N, Yamakawa K, Sasaki T, Saito I, Takakura K (1989) Intramedullary cavernous angioma with trigeminal neuralgia: a case report and review of the literature. Neurosurgery 25:97–101

14. Seifert V, Gaab MR (1989) Laser-assisted microsurgical extirpation of a brain stem cavernoma: case report. Neurosurgery 25:986–990
15. Seifert V, Trost HA, Dietz H (1989) Cavernous angiomas of the supratentorial compartment. Zentr Bl Neurochir 50:89–92
16. Sigmard M, Garcia Bengochea F, Ballinger WE, Mickle JP, Quisling RG (1986) Cavernous angioma: a review of 126 collected and 12 new clinical cases. Neurosurgery 18:162–172
17. Steiger HJ, Markwalder TM, Reulen HJ (1987) Clinicopathological relations of cerebral cavernous angiomas. Observations in eleven cases. Neurosurgery 21:879–884
18. Voigt K, Yasargil MG (1976) Cerebral cavernous hemangiomas or cavernomas: incidence, localization, diagnosis, clinical features and treatment. Review of the literature and report of an unusual case. Neurochirurgia 198:59–68

667 Histologically Verified Cavernous Hemangiomas of the CNS: Review of Localization, Symptoms, and Signs, Diagnosis, and Results of Operative Treatment

M. Hahn, A. Aschoff, and S. Kunze[1]

Cavernous hemangiomas are low-flow malformations that consist of ectatic, largely thrombosed and septated venous convolutions. There are only tiny arterial feeders whose walls usually lack elastic fiber; brain tissue is never interposed. Old hemorrhages and calcifications are frequent.

The first description of an intracerebral cavernous hemangioma goes back to Luschkae [2], in 1854. As early as in 1890, decades before other vascular malformations had been operated on, Bremer and Carson [1] successfully resected a parietal cavernous hemangioma and thus removed a focus of seizures.

Despite this early success, favorable conditions for operative treatment including lack of involution of brain tissue, good delimitation of the abnormality and minimal connection with normal blood vessels, and a considerable incidence in autopsy studies, these low-flow lesions remained little known until the mid 1970s. In the literature published up to 1970 we found only 45 cavernous hemangiomas.

With the advent of computed tomography (CT), cavernous hemangiomas became detectable. Seven years later, twice the number of cavernous hemangiomas had been operated upon (92 cases) than in the 70 years. The further advent of magnetic resonance imaging (MRI), with its superior sensivity and high specificity for cavernous hemangiomas, nearly solved remaining diagnostic problems. The term "cryptic" malformation was therefore rendered obsolete, and an almost logarithmic increase in operations on cavernous hemangiomas ensued.

The most reasoned and most complete survey by Simard et al. [5], in 1986, included 138 cases. We have reviewed 667 histologically verified cavernous hemangiomas reported in the literature, including 37 from our own department of neurosurgery at the University of Heidelberg. This high number of lesions allows us to give a representative overview of distribution in the CNS of these abnormalities. Nearly two-thirds of all cavernous hemangiomas (n = 392; 59%) are cortically or subcortically located. Lesions are most commonly located with the temporal lobes, the frontal lobes being second in frequency (Fig. 1).

A clinically special group concerns lesions of the middle cranial fossa. These have been described exclusively in female patients; they may enhance angiographically, and on CT they may appear like basal meningiomas. During operation they tend to bleed and are thus much more difficult to operate upon.

[1] Neurochirurgische Klinik, Universität Heidelberg, Im Neuenheimer Feld 400, W-6900 Heidelberg, FRG

Advances in Neurosurgery, Vol. 19
W. J. Bock, Ch. Lumenta, M. Brock, M. Klinger (Eds.)

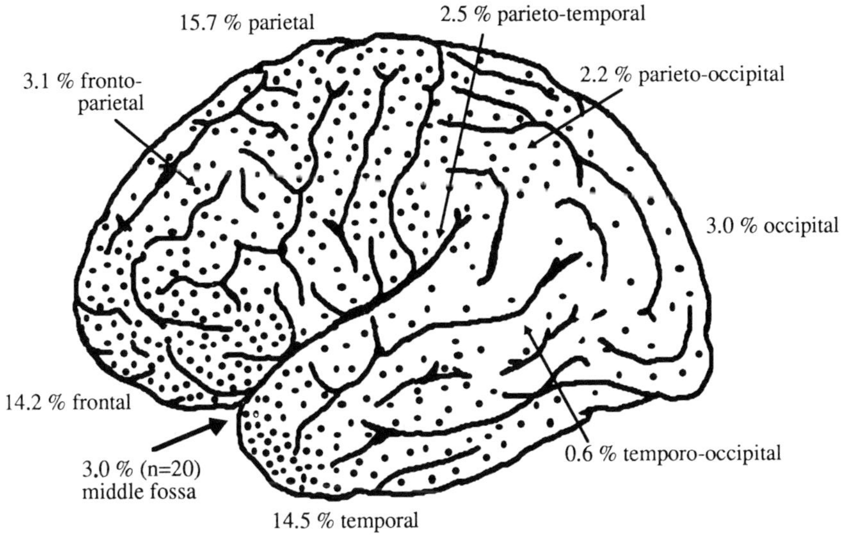

Fig. 1. Distribution of 390 cavernous hemangiomas located cortically or subcortically

Deeply located cavernous hemangiomas (Fig. 2) may occur in the basal ganglia ($n = 45$), in the ventricular system ($n = 15$), and within the pineal region ($n = 7$). Occasionally, cavernous hemangiomas have been found in the suprasellar region ($n = 8$) and in the pituitary gland ($n = 2$). Cavernous hemangiomas are particularly common in the posterior fossa, especially in the brainstem ($n = 129$, 19%; Fig. 3).

We believe that because cavernous hemangiomas in the brainstem are more frequently reported on than those in more usual locations of the cerebrum, the ratios given above are probably not representative for all cavernous angiomas.

Cavernous hemangiomas may also be found in the cerebellopontine angle, the fourth ventricle, and, comparatively rarely, within the cerebellum.

The age at which cavernous hemangiomas become critically manifest extends from birth to old age. There appears to be no gender preference, since 50.2% of cavernous hemangiomas are seen in males and 49.8% in females.

Supratentorial cavernous hemangiomas manifest clinically in seizures (33%), hemorrhages with or without mass effects (30%), and neurological deficits, usually caused by hemorrhage (37%). Microhemorrhages may develop without causing symptoms and are seen in all cases. Brainstem cavernous hemangiomas present with recurring hemorrhages and may progress to cause various cranial palsies; the pyramidal tracts may also be involved.

Thirty-two cases of spinal cavernous hemangioma have been published. The lesions may be located extradurally, intradurally, or within the spinal cord. Through hemorrhage they either cause acute paraplegia or a progressive paraparesis secondary to compression of the spinal cord.

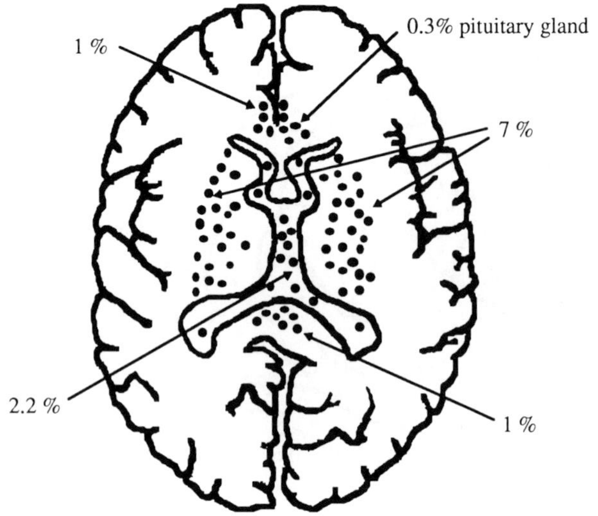

Fig. 2. Distribution of 78 cavernous hemangiomas located deeply

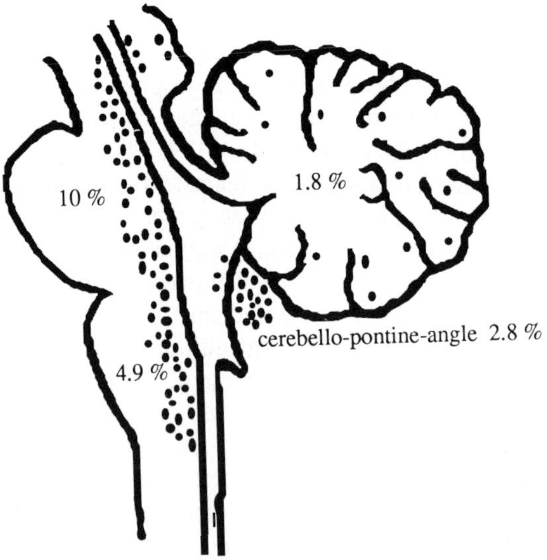

Fig. 3. Distribution of 129 cavernous hemangiomas in the posterior fossa

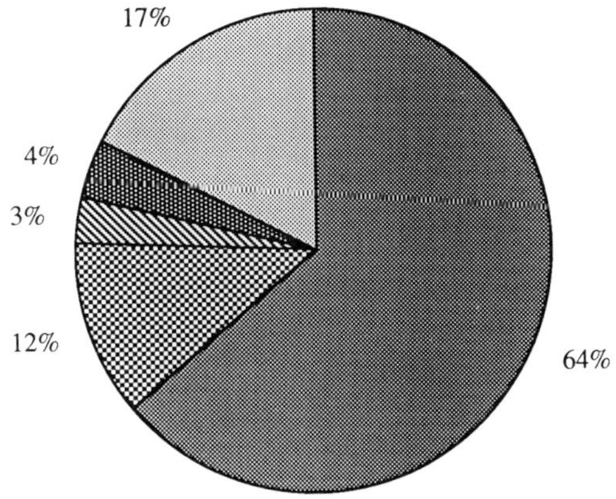

Fig. 4. Outcome in 505 patients operated upon for cavernous hemangiomas

The case material collected at the department of Neurosurgery of the University of Heidelberg includes 35 operated cases and 2 autopsy findings. We would like to stress that seven of the lesions were in a pontomesencephalic location and two were spinal cavernous hemangiomas.

The blood perfusion of cavernous hemangiomas is so slow that angiographic demonstration is usually unsuccessful. The exceptions to this, as we have mentioned, are lesions of the middle cranial fossa at the base of the skull. Characteristic CT findings include absence of mass effect and edema, slight enhancement or none upon contrast administration, and granular calcifications. The MRI appearance very closely mimics what is seen at autopsy, making this imaging modality the first choice for diagnosis. The specificity of MRI is also high, but in cases of acute hemorrhage a cavernous hemangioma may not be identified as such. In intraoperative ultrasonography, lesions are highly echogenic.

In 21 documented stereotactic biopsies (three from the University of Heidelberg), no histologic diagnosis could be arrived at. This is understandable if one looks at the histology of these abnormalities, for what is removed at biopsy is chiefly blood, not the characteristic tissue. We believe that stereotactic biopsy is contraindicated in these lesions, because of a high rate of postoperative hemorrhage (which may be fatal) and the very limited diagnostic success.

Out of 505 operations (Fig. 4) results were very good or good in 76%. In 3% neurologic deficits resulted, and in 4% patients died. However, this number includes historical cases as well as primary severe hemorrhages; 17% were without sufficient documentation. Surprisingly, in the 129 cavernous hemangiomas of brainstem, 90% of the postoperative results were either very good or good, and with 4% the mortality was surprisingly low.

In an extensive autopsy study [4] the incidence of cavernous hemangiomas has been determined as 0.4%. This number was confirmed by the recent MRI study [3], which put the rate at 0.44%.

Statistically reliable data about the natural history of these lesions are a present subject of interest in research, as so far little is known about it. The remarkable incidence of cavernous hemangiomas and their relatively rare clinical manifestation allows us to assume that the risk of spontaneous hemorrhage is considerably lower than the risk of bleeding in high-flow vascular malformations.

The clinical evolution of symptomatic cavernous hemangiomas and the epidemiologic data as known at present determine what should be done clinically. An absolute indication for surgery is given by severe or recurrent hemorrhage. Removal of the malformation is also indicated in patients with lesion-induced seizures resistant to anticonvulsive medication, because very often it is possible to eliminate focus of seizures. A relative indication exists in the case of lesions located cortically, outside of eloquent regions, because here the surgical risk is minimal. In cases where the lesion is located in eloquent parts of the brain and symptoms are mild or seizures can be controlled with anticonvulsive medication, the decision to operate may be more difficult.

In our opinion, surgery for asymptomatic lesions found only coincidentally is not warranted.

References

1. Bremer L, Carson NB (1890) A case of brain tumor (angioma cavernosum), causing spastic paralysis and attacks of tonic spasm: operation. Am J Med Sci 100:219–242
2. Luschkae H (1854) Kavernöse Blutgeschwulst des Gehirns. Virchows Arch [A] 6:458–470
3. Robinson JR, Little JR, Awad IA (1990) The natural history of cavernous angiomas. J Neurosurg 72:333 A
4. Sarwar M, McCormick WF (1978) Intracerebral venous angioma. Arch Neurol 35:323–325
5. Simard JM, Garcia-Bengochea F, Bollinger WE, Mickle P, Quisling RG (1986) Cavernous angioma: a review of 126 collected and 12 new clinical cases. Neurosurgery 18:162–172

Asymptomatic Cryptic Vascular Malformations

C. Gilliard, P. Laloux, C. Thiran, and S. Mourin[1]

From all large series of autopsies in addition to experience provided by current neurosurgical practice, it is well known that blood vessel hamartomas are rare. During recent years, the contribution of magnetic resonance imaging (MRI) [10, 19] to the diagnosis of cryptic vascular malformations has led to an increase in the recorded incidence of this type of malformation. Some problems are developing such as: what is the best neurosurgical option in cases of asymptomatic vascular malformations?

We present two cases of angiographically cryptic multiple vascular malformations, one of which (the symptomatic one) was histologically confirmed. After a review of the literature, we discuss the neurosurgical relevance of our cases.

Case Reports

Case 1

A 77-year-old women had been well until 2 months prior to admission, when she started to experience some difficulties in walking on her own. She had no previous medical record. The neurological examination revealed paraparesis with predominant proximal weakness. Slight hypesthesia was found at the TH 10 level. No urinary disturbances were found. MRI led to the diagnosis of an intramedullary hematoma with a cryptic vascular malformation at TH 9 level. Medullary angiography showed absolutely no vascular abnormality. On operation, a typical mulberry-like tumor was found and excised. Progressive improvement of the patient's neurological status was seen. MRI exploration of the central nervous system (CNS) showed a great number of the intraparenchymatous asymptomatic cryptic vascular malformations (Fig. 1).

The patient's daughter, 47-year-old, was also examined. MRI outlined the existence of a right frontal cryptic asymptomatic vascular malformation (Fig. 2); the angiogram was normal. She refused any surgical treatment.

[1] Department of Neurosurgery, University Clinics of Mont-Godinne, B-5530 Yvoir, Belgium

Advances in Neurosurgery, Vol. 19
W. J. Bock, Ch. Lumenta, M. Brock, M. Klinger (Eds.)

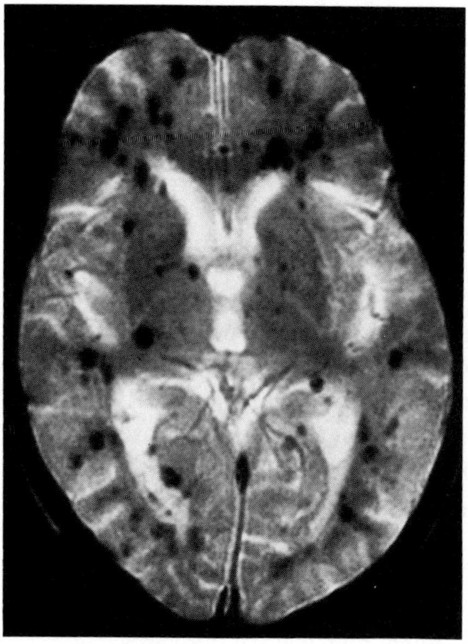

Fig. 1. Axial MRI (TR FFE 500 ms, TE 35 ms), showing numerous little intraparenchymatous hypointense "cryptic" vascular lesions

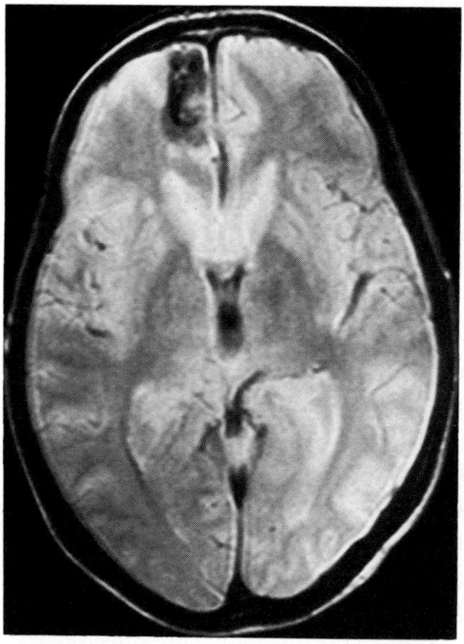

Fig. 2. Axial MRI (TR SE 2189 ms, TE 50 ms), showing a right frontal mixture of increased and decreased signal intensity with a prominent border of markedly decreased intensity

Case 2

A 20-year-old man was admitted after diagnosis of a left parietal expansive lesion. MRI showed multiple lesions with typical characteristics of cryptic vascular malformations in all parts of the CNS (Fig. 3). In the parietal region, an encapsulated hematoma with a peripheral vascular nidus could be seen. Parietal surgery confirmed the histological diagnosis of capillary telangiectasia in the walls of the hematoma. Further spontaneous evolution was seen in a dramatic tendency to hemorrhage in other localizations, with continuing good neurological status.

This patient's brother showed a normal CNS on MRI exploration and the family had no history of this type of problem.

Discussion

The first description of vascular hamartomas was given by Virchow in 1863. Crawford and Russell [6] in 1956 were the first to give the designation "cryptic" to a cluster of abnormal arteriovenous connections measuring less than 2–3 cm maximum [15]. The coming of angiography and MRI has made it possible to reduce the size by which this type of malformation is defined, and it would be better to replace the term "cryptic" by "angiographically occult" [16, 27].

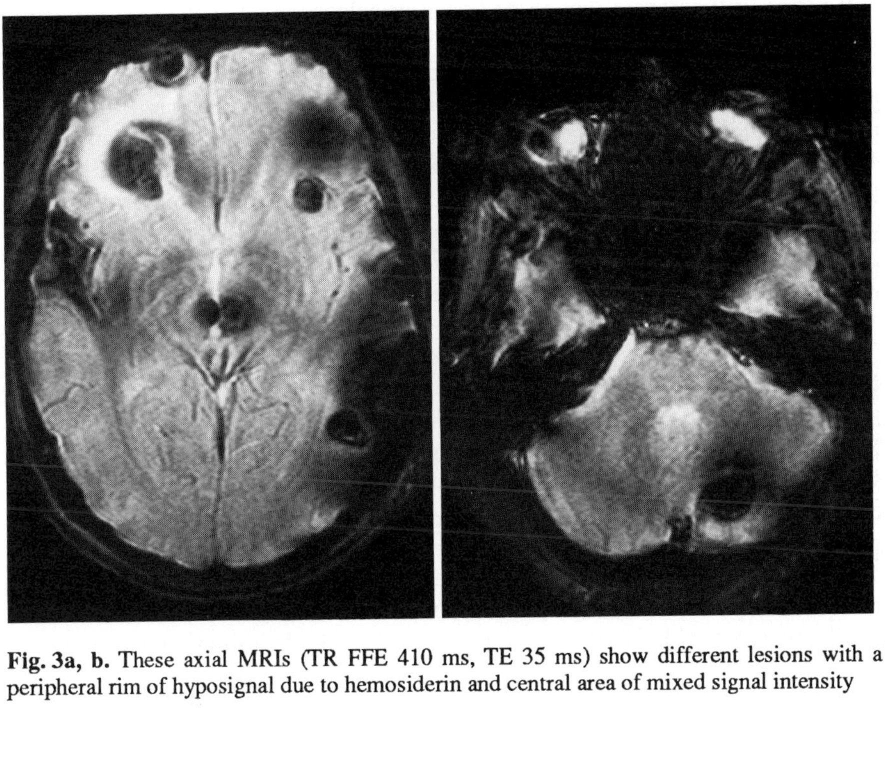

a b

Fig. 3a, b. These axial MRIs (TR FFE 410 ms, TE 35 ms) show different lesions with a peripheral rim of hyposignal due to hemosiderin and central area of mixed signal intensity

Russell and Rubinstein [21] separated this group of malformations into four subgroups: capillary telangiectasias, cavernomas, venous angiomas, and microarteriovenous malformations. The two first are difficult to distinguish and may be akin [9, 30]. This is one of the arguments of our presentation.

A lot of these malformations are asymptomatic [8], as in our cases. On the other hand, according to available literature for cavernomas [22, 23, 26], the clinical picture can be divided in three: one-third with epilepsy, one-third with hemorrhage, and one-third with a tumoral process.

According to Sigal [12], the MRI picture is quite precise but not pathognomonic: a thin rim of low signal intensity from hemosiderin surrounds a central area of variably high signal intensity due to methemoglobin. The other typical elements of hypo-signal intensity are due to calcifications and the edema mass effect. Both angiography and CT confirm the "cryptic" character related to the low vascular flow of this type of lesions [18].

The growth mechanism is presently not well understood [17], but a great tendency to bleed is often described, as particularly observed in case 2. This could explain the recurrent microhemorrhages with ensuing occlusion of contiguous vascular channels [9], followed by reorganization, fibrosis, and calcifications.

Multiple localizations are encountered and the autosomal dominant mode is well known in cavernomas, but familial [2–4, 11, 14] and intramedullary forms [1, 5, 24, 28, 29] such as case 1 are rare [7]. Telangiectasias [5] are usually solitary, but occasionally multiple [9], as seen in case 2. Associations of these two types of hamartomas and transitional phenomena have only occasionally been described [9].

It seems well accepted that an extensive or solitary accessible lesion is a good surgical option [12, 22, 26]. This is the only way to exclude the risk of hemorrhage, and it can also be helpful in ameliorating epilepsy. Asymptomatic lesions in multiple localization should be evaluated for both the natural and the surgical risks. A few publications discuss surgery of deep-seated lesions [23] such as thalamus [20] or brainstem localizations [13, 25], and also encourage the evolution of surgical technique. General agreement exists about the inefficiency of radiotherapy in these cases. Symptomatic medullary localization is also a good surgical indication [5, 29]. Our case 1 seems to be the first case report of an operated intramedullary cavernoma in a patient with multiple localizations [7].

Conclusion

More accurate diagnosis of a rare pathological condition is possibly by MRI. This should permit more appropriate treatment of symptomatic cases of angiographically occult vascular malformations. The hypothesis of a familial form should prompt detailed observation of all first-degree relatives by a noninvasive procedure. Genetic counseling should be offered in case of positive findings. The final decision to operate on an asymptomatic patient should depend on factors such as localization, risk of hemorrhage, the presence of multiple lesions, and also the experience and technical limits of neurosurgeon himself.

References

1. Bergstrand A, Höök O, Lidvall H (1964) Vascular malformations of the spinal cord. Acta Neurol Scand 40:169–183
2. Bicknell J (1989) Familial cavernous angioma of the brain stem dominantly inherited in Hispanics. Neurosurgery 24:102–105
3. Bicknell J, Carlow T, Kornfeld M, Stovring J, Turner P (1970) Familial cavernous angiomas. Arch Neurol 35:746–749
4. Combelles G, Blond S, Biondi A, Combelles-Pruvot M, Szikla G, Christiaens J (1983) Formes familiales des hémangiomes caverneux intracrâniens. Neurochirurgie 29:263–269
5. Cosgrove G, Bertrand G, Fontaine S, Robitaille Y, Melanson D (1988) Cavernous angiomas of the spinal cord. J Neurosurg 68:31–36
6. Crawford J, Russel D (1956) Cryptic arteriovenous and venous hamartomas of the brain. J Neurol Neurosurg Psychiatry 19:1–11
7. Feve J, Rey A (1989) Epilepsie, hémorragie, méningée, paraparésie et calcification intra-crâniennes. Rev Neurol (Paris) 145:169–173
8. Giombini S, Morello G (1978) Cavernous angiomas of the brain. Acta Neurochir (Wien) 40:61–82
9. Greenfield's Neuropathology (1984) Blood-vessel hamartomas. Arnold, London, pp 127–134
10. Griffin C, De La Paz R, Enzmann D (1987) Magnetic resonance appearance of slow flow vascular malformations of the brain stem. Neuroradiology 29:506–511
11. Hayman L, Evans R, Ferrell R, Fahr L, Ostrow P, Riccardi M (1982) Familial cavernous angiomas. Am J Med Genet 1:147–160
12. Houtteville JP (1989) Les cavernomes intra-crâniens (Table ronde). Neurochirurgie 35:73–131
13. Kashiwagi S, Van Loveren H, Tew J, Wiot J, Weil S, Lukin R (1990) Diagnosis and treatment of vascular brain-stem malformations. J Neurosurg 72:27–34
14. Mason I, Aase J, Orrison W, Wicks J, Seigel R, Bicknell J (1988) Familial cavernous angiomas of the brain in an Hispanic family. Neurology 38:324–326
15. McCormick W, Nofzinger J (1966) Cryptic vascular malformations of the central nervous system. J Neurosurg 24: 865–875
16. Ogilvy C, Heros R, Ojemann R, New P (1988) Angiographically occult arteriovenous malformations. J Neurosurg 69:350–355
17. Pozzati E, Giuliani G, Nuzzo G, Poppi M (1989) The growth of cerebral cavernous angiomas. Neurosurgery 25:92–97
18. Prakash B, Beohar P, Misra R, Low flow (cryptic) arteriovenous malformation and spontaneous haematoma. Acta Neurochir (Wien) 69:61–67
19. Rigamonti D, Drayer B, Johnson P, Hadley M. Zabramski J, Spetzler R (1987) The MRI appearance of cavernous malformations (angiomas). J Neurosurg 67:518–524
20. Roda J, Alvarez F, Isla A, Blazquez M (1990) Thalamic cavernous malformation. J Neurosurg 72:647–649
21. Russell D, Rubinstein L (1959) Pathology of tumors of the nervous system. Arnold, London, pp 77–92
22. Simard J, Garcia-Bengochea F, Ballinger W, Mickle J, Quisling R (1986) Carvernous angioma: a review of 126 collected and 12 new clinical cases. Neurosurgery 18:162–172
23. Vaquero J, Salazar J, Martinez R, Martinez P, Bravo G (1987) Cavernomas of the CNS: clinical syndromes, CT scan diagnosis, and prognosis after surgical treatment in 25 cases. Acta Neurochir (Wien) 85:29–33
24. Vaquero J, Martinez R, Martinez P (1988) Cavernomas of the Spinal Cord. Neurosurgery 22:143–144
25. Veerapen R, Sbeih I, O'Laoire S (1986) Surgical treatment of cryptic AVM's and associated hematoma in the brain stem and spinal cord. J Neurosurg 65:188–193

26. Voigt K, Yasargil M (1976) Cerebral cavernous haemangiomas or cavernomas. Neurochirurgia (Stuttg) 19:59–68
27. Wakai S, Ueda Y, Inoh S, Nagai M (1985) Angiographically occult angiomas: a report of thirteen cases with analysis of the cases documented in the literature. Neurosurgery 17: 549–556
28. Wang A, Morris J, Fischer E, Peterson R, Lin J (1988) Cavernous hemangioma of the thoracic spinal cord. Neuroradiology 30:261–264
29. Zentner J, Hassler W, Gawehn J, Schroth G (1989) Intramedullary cavernous angiomas. Surg Neurol 31:64–68
30. Zülch KJ (1986) Vascular malformations. In: Zülch KJ (ed) Brain tumors. Their biology and pathology, 3rd edn. Springer, Berlin Heidelberg New York, pp 451-460

Supratentorial Tumors in Childhood

Pediatric Brain Tumors

R.W. Oberbauer[1]

Introduction

Whether brain tumors in childhood can be regarded as a district entity remains a subject of controversy, as in terms of histological and topical aspects altogether there is no significant difference between brain tumors in children and adults. Koos and Miller [3] put down this insignificant difference (Table 1), comparing their series of 700 pediatric brain tumors with the statistical data on 6000 brain tumors in patients of all ages collected by Zülch [7]. In terms of histological grading and location, there is no substantial difference between the two age groups.

However, because a child's brain is still incompletely developed, and because of the natural hope for an almost full human life, pediatric brain tumors have been dealt with separately for about a century. A huge number of publications on the subject exist: Table 2 lists only a small proportion of the larger series. All this reflects the presently accepted attitude to consider children as more than simply smaller adults, and in all aspects of treatment to be anxiously aware of the developing brain.

Table 1. Comparison of brain tumors in children and in all age groups

Tumor classification	Children (700, [3]) %		All ages (6000, [7]) %	
Neuroectodermal tumors	68.4		52.7	
Medulloblastoma		19.0		4.0
Glioma		38.0		35.3
Paraglioma		11.4		13.0
Gangliocytoma		0.0		0.4
Mesodermal tumors	8.1		22.5	
Ectodermal tumors	9.7		1.3	
Congenital + embryonic tumors	1.3		1.9	
Vascular malformations	0.3		2.1	
Others	12.2		10.9	

[1] Neurochirurgische Klinik, Universität Graz, A-8036 Graz, Austria

Advances in Neurosurgery, Vol. 19
W. J. Bock, Ch. Lumenta, M. Brock, M. Klinger (Eds.)

Table 2. Selection of large studies on brain tumors in childhood

Authors	Year	No. of cases
Star	1889	300
Cushing	1926	154
Davis	1933	209
Förster	1937	101
Bailey et al.	1939	102
Zülch	1940	234
Keith et al.	1949	427
Walker-Hopple	1949	100
Boldrey et al.	1950	220
Bodian-Lawson	1953	129
Ingraham-Matson	1954	313
Korniansky	1954	764
Odom	1956	164
Hertz	1956	153
Bergstrand et al.	1958	248
Grant-Jones	1958	200
Arendt-Nevsesianta	1959	1516
French	1959	273
Katsura et al.	1959	618
Umbach	1963	243
Tönnis-Friedman	1964	457
Bergamini	1965	100
Isler	1965	429
Klein	1966	357
Bushe	1967	362
Gerlach et al.	1967	600
Grote	1967	438
Koos-Miller	1968	700
Maatson	1969	751
Tomita-Raimondi	1979	310
Yates et al.	1979	689
Iooma et al.	1984	100
ISPN	1988	876

Being relatively rare entities some 15 pediatric brain tumors are encountered in the average-size neurosurgical department every year. If infants (< 1 year) are counted separately, because of their very rapid brain evolution and their closeness to embryonic development, this specialty of brain tumors in the 1st year of life is found once a year or even less. This fact, together with the new imaging facilities leading to earlier diagnosis, prompted a cooperative study on brain tumors in the 1st year of life [1] via the educational committee of the International Society for Pediatric Neurosurgery (ISPN).

Results

In total, 876 cases of brain tumors in the 1st year of life, from four geographical areas (North America, Central and South America, Europe, and Asia) were evaluated. The sexes were almost equally represented (465 males, 404 females), which is in contrast to later childhood – according to a number of large series, there is later a significant predominance of boys. The age distribution revealed two peaks, at the beginning and the end of the 1st year respectively, in particular the first appears remarkable (Fig. 1). As was to be expected, the diagnosis was established by CT in the vast majority (771) of cases. The relatively high incidence of angiography (305 cases) and air studies/pneumencephalography (56 cases) reflect the lack of new imaging facilities in some countries. As to symptoms, elevation of intracranial pressure (68%) is by far the leading symptom in this age group, followed by cranial nerve deficit (22%), and impaired consciousness (19%). Seizures were encountered in about 12%, other symptoms are partly related to tumor localization.

Supratentorial tumors (65.4%) are about twice as frequent as infratentorial (29%); both compartments are affected in 1.5% of patients. The 2.1:1 ratio between the incidences of tumors in the two compartments agrees roughly with other studies – Raimondi and Tomita 1.8:1, Tooma and Kendall 1.5:1, Zuccaro et al.4:1 [2, 4, 6]. The anatomical locations are shown in Table 3; almost one-third were found within the ventricular system.

Histologically, the most common tumors are astrocytomas (28%), ependymomas (11.4%), medulloblastomas (11.3%), and plexus papillomas (10.6%; Table 4). There are 6.2% primitive neuroectodermal tumors (PNET), which belong to the first group of "not other specified" PNETs in the terminology of Rorke [5]. Craniopharyngiomas in this age are almost negligible, there being only 4 out of 876 cases (0.4%).

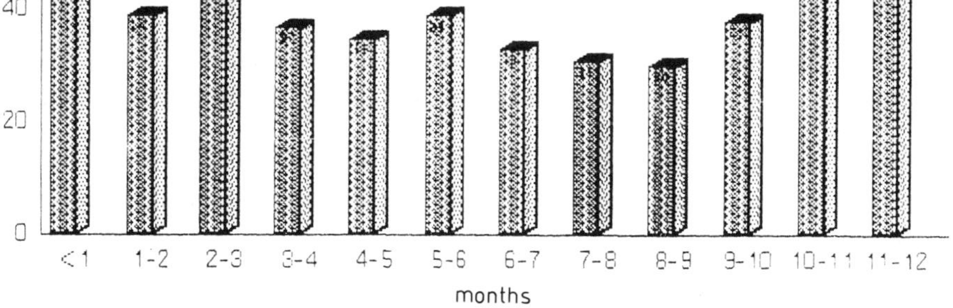

Fig. 1. Tumors in the 1st year of life; distribution by months

Table 3. Anatomical location of tumors in ISPN study

Location	%
Cerebral hemispheres	29
Intraventricular	29
Basal nuclei	18
Cerebellum	16
Brain stem	4.5
Pineal	1.5
Cerebral and cerebellar hem.	1.5
Others	0.5

Table 4. Histological classification of tumors in ISPN study ($n = 876$)

Astrocytoma	249
Ependymoma	100
Medulloblastoma	99
Plexus papilloma	93
PNET	55
Teratoma	44
Sarcoma	18
Meningioma	16
Gangiglioma	13
Neuroblastoma	11
Dermoid	10
Plexus carcinoma	8
Pineoblastoma	7
Hamartoma	5
Not reported	78
Other	70

PNET, primitive neuroectodermal tumors

Complete tumor removal was accomplished in 383 cases (43.7%), resection in 32%, 85 patients underwent biopsies, and 52 remained without any neurosurgical procedure. Hydrocephalus occurred in 68%; in 28.5% a CSF diversion procedure was employed. Radiation therapy was given in 122 cases, out of which these were 36 astrocytomas, 25 medulloblastomas, and 23 pineal tumors; the rest were either undifferentiated tumors or sarcomas. This figure of 122 patients undergoing irradiation appears relatively low, but considering the consequences of radiation to the developing brain, it should really be regarded as very high. One hundred and seventy infants had undergone chemotherapy; medulloblastomas, astrocytomas, ependymomas, and PNETs were again the leading types of tumor.

Table 5. Distribution of tumors by histological classification

	ISPN %	Graz %
Astrocytoma	31.1	43.7
Ependymoma	12.5	7.5
Medulloblastoma	12.4	15.0
Plexus papilloma	11.6	3.7
PNET	6.9	7.5
Sarcoma	2.2	3.7
Craniopharyngioma	0.4	3.2
Others	22.9	15.7

The follow-up period ranged between 6 months and 6.5 years, with a mean of 4.3 years. At the time of the study, 352 infants had died and 56 were lost to follow up. Of the remaining 468, 110 (12.5% of the entire study, or 23.5% of the survivors) are reported to be normal; there is mild retardation in 30.1% and severe retardation in 19.7%. Moderate to severe neurological disorders are found in 43.1%, frequently in combination with psychomotor retardation. Seizures have occurred in 27%.

With regard to the topic of supratentorial tumors in childhood it is interesting to compare the data from this large series with studies on the entire period of childhood. Table 5 shows a histological comparison of the ISPN study with data from the University of Graz (1980–1989) on all pediatric age groups, which are quite similar to those from most other series. There are differences in some subgroups like astrocytomas, and craniopharyngiomas are definitely more frequent in later childhood. However, some discrepancies may well be related to variable histological classification at different institutions. The supra-/infratentorial ratio revealed no substantial difference, and with regard to tumor location, there is a 5% lower incidence of intraventriculor tumors if all pediatric age groups are considered.

Conclusion

The data from this international cooperative study do not only focus on the 1st year of life, but seem to reflect the following years in childhood quite well. Principally, the difference in dignity of brain tumors with regard to age is surprisingly low. What makes the difference in pediatric brain tumors is the continuous evolution of the brain, which with the numerous new achievements in surgery and adjuvant therapy, deserves a new orientation in treatment.

References

1. Di Rocco C, Jannelli A, Ceddia A (1990) Intracranial tumors in the first year of life. Child's Nerv Syst
2. Iooma R, Kendall BE (1982) Intracranial tumors in the first year of life. Neuroradiol 23:267–274
3. Koos WT, Miller MH (1971) Intracranial tumors of infants and children. Thieme, Stuttgart
4. Raimondi AJ, Tomita T (1983) Brain tumors during the first year of life. Child's Brain 10:193–207
5. Rorke LB (1983) The cerebellar medulloblastoma and its relationship to primitive neuroectodermal tumors. J Neuropathol Exp Neurol 42:1–15
6. Zuccaro G, Taratuto AL, Monges K (1986) Intracranial neoplasms during the first year of life. Surg Neurol 26:29–36
7. Zülch KJ (1956) Die Hirngeschwülste. Barth, Leipzit

Multidisciplinary Approach to the Treatment of Supratentorial Tumors in Children

J.J.A. Mooij[1], J.H. Begeer[2], R. le Coultre[2], J. Leeuw[3], R. Tamminga[3], A. Kingma[3], D.M. Mehta[4], and L. Vencken[5]

Introduction

Brain tumors can only be treated by the combined efforts of neurosurgeons, radiotherapists, and medical oncologists. This holds especially true in children, where close cooperation with other specialists in mandatory, i.e., the child neurologist for timely diagnosis and follow-up, the neuropsychologist for assessment of treatment effects, and so on. Since standard treatment – surgery and radiotherapy – is not sufficient in a lot of cases, while on the other hand the results of chemotherapy in brain tumors are far from satisfactory, multimodality treatment protocols become more and more necessary for adequate management of brain tumors.

Based on these and other considerations, a Pediatric Neuro-oncology Group was founded some 13 years ago at the University Hospital in Groningen, for multidisciplinary treatment and management of infants and children with brain tumors. The hard core of the group consists of specialists from the departments of child neurology, neurosurgery, pediatric oncology, neuroradiology, and radiotherapy. Close cooperation exists with the departments of neuropathology, endocrinology, and ophthalmology. This report deals with the group's experience in children with supratentorial brain tumors seen during the last 13 years.

Patients and Results

In 13 years, 172 infants and children (up to 16 years) with a brain tumor were seen; 72 tumors were located supratentorially (42%). A broad spectrum of histolgical types was encountered (Fig. 1).

Hemispheric Tumors

The tumors located in a cerberal hemisphere (the first three rows in Fig. 1) were treated by total or subtotal surgical removal and radiotherapy. The only patient with

[1] Department of Neurosurgery, University Hospital, Groningen, The Netherlands
[2] Department of Child Neurology, University Hospital, Groningen, The Netherlands
[3] Department of Pediatric Oncology, University Hospital, Groningen, The Netherlands
[4] Department of Radiotherapy, University Hospital, Groningen, The Netherlands
[5] Department of Neuroradiology, University Hospital, Groningen, The Netherlands

Advances in Neurosurgery, Vol. 19
W. J. Bock, Ch. Lumenta, M. Brock, M. Klinger (Eds.)

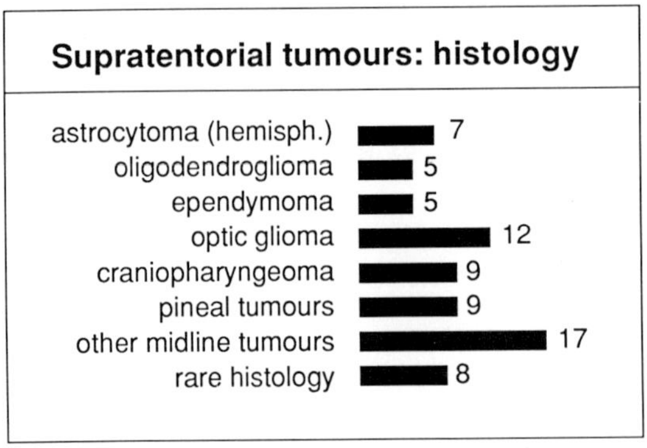

Fig. 1. Histological classification of 72 supratentorial brain tumors in infants and children up to 16 years of age

high grade malignant astrocytoma died within 9 months. Of the six low grade astrocytoma patients, two died and four survived for periods between 1 and 13 years.

In the patients with oligodendroglioma no relation could be demonstrated between grade of histological malignancy and survival. Two patients died and three survived. All patients with an ependymoma (three high grade malignant, two low grade) died within 30 months following the establishment of their diagnosis.

Optic Gliomas

All patients in this series had mixed optic nerve and chiasm tumors. A rather conservative attitude was assumed in the treatment (or even diagnostic procedures) of these patients (Table 1). The majority of the patients remained stable over the years; the only death was encountered in the partial resection group, as an immediately postoperative fatal complication.

Table 1. Diagnostic procedures in 12 optic glioma patients; relation with von Recklinghausen's disease, radiotherapy, and outcome (deterioration)

	n	Von Recklinghausen's		Radiotherapy		Deterioration	
		+	−	+	−	+	−
CT/MRI	5	4	1		5	1	4
Craniotomy no histology	1		1	1		1	
Minor biopsy	1	1			1		1
Partial resection	5	2	3	1	4	1	3

In one patient diagnosis was made on the basis of the swollen aspect of the optic nerve only, without histological proof. A recurrence with spinal metastases showed the tumor to be a germinoma instead of an optic glioma! Subsequent treatment with radiotherapy was successful.

Craniopharyngioma

In four patients apparently total surgical removal was achieved. One patient, however, had a recurrence of the cyst after 2 years. She was successfully treated by surgery once more and subsequent radiotherapy. In three patients partial resection was followed by external irradiation; the disease was then stable for 3–8 years. In two other patients aspiration of the cystic component of the tumor was followed by instillation of radioactive yttrium. The beneficial effect of this compound on the tumor was counteracted by its deleterious action on the adjacent vessels in the thalamus: progressive thalamic infarction led to death in both patients within 2 years.

Pineal Tumors

In the pineal region a preponderance of dysgerminomas was found (5/9). Two of these patients died despite appropriate radiotherapy.

Of two patients with embryonic cell carcinoma, one died within 5 months, the other is stable for the moment (6 months). Histological specimens from stereotactic biopsies were sometimes difficult to interpret: for example, one of the dysgerminomas proved later to be a pinealoblastoma. Shunts were necessary in all patients; radiotherapy was applied in all patients except one, whose tumor (low grade astrocytoma) was partially resected in another institution.

Other Midline Tumors

Other tumors in the midline region consisted of thalamic, hypothalamic, and hypophyseal tumors (Table 2). All patients were treated by stereotactic or open surgery and radiotherapy. The patients with low grade astrocytomas did remarkably well. A shunt was necessary in most of these patients.

Histological Types

Survival in the single cases of rare tumors encountered is presented in Table 3. Treatment consisted of surgical resection followed by radiotherapy. Chemotherapy was tried in the patients with lymphoma and primitive neuroectodermal tumor.

Table 2. Histological diagnosis and mortality in 17 patients with midline tumors other than optic glioma, craniopharyngioma, or pineal region tumors

	n	Deaths
Low grade astrocytoma	10	1
Malignant astrocytoma	3	3
Hypophyseal adenoma	2	1
Dysgerminoma	2	1

Table 3. Histological diagnosis and survival in 8 patients with unusual histology

	Survival (years)
Fibrosarcoma	6
Hamartoma	0[a]
Malignant schwannoma	1[a]
B-cell lymphoma	1.5
PNET, supratentorial	2[a]
Ganglioma uncus	3
Bourneville glioma	5
Plexus papilloma	5

[a] Dead
PNET, primitive neuroectodermal tumor

Discussion

The series of infants and children with supratentorial tumors presented here had a survival of about 64%. Survival was highest in optic glioma and low grade astrocytoma cases.

For low grade astrocytoma, biopsy or partial resection followed by radiotherapy seems to be the most appropriate way of treatment today. However, close follow-up with high quality MRI might be an alternative to immediate postoperative irradiation in some cases. In optic glioma patients with von Recklinghausen's disease, imaging seems to be sufficient for making the diagnosis, in other cases histological specimens should be obtained because of the variety in tumors possible in this region. Radiation therapy should be preserved for high grades of malignancy and/or progressive disease.

Bad results were obtained especially in the ependymomas, in some of the dysgerminomas, and in various other cases dispersed among the other subdivisions of this series. Chemotherapy, applied in some of these cases, was rather unsuccessful. The number of patients newly admitted to the study of the Pediatric Neuro-oncology Group is about 10–15 each year, which is far too low a number to accumulate any reliable experience with new forms of chemotherapy. Therefore, the Group recently joined one of the children's cancer consortiums in the United States, the Pediatric Oncology Group (POG). The major goals of the POG are to study the clinical features of CNS tumors, to design and study specific treatment regimes for CNS tumors, and to evaluate functional integrity and quality of life [1].

The bad effects of radiotherapy on the developing brain are well known. For this reason, radiation therapy is postponed more and more in the various treatment regimens, to at least after the age of 3, and in the near future possibly to an even later stage. It is here that the role of chemotherapy will become clear first, being a possible solution of the "waiting period."

Preservation or restoration of quality of life should be the major goal of any treatment for children with brain tumors. In our series, as in many others, this was not fully achieved. Of 23 children in our series who could be followed by frequent neuropsychological evaluation for more than 3 years, almost all scored significantly lower than age-matched normal children in the fields of intelligence, verbal auditory memory, verbal motor integration, and fine motor function. No special correlation was found between test scores and specific tumor type or localization.

Conclusion

The results presented here once more underline the necessity of developing better treatment regimens for many supratentorial brain tumors in infants and children. Options are more aggressive surgery, and multimodality chemotherapy in sandwich form with radiation therapy, this all in well-designed prospective multi-center protocols.

References

1. Cohen ME, Duffner PK (1989) Treatment of CNS neoplasms in childhood by the pediatric oncology group. Brain Dev 11:360–367

Treatment and Course of Malignant Supratentorial Brain Tumors in Childhood

A.M. Messing[1], Ch. Lumenta[1], W. Otten[1], R. Schober[2], and U. Göbel[3]

It is well known that brain tumors represent the second most common neoplastic disease in childhood, with an incidence of 1.8–3.1 cases per 100.000 children [7, 10]. However, no positive changes in the treatment of these tumors have yet been achieved as they have in other forms of childhood cancer [2]. The aim of the following study is to demonstrate the current treatment of malignant supratentorial brain tumors in childhood at the University Hospital in Düsseldorf.

Patients

Between 1984 and 1989 a total of 33 children with supratentorial brain tumors were operated upon. They were treated by both neurosurgeons and pediatricians. Radiotherapists and neuropathologists were also involved. Sixteen of the children were suffering from a malignant process, defined as WHO grade III or IV. The age at time of first diagnosis was from 1 day up to 14 years, the registration limit being 16 years (Fig. 1). Boys were more frequently affected than girls, with a ratio of 10:4. The commonest histological diagnoses were primitive neuroectodermal tumor (PNET; five cases) and anaplastic astrocytoma (four cases). A quite rate tumor, malignant fibrous histiocytoma, had been diagnosed in one child.

Course and Treatment

In ten cases the history started less than 6 months previously. In ten cases the primary symptom was a motor dysfunction. In nine cases headache, nausea, and visual dysfunction were mentioned. At the time of investigation none of the children gave signs of another malignant disease. In one case two siblings died after an unknown tumorous disease of infancy.

---

[1] Neurochirurgische Klinik, Medizinische Einrichtungen der Heinrich-Heine-Universität, Moorenstr. 5, W-4000 Düsseldorf, FRG
[2] Abteilung Neuropathologie, Medizinische Einrichtungen der Heinrich-Heine-Universität, Moorenstr. 5, W-4000 Düsseldorf, FRG
[3] Abteilung Pädiatrische Onkologie, Medizinische Einrichtungen der Heinrich-Heine-Universität, Moorenstr. 5, W-4000 Düsseldorf, FRG

Advances in Neurosurgery, Vol. 19
W. J. Bock, Ch. Lumenta, M. Brock, M. Klinger (Eds.)

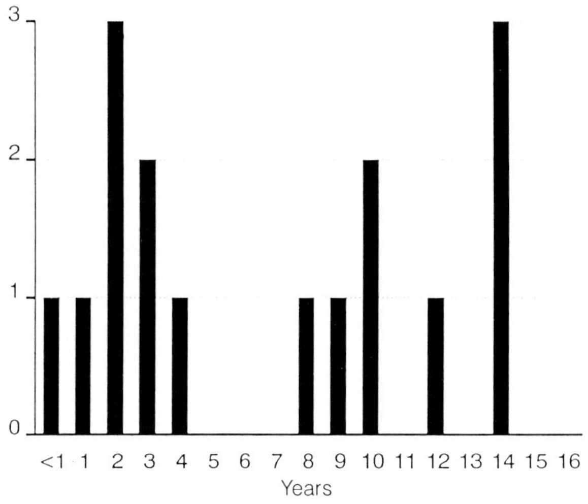

Fig. 1. Age at diagnosis ($n = 16$)

Computed tomography before and after contrast were performed in all cases prior to operation. Since magnetic resonance imaging is easily available it was also used. Only two children underwent angiography.

Table 1. Histological diagnosis, treatment, and tumor size

Histological diagnosis	Treatment	Tumor size
PNET	2 x PR + RA + C	
PNET	2 x TR + RA + C	> 2 BR
PNET	B + RA + C	> 2 BR
PNET	TR	> 2 BR
PNET	PR	> 2 BR
Astrocytoma	PR + RA + C	
Astrocytoma	1 x TR, 1 x PR + C	> 2 BR
Astrocytoma	2 x PR + RA	> 2 BR
Astrocytoma	PR + RA	
Plexus papilloma	2 x PR	> 2 BR
Plexus papilloma	TR	> 2 BR
Glioma	B	> 2 BR
Glioma	B	> 2 BR
Ependymoma	2 x TR + RA + C	
Oligodendroglioma	PR + RA + C	
Malig. fibr. histiocytoma	TR	

PNET, primitive neuroectodermal tumor; *PR*, partial resection; *TR*, total resection; *B*, biopsy; *RA*, radiotherapy, *C*, chemotherapy; *BR*, brain region.

Table 2. Treatment and results

Treatment	Results	Survival time (months)	Recur.
1 x TR, 1 x PR + C	Unchanged, moderate deficits	8	R
2 x TR + RA + C	Improved, mild deficits	23	R
2 x TR + RA + C	Improved, mild deficits	20	R
2 x PR + RA + C	†	26	RR
PR + RA + C	Improved, mild deficits	28	R
PR + RA + C	†	13	RR
2 x PR + RA	†	12	R
PR + RA	†	6	R
B + RA + C	Unchanged, severe deficits	28	
TR	Improved, healthy	46	
TR	†	< 1	
TR	†	< 1	
2 x PR	Unchanged, moderate deficits	33	R
PR	†	< 1	
B	†	< 1	
B	†	< 1	

TR, total resection; *PR*, partial resection; *RA*, radiotherapy; *C*, chemotherapy; *B*, biopsy; *R*, one recurrence; *RR*, two recurrences; †, died.

At the time of diagnosis as many as ten out of 16 tumors involved more than two brain regions.

Five children had combined chemo- and radiotherapy after surgical extirpation of the tumor, in two cases total. In one further case combined adjuvant therapy followed a stereotactic biopsy. Three of these children suffered from a PNET, two of which showed glial differentiation. The remaining three suffered from an astrocytoma WHO grade III, an oligodendroglioma WHO grade III, and a secondarily dedifferentiated ependymoma WHO grade III–IV that had been totally extirpated and diagnosed as WHO grade I–II 7 months previously. In two cases, both anaplastic astrocytomas, partial tumor excision was followed by radiotherapy (Table 1). One of these children had a recurrence after 5 months during radiotherapy. The tumor in the second developed large areas of necrosis and calcifications so that the grading became WHO grade III–IV instead of remaining WHO grade III. A 9-year-old boy who was also operated on for an anaplastic astrocytoma was treated with chemotherapy during which he suffered a recurrence. In his case grading also changed from WHO grade III to WHO grade III–IV.

The other patients were operated without further treatment. In three cases the extirpation was considered total. Two other children underwent only stereotactic biopsy and a palliative shunt operation.

The mean radiation dosage was 35 Gy, with an additional focal boost of 15 Gy.

At present children with a malignant brain tumor are treated at the University Hospital in Düsseldorf with a GPO (Gesellschaft für Pädiatrische Onkologie) chemotherapy scheme consisting of four elements. Recurrences after a course of chemotherapy are treated with a combination of carboplatinum and VP 16 [6].

Results (Table 2)

The follow-up ranged from 3 days up to 46 months. The longest surviving patients were a child with a plexus papilloma WHO grade III, who is still alive after 33 months, and two children who have both survived for 28 months so far, one with an oligodendroglioma WHO grade III and one with a PNET of the pineal region. These three children show mild, moderate, and severe neurological deficits respectively without evidence of a deterioration in comparison with the status on admission.

The longest survival time of 46 months is in the boy with the malignant fibrous histiocytoma, there being no signs of a recurrence and the patient in a condition of complete health.

In summary, the following results were found. Nine children died during the period of observation, having survived for a mean of 6.3 months. Four of them died during the immediate postoperative period. Seven of them had suffered from a WHO grade IV tumor which in six had involved more than two brain regions. During or after therapy the remaining children showed mild deficits in three cases, moderate deficits in two, and severe deficits in one. One child is healthy. In the surviving children there has been no case of deterioration from the status at admission; four children improved and the rest are unchanged. Seven patients have developed a recurrent tumor and two a second. We defined recurrence as a clear increase in tumor size or reappearance of the tumor after total removal during or after therapy. Five of these children have been subjected to another operation.

Four of the six patients who underwent a combination of surgery, or biopsy, chemotherapy, and radiotherapy have survived for 23–33 months. Their clinical state of health is described as with mild deficits in three cases and severe deficits in one. The mean survival time of the children with WHO grade III tumors was 24 months, and of those with WHO grade IV tumors only 11 months.

Discussion

Since the group of patients presented is rather small and the range of histological diagnoses is wide, treatment can only be evaluated to a limited extent. It appears reasonable, however, to conclude active surgical intervention together with adjuvant chemo- and radiotherapy seems to be the treatment of choice. Comparing the results of combined therapy with those of operation alone, prolonged survival and improved quality of life are obvious with the combined therapy, as recent clinical studies, e.g., that of the Children's Cancer Study Group, have proved [1, 7, 11]. Total tumor extirpation if possible is the first requirement [2]. A second surgical intervention in the case of recurrence is also meaningful.

Nevertheless, the results depend on the biological features of the individual tumor, which are very difficult to evaluate in childhood [5, 8]. In addition, tumor size at the time of diagnosis is of importance. A further point of discussion is whether the histological dedifferentiation that was observed in single cases during adjuvant therapy is the consequence of the treatment or merely the natural biological behavior of the tumor.

At present there is no treatment promising long-term success for malignant supratentorial brain tumors in childhood. In order to provide the best possible treatment neurosurgeons must cooperate with pediatric oncologists, radiotherapists, and neuropathologists to provide individualized management that takes account of the particular features of the tumor, the course of the disease, the age of the child, and the child's tolerance of treatment [3, 4, 6, 9].

References

1. Allen J, Bloom J, Ertel J, Evans A, Hammond D, Jones H, Levin V, Jenkin D (1986) Brain tumors in children: current cooperative and institutional chemotherapy trials in newly diagnosed and recurrent disease. Semin Oncol 13:110–120
2. Cohen ME, Duffner PK (1985) Current therapy in childhood brain tumors. Neurol Clin 3(1): 147–164
3. Duffner PK, Cohen ME (1983) Long-term effects of treatment on endocrine function in children with brain tumors. Ann Neurol 14:528–532
4. Duffner PK, Cohen ME (1985–86) Treatment of brain tumors in babies and very young children. Pediatr Neurosci 12:304–310
5. Giuffre R (1989) Biological aspects of brain tumors in infancy and childhood. Childs Nerv Syst 5:55–59
6. Kühl J (1988) Chemotherapie bei Hirntumoren im Kindesalter. Literaturübersicht und Pilotprotokoll. Klin Padiatr 200: 214–220
7. Prados M, Levin V (1987) Malignant supratentorial gliomas in childhood. Pediatr Neurosci 13:144–151
8. Schiffer D, Giordanna MT, Vigliani MC (1989) Brain tumors of childhood: nosological and diagnostic problems. Childs Nerv Syst 5(4):220–229
9. Schulte FJ, Herrmann HD (1988) Brain tumors in children. Acta Neurochir (Wien) 94:42–46
10. Surveillance Epidemiology End Result (SEER) (1987) Registry data 1978–1984. Pediatr Neurosci 13:144–151
11. van Eys J, Baram TZ, Cangir A, Brunner JM, Martinez-Prieto J (1988) Salvage chemotherapy for recurrent primary brain tumors in children. J Pediatr 113:601–606

Interstitial Irradiation of Supratentorial Cerebral Gliomas in Childhood with Permanently Implanted Iodine 125: Preliminary Results

J. Voges, H. Treuer, W. J. Schlegel, O. Pastyr, and V. Sturm[1]

Introduction

Local cure of a cerebral glioma by surgery alone is often precluded by the invasion of tumor cells into surrounding macroscopically healthy brain tissue. In patients with brainstem gliomas, which account for 10%–25% of all intracranial neoplasms in children [5], cerebral areas are involved which are functionally more or less impossible.

For patients with unresectable grade I or grade II tumors, irradiation is the only possible therapy. However, the risk of radiation damage to normal brain tissue limits the dose that can be delivered by external X-ray sources. Moreover, high radiation doses delivered to the brain of children has been shown to cause pituitary dysfunction and a decrease in intellectual ability [19].

To achieve the local control with optimal sparing of the surrounding healthy tissue, interstitial irradiation with implanted isotopes has been established during the last 30 years [15, 17]. Considering that most gliomas do not metastasize within the central nervous system [2] and grow in a circumscribed area of the brain [9], this modality of local treatment is logical.

The steep dose gradient achieved with interstitial irradiation and the development of an integrated system of computerized sterotactic operation and irradiation planning, guided by computed tomography (CT), allows highly precise local irradiation of unresectable or partly removable low grade gliomas even in functionally important or deep areas of the brain at doses potentially sufficient for tumor destruction [1, 16, 18].

Patients and Methods

From 1982 through 1987, 61 patients with a cerebral glioma were treated with permanent implantation of low-dose-rate seeds of ^{125}I. Twelve of these patients were selected out according to the following criteria:

- The age of the patients at the date of stereotactic surgery had been below 16 years.
- The tumors had been inoperably or only partly resectable.

[1] Abteilung für Stereotaxie und funktionelle Neurochirurgie, Neurochirurgische Universitätsklinik Köln, Joseph-Stelzmann-Str. 9, W-5000 Köln 41, FRG

Advances in Neurosurgery, Vol. 19
W. J. Bock, Ch. Lumenta, M. Brock, M. Klinger (Eds.)

- The lesions had been sufficiently demarcated in contrast-enhanced CT scans, the maximal diameter not exceeding 5 cm.
- The histopathological diagnosis was established before seed implantation, by either stereotactic biopsy or partial microneurosurgical resection.

After fixation of a modified, CT-compatible Riechert-Mundinger stereotaxic frame [18] and administration of contrast medium (Solutrast 300/Byk-Gulden-Lomberg, Konstanz, FRG), CT scanning was performed. CT data were transferred by magnetic tape into a computer (VAX 11/700 Computer, Digital Equip. Corp., USA) and the tumor borders demarcated manually at the computer screen. Determination of target points and the planning of interstitial irradiation treatment were carried out with a special computer program described elsewhere [1, 16]. Measurement of tumor volume was an option of the program.

The activities (0.9–26.5 mCi) of the permanently implanted seeds were chosen to allow an accumulated dose of 55–100 Gy to the tumor surface (mean 78 Gy), the dose rate ranging from 3.0–5.5 cGy/h (mean 3.75 cGy/h; Table 1). The iodine sources were implanted under general anesthesia. Immediately before implantation and during the first days after the stereotactic operation, dexamethasone was administered orally. None of the patients treated with interstitial irradiation received systemic or local chemotherapy.

Three and 9 months after implantation and then at yearly intervals, CT scanning with and without contrast medium and neurological examinations were performed.

Table 1. Characteristics of 12 patients treated with interstitial irradiation

Age (years)	
range	1–15
mean	8.8
Sex (no. of pat.)	
male	7
female	5
Sites (no. of pat.)	
cortex	3
basal ganglia	6
hypothalamus	3
Histology (no. of pat.)	
pilocytic astrocytoma	8
astrocytoma G II	4
^{125}I activities (mCi)	
range	0.9–26.5
mean	10.4
Implanted volume (cm^3)	
range	1.0–63.2
mean	18.3

Results

From October 1982 through September 1987 12 children (5 girls and 7 boys) with a supratentorial cerebral glioma were treated with interstitial irradiation. At the time of seed implantation the children ranged in age from 1 to 15 years, with a mean age of 8.8 years. Eight had a pilocytic astrocytoma and four an astrocytoma grade II (Kernohan classification; Table 1). The tumors were diagnosed histopathologically [14] by previously resected material (microsurgical biopsy in five patients) or by stereotactic biopsies taken before ^{125}I seed implantation. In five patients hydrocephalus necessitated the implantation of a CSF shunt system before interstitial irradiation began.

The Karnofsky performance status [13] of all patients was in the range of 85%–90% (mean 88%).

CT scanning 3 months postoperatively showed tumor regression in all patients. The mean volume reduction was to 72.8% of preoperative tumor volumes.

One patient with a grade II lesion had a cystic tumor relapse after initial response. The relapse-free interval of this patient was 36 months. Another patient (pilocytic astrocytoma thalamus) had initial tumor shrinkage but died 14 months postoperatively. The death was most probably caused by tumor hemorrhage (CT examination on admission to hospital; an autopsy was not allowed). All other patients are stable without clinical or radiological signs of tumor regrowth.

Figure 1 shows the survival curves estimated by the method of Kaplan and Meier [12]. Survival was defined as the time span between interstitial irradiation and the end of the retrospective analysis (November 1989) or death. With a mean follow-

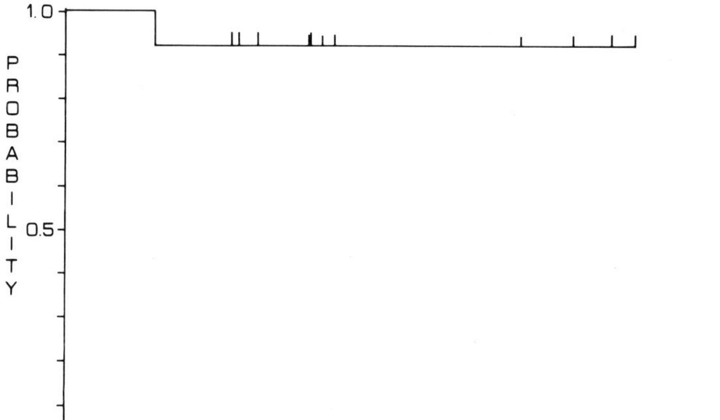

Fig. 1. Kaplan-Meier representation of the probability of survival after interstitial irradiation with ^{125}I. Twelve patients with a low grade cerebral glioma. *Ticks* represent censored patients

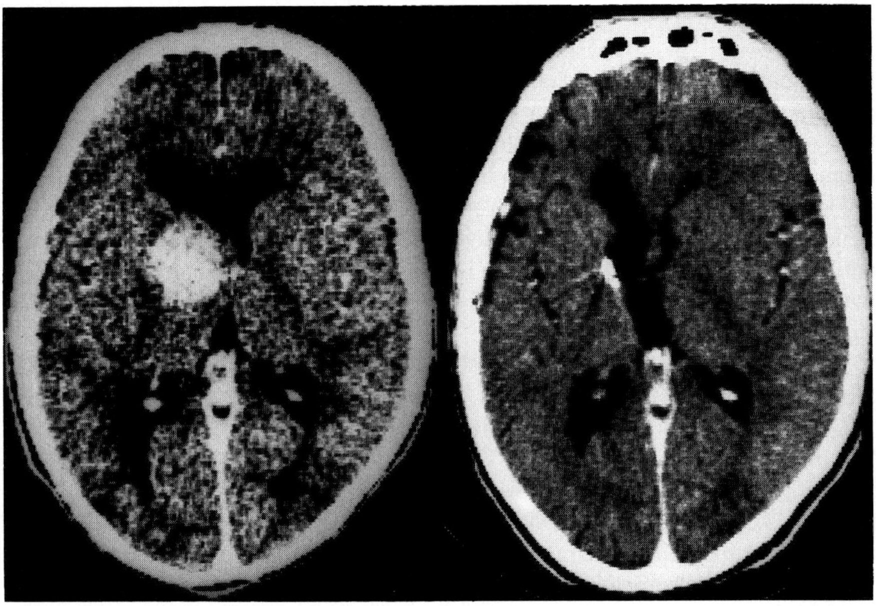

Fig. 2. CT examination of a patient with a pilocytic astrocytoma, *left* preoperatively and *right* 7 years after interstitial irradiation

up of 51.5 months, the estimated 4-year survival probablity is 92%. Figure 2 demonstrates a long-term follow-up.

There was no operative and perioperative morbidity or mortality. Nine to 18 months (mean 11.2 months) after the implantation procedure the CT scan of five patients showed radiation-induced changes around the ^{125}I seeds (contrast enhancement: two patients; edema: one patient; contrast enhancement and edema: two patients). In four patients these alterations could be observed 5–7 months after implantation and were interpreted as limited radiation necrosis. The CT examination of one patient (pilocytic astrocytoma) revealed a permanent hypodense lesion in the hypothalamus. Two years before ^{125}I seed implantation this patient had been treated with conventional radiotherapy (55 Gy).

At the end of the retrospective analysis the Karnofsky performance status had increased in four patients and remained stable in six. The Karnofsky score of the patient with a radiation-induced lesion in the hypothalamus decreased irreversibly (hormone dysregulation, one-sided amaurosis, psychomotor seizures).

Discussion

With a mean follow-up time of 51.5 months the estimated survival probability of the patients analyzed in this study is 92%. In cases where a conventional treatment schedule (cytoreductive surgery and external radiation) was not feasible, local tumor control was achieved with a mean tumor surface dose of 78 Gy. The survival times of our patients are slightly better than those reported by Etou et al., who described their experiences with interstitial irradiation of gliomas located in the diencephalon, basal ganglia, thalamus, and midbrain [4]. Over a 10-year-period their 5-year survival rate was 22.2% in patients with an astrocytoma grade I ($n = 36$) and 21.4% in patients with an astrocytoma grade II ($n = 14$).

The overall estimated 5-year survival after external beam irradiation as reported in the literature ranges from 22.8% to 40% [6, 8]. However, three points make direct comparison of our results with data from midline tumors in children treated with conventional external radiotherapy difficult [3, 6, 8]. First most of the lesions evaluated in different studies were not diagnosed histopathologically before treatment. Secondly, some of the patients were treated with systemic chemotherapy. Thirdly, tumors were located not only supratentorially but also in the midbrain and pons. Some authors have defined tumor location as a significant factor influencing survival. A literature overview ranges the estimated 5-year survival probability of patients with neoplasms in thalamus and mitbrain between 50% and 73% [8].

Both seed implantation and interstitial irradiation were well tolerated in our series (no operative or perioperative mortality or morbidity). As a result of radiation-induced tumor regression the Karnofsky performance status improved in four patients. Side effects occurred in one of our 12 patients, whose Karnofsky index decreased by 20% due to localized radiation necrosis.

The following facts make the interpretation of these favorable results difficult: (a) the study is retrospective and lacks a control group, (b) the number of patients and the observation periods are small, considering the natural course of low grade gliomas, and (c) the patients have relatively high Karnofsky scores. The last point could have influenced the results positively. On the other hand, location of the tumors in functionally important areas of the brain must be considered negative with regard to prognosis.

Despite the possible bias due to the drawbacks of this study which we have just mentioned, our data show the effectivity and benignity of low-dose-rate interstitial irradiation in clearly defined low grade gliomas. An indispensable requirement is the use of modern stereotactic treatment planning and implantation techniques, which enable the administration of any radiation dose to any intracranial target volume with the highest precision, thus optimally sparing the surrounding tissue [1, 16, 18]. The optimal surface dose, dose-rates and duration of interstitial irradiation are not yet known. The treatment parameters are chosen on an empirical basis and vary between the various centers using this method.

Considering the estimated cell cycle time of low-grade astrocytomas (30–45 days) [10], and a mean dose rate of 3.75 cGy/h, delivered by permanently implainted ^{125}I, each tumor cell should have received at least 2700–4050 cGy per cell cycle. Results of multiple in vitro and in vivo studies have shown that the critical factor for the inhibition of mitosis is the amount of radiation absorbed per cell cycle rather than the fixed dose rate per minute. The minimum dose seems to be 720–990 cGy/cell cycle [7]. With doses as low as 4000–5000 cGy accumulated at the tumor surface (100% isodose) after permanent implantation of sources of ^{125}I, a dose rate per cell cycle of 1840–2300 cGy would be achieved. From a theoretical point of view, these values should be sufficient for local tumor control and could simultaneously lower the incidence of treatment-related side effects.

Hoshino et al., who labeled S-phase cells of low grade astrocytomas with intravenously administered bromodeoxyuridine (BUdR), analyzed the survival times after tumor extirpation according to BUdR-labeling indices (BUdR-LIs) [11]. Forty percent of the labeled astrocytomas had LIs of 1% or more, reflecting a higher proliferative potential than histologically similar tumors with BUdR-Lis below 1%. The estimated survival curves (nonparametric analysis of Kaplan-Meier) demonstrated a significantly higher 3-year survival in patients with low BUdR-LIs than in patients whose tumors had higher LIs. With one exception, all patients in the group with LIs above 3% developed tumor regrowth or died during follow up. This demonstrates that within the same tumor histologically diagnosed as a benign glioma, parts with high proliferative potential can exist. In these areas the cell cycle times are shorter than estimated for a benign astrocytoma, and a low dose rate of permanently implanted ^{125}I would not be sufficient to achive 100% cell death.

Therefore even a high number of standardized treated patients and/or randomized prospective studies can show the minimum effective dose in relation to the different histopathological diagnosis.

References

1. Bauer-Kirpes B, Sturm V, Schlegel W. Lorenz WJ (1988) Computerized optimization of 125-I implants in brain tumors. Int J Radiat Oncol Biol Phys 14:1013–1023
2. Ehrlich SS, Davis RL (1978) Spinal subarachnoid metastasis from primary intracranial glioblastoma multiforme. Cancer 42:2854–2864
3. Eifel PJ, Cassady JR, Belli JA (1987) Radiation therapy of tumors of the brainstem and midbrain in children: experience of the Joint Center for Radiation Therapy and Children's Hospital Medical Center (1971–1981). Int J Radiat Oncol Biol Phys 13:847–952
4. Etou A, Mundinger F, Mohadjer M, Birg W (1989) Stereotactic interstitial irradiation of diencephalic tumors with iridium 192 and iodine 125: 10 years follow-up and comparison with other treatments. Childs Nerv Syst 5:140–143
5. Farwell JR, Dohrmann GJ, Flannery JT (1977) Central nervous system tumors in children. Cancer 40:3123–3132
6. Freeman CR, Suissa S (1986) Brain stem tumors in children: results of a survey of 62 patients treated with radiotherapy. Int J Radiat Oncol Biol Phys 12:1823–1828
7. Hall EJ (1978) Radiobiology for the radiologist, 2nd edn. Harper and Row, Hagerstown/Maryland
8. Halperin EC, Wehn St M, Scott JW, Djang W, Oakes WJ, Friedman HS (1989) Selection of a management strategy for pediatric brainstem tumors. Med Pediatr Oncol 17:116–125
9. Hochberg FA, Pruitt A (1980) Assumptions in the radiotherapy of glioblastomas. Neurology 30:907–911
10. Hoshino T, Barker M, Wilson CB, Boldrey EB, Fewer D (1972) Cell kinetics of human gliomas. J Neurosurg 37:15–26
11. Hoshino T, Rodriguez LA, Cho KG, Lee KS, Wilson CB, Edward MSB, Levin VA, Davis RL (1988) Prognostic implications of the proliferative potential of low grade astrocytomas. J Neurosurg 69:839–842
12. Kaplan EL, Meier P (1958) Nonparametric estimation from incomplete observations. J Am Statist Assoc. 53:457–481

13. Karnofsky DA, Abelmann WH, Carver LF, Burchenal JH (1948) The use of nitrogen mustards in the palliative treatment of carcinoma with particular reference to bronchogenic carcinoma. Cancer 1:634–656
14. Kernohan JW, Mabon RF, Svien HJ, Adson AW (1949) A simplified classification of the gliomas. Proc Mayo Clin 24:71–75
15. Mundinger F (1966) The treatment of brain tumors with radioisotopes. Prog Neurol Surg 1:220–257
16. Schlegel WJ, Scharfenberg H, Sturm V, Penzholz H, Lorenz WJ (1981) Direct visualization of intracranial tumours in stereotactic and angiographic films by computer calculation of longitudinal CT-sections: a new method for stereotactic localization of tumor outlines. Acta Neurochir (Wien) 58:27–35
17. Szikla G, Peragut JC (1984) Irradiation interstitielle des gliomes. Neurochirurgie 21 [Suppl 2]:187–228
18. Sturm V, Pastyr O, Schlegel W, Scharfenberg H, Zabel HJ, Netzeband G, Schabbert S, Berberich W (1983) Stereotactic computer tomography with a modified Riechert Mundinger device as the basis for integrated stereotactic neuroradiological investigations. Acta Neurochir (Wien) 68:11–17
19. Wara WM (1985) Radiation therapy for brain tumors. Cancer 55:2291–2295

Radiological Results of Intracavitary Brachytherapy of Cystic Craniopharyngioma in Childhood and Adolescence

G. Blaauw[1] and J.H. van den Berge[2]

Introduction

In 43%–74% of cases, craniopharyngiomas are mainly cystic in nature [1, 2, 3]. Intracavitary brachytherapy (IB) may be indicated in such cases, because the cyst can often be obliterated or its volume effectively reduced by this treatment. In this paper we report the radiological results of stereotactic intracavitary irradiation using yttrium 90.

Patients and Methods

Our patients were 16 children who received 18 injections of yttrium by the stereotactic procedure and for whom follow-up data are available. The series is derived from a total of 35 patients including adults.

The age distribution at the time of IB was 4–18 years (Fig. 1). The follow-up period ranged from 6 to 73 months. Four patients died; in one, death was the result of bacterial infection, while in the other three it was directly related to the tumor. In all patients, IB was the primary treatment focused on the lesion.

We aimed at a radiation dose of at least 200 Gy at the inner surface of the cyst wall, following Backlund's procedure [4, 5]. Multiple simultaneous yttrium injections were administered to one of the patients with multycystic craniopharyngioma. In the second and third multicystic cases, an initially small second cyst left untreated at the time of the first injection increased in size so much that a second injection became necessary. This was again successful in both instances, but in one patient who eventually died a third cyst developed which was left untreated. Only one injection was performed in the fourth and fifth multicystic cases.

Three-quarters of the cases had solitary cysts (Fig. 2). Cyst volume varied between 1.38 and 180 ml before treatment (Fig. 3), as determined by the computer tomography (CT) scanner's standard software for 1.5-mm-thick slices [6].

[1] Department of Neurosurgery, De Wever Hospital, Heerlen, The Netherlands
[2] Department of Neurosurgery, Erasmus University Hospital, Rotterdam, The Netherlands

Advances in Neurosurgery, Vol. 19
W. J. Bock, Ch. Lumenta, M. Brock, M. Klinger (Eds.)

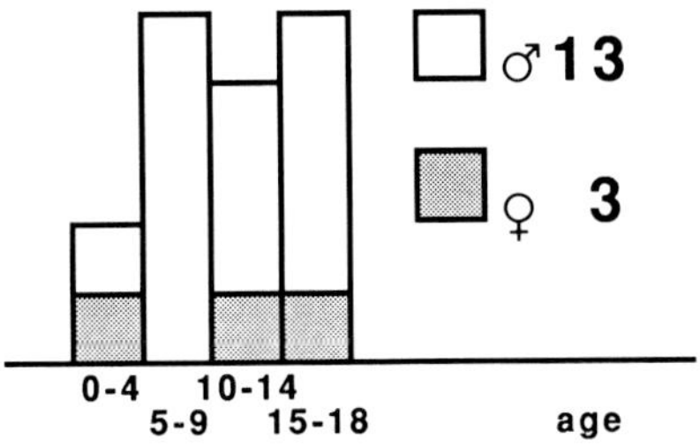

Fig. 1. Age and sex of patients. There is a significant preponderance of male patients

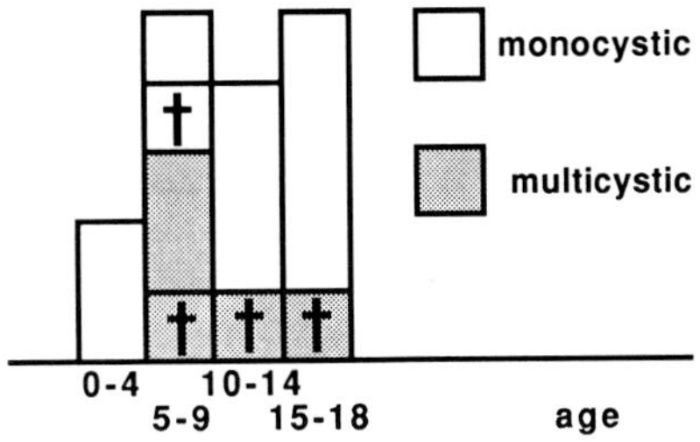

Fig. 2. Age, monocystic vs. multicystic diagnosis, and death. Death occurred mainly in patients with multicystic craniopharyngioma

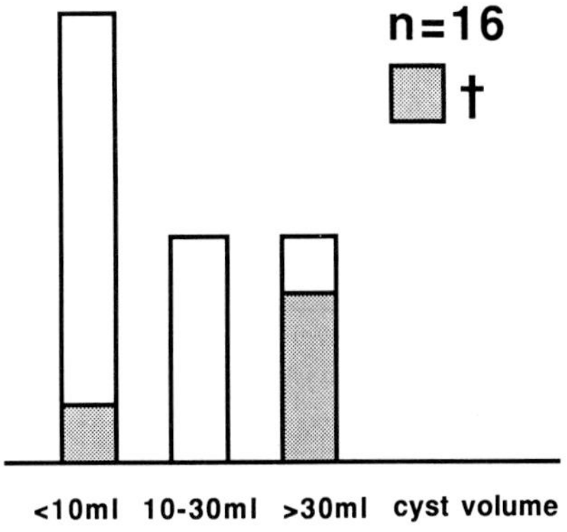

Fig. 3. Cyst volume and death. A possible relation between volume and prognosis is suggested by the deaths of patients with large cysts

Results

CT stereotactic puncture of the cyst and injection of yttrium was performed using the fine needle technique, to diminish leakage of the isotope [5]. Biopsies were not carried out, but the diagnosis was established by examining the cyst fluid, especially by demonstrating the presence of cholesterol crystals using polarized light microscopy. The ophthalmological and endocrinological results after IB in the complete series will be published in a separate paper.

Follow-up CT showed in most cases gradual cyst regression, which commenced a few months after the IB procedure. In three patients the cyst resolved completely after treatment. In ten patients the cysts decreased in size. Reduction was significant (more than 50%) in seven of these, while a reduction of less than 50% occurred in three cases. In three patients the cyst increased in size; this was treated by repeated aspirations, resulting in a fatal bacterial infection in one patient. In one patient the solid tumor component enlarged, requiring external fractionated radiotherapy.

Discussion

The results of this study signify that in 80% of cases yttrium injection influenced the size of the craniopharyngioma cyst, although the treatment was significantly efficacious in only 60% of the cases. In one patient the solid part of the tumor increased in size.

The prognosis of cystic craniopharyngioma may be volume-related, as three of the four patients who had large cysts eventually died (Fig. 3). One patient whose

Table 1. Published results of intracavitary brachytherapy with different radionuclides in children and adults[a]

Authors and year	No. of patients	Radionuclide and no. of injections				Stabilization or reduction of cyst vol.	Increase of cyst vol.	Lost to follow-up
		P	Au	Yt	Rh			
Sturm et al. 1981 [7]	15			25		15 Patients		
Kobayashi et al. 1981 [8]	8	4	6			10 Cysts		
Kodama et al. 1981 [9]	16		20			14 Patients	1 Pat.	1
Netzeband et al. 1984 [10]	33			33	7	33 Cysts	7 Cysts	
Szikla et al. 1984 [11]	13				15	13 Patients		
Musolino et al. 1985 [12]	16		2	1	17	14 Patients		2
Strauss et 1985 [13]	18			18		10 Patients	1	7
Guevara et al. (1988) [14]	17			17		12 Patients	4	1
Julow et al. (1988) [15]	20			25		25 Cysts		
Pollock et al. (1988) [16]	9	9				9 Patients		
Backlund et al. 1989 (17)	21			28		21 Patients		

[a] Only patients who were followed up were included.

cyst volume was less than 10 ml died in connection with uncontrollable epileptic seizures. A prognostic correlation probably also exists in multicystic cases, as three of the four deaths occurred in this group. We could not detect a relationship with age (Fig. 2).

Some results from the literature are presented in Table 1. A total of 227 isotope injections were performed in 186 patients using phosphorus 32, yttrium 90, rhenium 186, or gold Au 198. These are the most suitable β-radiation-emitting isotopes for this purpose, although both rhenium and gold also emit a considerable amount of γ-radiation. The rhenium sulfide compound tends to convert to water-soluble perrhenate, whereas the remaining isotopes are stable colloids, resulting in less leakage. Yttrium has the shortest half-life. It is, therefore, most frequently regarded as the most suitable isotope for IB. It is apparent from the literature results that IB is generally successful in arresting the progression of the growth of craniopharyngioma cysts. In the majority of cases reported significant reduction of the cyst volume was achieved, some cysts remained stable, and only a minority enlarged.

Intracavitary brachytherapy is a safe and efficacious treatment which should be considered as a primary surgical modality in cases of solitary cystic or multicystic craniopharyngiomas. The treatment obviates the need for craniotomy and resection in the majority of patients. In our series it resulted in stabilization or reduction of cyst size in 80% of cases.

References

1. Cabezudo JM, Vaquero J, Garcia-de-Sola R et al. (1980) Computed tomography in craniopharyngiomas: a review. Surg Neurol 15:422–427
2. Fitz CR, Wortzman G, Harwood-Nash DC et al. (1978) Computed tomography in craniopharyngiomas. Radiology 127:687–691
3. Miller JH, Pena AM, Segall HD (1980) Radiological investigation of sellar region masses in children. Radiology 134:81–87
4. Backlund E-O, Johansson L, Sarby L (1972) Studies on craniopharyngiomas II. Treatment by stereotaxis and radiosurgery. Acta Chir Scand 138:749–759
5. Backlund E-O (1973) Studies on craniopharyngiomas III. Stereotaxic treatment with intracystic yttrium-90. Acta Chir Scand 139:237–247
6. Lunsford LD, Levine G, Gumerman LW (1985) Comparison of computerized tomographic and radionuclide methods in determining intracranial cystic tumor volumes. J Neurosurg 63:740–744
7. Sturm V, Scheer KE, Schlege W et al. (1981) Intrakavitäre Kontaktbestrahlung von zystischen Kraniopharyngiomen durch stereotaktisch appliziertes Y-90. Strahlentherapie [Sonderb] 76:113–118
8. Kobayashi T, Kageyama N, Ohara K (1981) Internal irradiation for cystic craniopharyngioma. J Neurosurg 55:896–903
9. Kodama T, Matsukado Y, Uemara S (1981) Intracapsular irradiation therapy of craniopharyngiomas with radioactive gold: indication and follow-up results. Neurol Med Chir (Tokyo) 21:49–58
10. Netzeband G, Sturm V, Georgi P et al. (1984) Results of stereotactic intracavitary irradiation of cystic craniopharyngiomas. Comparison of the effects of yttrium-90 and rhenium-186. Acta Neurochir [Suppl] (Wien) 33:341–344

11. Szikla G, Musolino A. Miyahara S et al. (1984) Colloidal rhenium-186 in endocavitary beta irradiation of cystic craniopharyngiomas and active glioma cysts. Acta Neurochir [Suppl] (Wien) 33:331–339
12. Musolino A. Munari C, Blond S et al. (1985) Traitement stéréotaxique des kystes expansifs de cranio-pharyngiomas par irradiation endocavitaire beta (Re 186; Au 198; Y 90). Neurochirurgie 31:169–178
13. Strauss L, Sturm V, Georgi P et al. (1982) Radioisotope therapy of cystic craniopharyngiomas. Int J Radiat Oncol Biol Phys 8:1581–1585
14. Guevara JA, Bunge HJ, Heinrich JJ et al. (1988) Cystic craniopharyngioma treated by 90-yttrium silicate colloid. Acta Neurochir [Suppl] (Wien) 42:109–112
15. Julow J, Lányi F, Hajda M et al. (1988) Further experiences in the treatment of cystic craniopharyngiomas with yttrium 90 silicate colloid. Acta Neurochir [Suppl] (Wien) 42:113–119
16. Pollack IF, Lunsford LD, Slamovits TL et al. (1988) Stereotaxic intracavitary irradition for cystic craniopharyngiomas. J Neurosurg 68:227–233
17. Backlund E-O, Axelsson B, Bergstrand C-G et al. (1989) Treatment of craniopharyngiomas – the stereotactic approach in a ten to twenty-three years' prospective. I. Surgical, radiological and ophthalmological aspects. Acta Neurochir (Wien) 99:11–19

Long-Term Results of Combined Surgery and Radiotherapy of Pilocytic Astrocytomas in the Middle Cranial Fossa

F. Rauhut[1], V. Reinhardt[2], H. Wiedemayer, and V. Budach[3]

Introduction

The incidence of pilocytic astrocytomas (WHO astrocytoma grade I) among brain tumors amounts to 6.5% [1, 2, 11]. In children this type of tumor is the most frequent orbital neoplasm [10, 12]. Radical extirpation is not possible because of extension into the optic system and infiltration of the neighboring brain substance, especially the hypothalamus. According to the literature, 25% of optic gliomas involve one optic nerve, 50% are located in the optic chiasm, and in 25% of cases there is infiltration of the hypothalamus [4, 6]. Where subtotal extirpation has been carried out, postoperative radiotherapy can prevent tumor progression [1, 5, 9].

Patients and Methods

Thirty-six patients (27 female, 9 male) with pilocytic astrocytomas of the optic nerve or chiasm were studied retrospectively. The mean age was 12 years (range: 1–17 years). The extent of tumor growth is shown in Fig. 1. In six cases (17%) tumors were localized in one optic nerve; in the rest, infiltration of the chiasm had occurred. Concurrent infiltration of the hypothalamus was seen in 11 patients (31%). Surgery alone was carried out on 15 patients, but radical extirpation of the tumor was possible in only four cases (12% of all cases). By contrast, 21 patients received radiotherapy directly after surgery (high voltage therapy, total dose 50 Gy, 5 fractions of 1.8 Gy per week). Three criteria are of importance for evaluating the outcome of therapy: (a) vision, (b) neurological status, (c) endocrinological functions.

[1] Neurochirurgische Klinik, Universitätsklinikum Essen, Hufelandstr. 55, W-4300 Essen, FRG
[2] Abteilung Neuropathologie, Universitätsklinikum Essen, Hufelandstr. 55, W-4300 Essen, FRG
[3] Abteilung Radiotherapie, Westdeutsches Tumorzentrum, Universitätsklinikum Essen, Hufelandstr. 55. W-4300 Essen, FRG

Advances in Neurosurgery, Vol. 19
W. J. Bock, Ch. Lumenta, M. Brock, M. Klinger (Eds.)

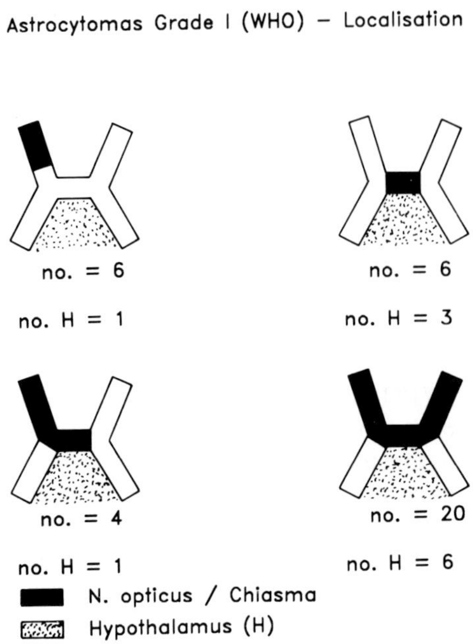

Fig. 1. Localization of pilocytic astrocytomas in 36 patients

Results

Preoperatively, vision tests in 14 patients of the surgical group showed various visual defects. After surgery, vision was unchanged in seven cases but was found to have improved in four and deteriorated in the rest. The neurological and endocrinological studies showed no change to the preoperative status in seven cases. An improvement in neurological and/or endocrinological disturbances was seen in three, while the rest showed deterioration or died.

The follow-up times in the surgical group are shown in Fig. 2. Four children died due to further extension with infiltration of the hypothalamus and tumor recurrence occurred in a 6-year-old child.

In the group treated with surgery and radiation, vision tests in 17 patients also showed a variety of visual defects before surgical intervention. After treatment, vision improved in five cases, remained unaltered in nine, and deteriorated in three. Functionally sigfnificant vision was preserved in 11 patients (78%).

Neurological and/or endocrinological disturbances found before and after combined therapy are illustrated in Fig. 3. Symptoms and signs improved in three cases, whereas five patients showed signs of deterioration or died.

The follow-up times after combined surgery and radiotherapy ranged from 3 months to 15 years (median 5.8 years; Fig. 4).

No tumor recurrence has yet occurred in the surviving patients. The two infants who died suffered from a large tumor involving the hypothalamus.

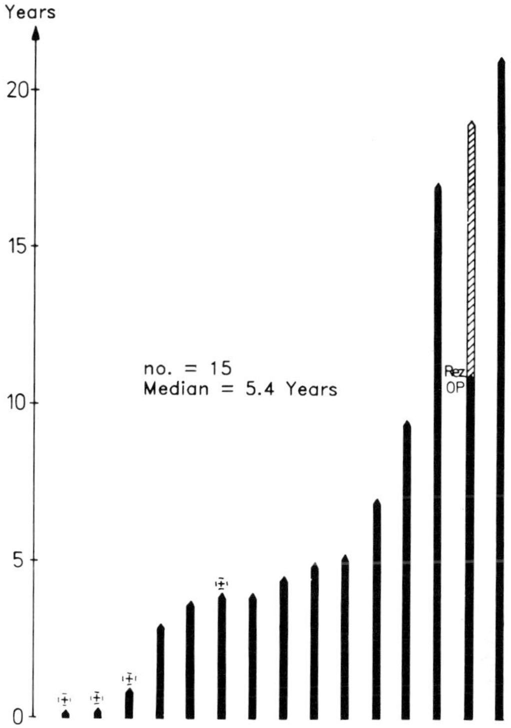

Fig. 2. Follow-up times after surgery

Discussion

Our treatment results so far do not allow exact evaluation of the efficacy of radiotherapy. For this, follow-up times of over 5 years are necessary, because pilocytic astrocytomas of the optic nerve grow very slowly. In our group treated with combined surgery/radiotherapy, only 14 patients have been under follow-up for such long periods. Due to different initial conditions it is not possible to compare the two treatment groups. In the group treated with surgery alone, more small tumors were found, which after radical extirpation have a 100% chance of recovery. Long follow-up times are also known in patients with subtotally extirpated tumors [8, 10]. In these cases periodic pattern of tumor growth has been discussed [6].

There are many reports in the literature on the efficacy of radiotherapy in the treatment of subtotally removed optic nerve gliomas [1]. Follow-up times of up to 35 years have been reported [3]. Montgomery (1977) and Horwich (1985) reported median follow-up times ranging from 6.3 to 8.2 years [5, 9]. In 37% of cases an improvement in visual defects was seen, whereas 50% showed cessation of progressive deterioration of visual acuity [2, 5, 9]. These reports agree with our experiences. From the radiobiological point of view, few dividing cell clones are found in low malignancy pilocytic astrocytomas. The aim of radiotherapy is to kill these cell formations. The selection of appropriate irradiation fields can be difficult because tumor infiltration can be more extensive than appears from computed tomog-

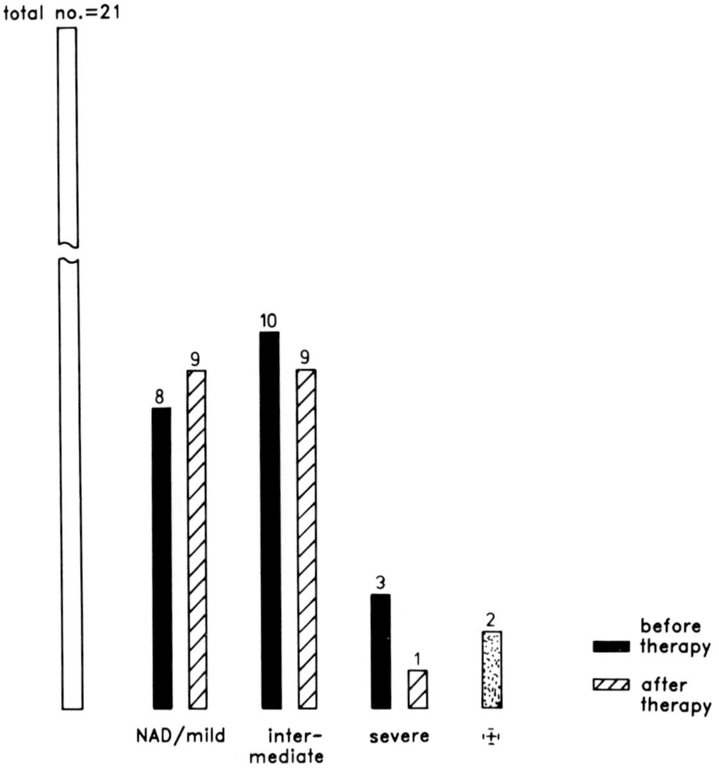

Fig. 3. Neurological and/or endocrinological disturbances before and after combined surgery and radiotherapy

raphy (CT) and magnetic resonance imaging (MRI). To avoid damage to the optic nerve, it is important that each single dose does not exceed 1.8 Gy. To date we have detected no neuroradiologically (CT, MRI) recognizable shrinkage after radiotherapy.

Prior to irradiation histological diagnosis of tumor status is essential, because CT and MRI do not give an exact morphological picture [7].

From the literature and our experiences the following treatment rationale appears to be the best:

1. Surgery is the therapy of choice in cases of isolated optic nerve involvement.
2. After histological diagnosis (biopsy, subtotal tumor removal), radiotherapy should be employed:
   (a) where there is chiasm or chiasm and hypothalamus infiltration and (b) where there is isolated optic nerve involvement with no tumor free area in the chiasma and margin of the optic nerve associated with a mild visual disturbance; (c) constitutes only a relative indication for irradiation, depending on the general conditions and wish of the patient.

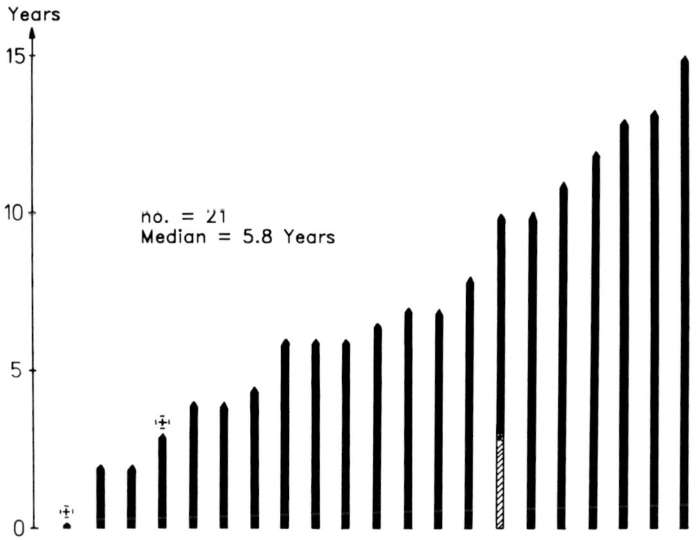

Fig. 4. Follow-up times after combined surgery and radiotherapy

References

1. Bamberg M (1987) Tumoren des Gehirns: In: Scherer E (ed) Strahlentherapie, 3rd edn. Springer, Berlin Heidelberg New York, pp 987–992
2. Danoff BF, Kramer S, Thompson N (1980) The radiotherapeutic management of optic nerve gliomas in children. Int J Radiat Oncol Biol Phys 6:45–50
3. Dosoretz DE, Blitzer PH, Wang CC, Lingwood RM (1980) Management of glioma of the optic nerve and/or chiasm. Cancer 45:1467–1471
4. Hoffmann JH (1982) Supratentorial brain tumors in children. In: Youmans JR (ed) Neurological surgery, vol 5, 2nd edn. Saunders, Philadelphia, pp 2702–2732
5. Horwich OP, Bloom HJG (1985) Optic gliomas: radiation therapy and prognosis. Int J Radiat Oncol Biol Phys 11:1067–1079
6. Housepian EM, Trokel SL, Jakubiec FO, Hildal SK (1982) Tumors of the orbit. In: Youmans JR (ed) Neurological surgery, vol 5, 2nd edn. Saunders, Philadelphia, pp 3042–3046
7. Kazner E, Wende S, Grumme TH, Lanksch W, Stochdorph O (1981) CT intrakranieller Tumoren. Springer, Berlin Heidelberg New York
8. Köning W, Frowein RA (1988) Therapie der Optikus-Gliome. In: Bamberg M, Sack H (eds) Therapie primärer Hirntumoren. Zuckschwerdt, Munich, pp 227–232
9. Montgomery AB, Griffin T, Parker RG, Gerdes AJ (1977) Optic nerve glioma: the role of radiation therapy. Cancer 40:2079–2080
10. Russel DS, Rubinstein LK (1989) Pathology of tumors of the nervous system. Arnold, London, pp 370–376
11. Zülch K (1986) Brain tumors. Their biology and pathology, 3rd edn. Springer, Berlin Heidelberg New York, pp 221–232
12. Zülch KJ, Wechsler W (1968) Pathology and classification of gliomas. Prog Neurol Surg 2:1–84

Discussion: PNET – A Melting-Pot of Unspecified Tumors?

W. Wechsler[1]

As a contribution to the main topic "Supratentorial tumors of childhood," a podium discussion on *primitive neuroectodermal tumors* (PNETs) was organized by the Congress Committee. The discussion was chaired by Professor Kleihues (Department of Neuropathology, Zurich) with comments by invited speakers Professor Rorke (Department of Pathology, The Children's Hospital, Philadelphia), Professor Jänisch (Department of Neuropathology, Charité, East Berlin), Professor Schulte (Department of Pediactrics, Hamburg), and Professor Wechsler (Department of Neuropathology, Düsseldorf).

In his introduction the chairman outlined the importance of the concept of primitive neuroectodermal tumors, as originated by Rorke in 1984 [4] and presented in detail 2 years later [5]. Kleihues expressed the view that many neuropathologists are attracted by the possibility of using the diagnosis of PNET. The question is, should the neuropathologists follow the original concept of Rorke, or should the diagnosis of PNET be reserved for special primary neuroepithelial tumors of the central nervous system. At the present time we cannot answer this question precisely. Nevertheless, it is necessary to outline the concept of PNETs for clinicians from the neuropathological point of view.

The WHO Brain Tumor Classification of 1979 [6] is now widely used in many countries of the world and fairly well accepted in Europe. This classification included PNET neither as a diagnosis nor as a concept. Under the guidance of Professor Zülch (Cologne, FRG) and Professor Rubinstein (Charlottesville, USA) a WHO-sponsored symposium in Houston in 1988 discussed modern trends in neuro-oncology and the question whether or not a revision of the 1979 WHO Classification is justified. Among the topics of this conference was the question whether or not PNET should be incorporated as a special entity. The proceedings of this meeting have been published by Fields [1] and it was agreed to organize another conference 2 years later. Kleihues took the initiative and in collaboration with Burger (Duke University, Durham, USA) and Scheithauer (Mayo Clinic, USA) organized a "WHO Meeting on Histological Typing of Tumors of the Central Nervous System" in Zurich, March 27–31, 1990, in which a group of 25 experts agreed upon the revision of the WHO Classification of 1979.

---

1 Abteilung Neuropathologie, Medizinische Einrichtungen der Heinrich-Heine-Universität, Moorenstr. 5, W-4000 Düsseldorf, FRG

Advances in Neurosurgery, Vol. 19
W. J. Bock, Ch. Lumenta, M. Brock, M. Klinger (Eds.)

As far as PNETs were concerned, the Zurich group wanted to introduce this name in the first revision of the WHO Classification, which will be published by the end of 1990. The following scheme was proposed:

Classification proposal for embryonal tumors of neuroepithelial tissue:

1. Medulloepithelioma
2. Neuroblastoma
   Variant: ganglioneuroblastoma
3. Ependymoblastoma
4. Retinoblastoma
5. *Primitive neuroectodermal tumors (PNETs)*
   with multipotent differentiation: neuronal, astrocytic ependymal, muscle, melanotic, etc.
   a. *Medulloblastoma*
      Variants: desmoplastic medulloblastoma, medullomyoblastoma, melanocytic medulloblastoma
   b. *Cerebral or spinal PNETs*

Rorke presented an excellent review of the history and present state of the study of PNETs. Modern immunohistochemistry has made it possible to study a great number of differentiation antigens in this group of tumors, which reveals that these tumors present a complex and variable intermediate filament pattern and express various neuroendocrine differentiation markers, "suggesting that central nervous system PNETs comprise a distinct, albeit heterogeneous group of neoplasms" [2, 3]. Contributions by Jänisch, Schulte, and Wechsler added details concerning the histopathology, the question of tumor grading, the application of modern neuropathological techniques for the evaluation of uni-, bi- or multipotent differentiation patterns, the determination of the proliferative potential with proliferation-associated antigens such as Ki-67, and the variable patterns of receptor expression for a number of growth factors, e.g., epidermal growth factor or nerve growth factor. As far as age and location are concerned, PNETs in supratentorial locations do occur during childhood and adolescence, but also in adult patients of both sexes.

While Rorke includes medulloblastoma of the cerebellum in the PNET category, the tendency favored by Kleihues, Jänisch, and Wechsler is to continue to use the name medulloblastoma for the cerebellar tumors and apply the PNET diagnosis preferentially to tumors of his histo- and cytopathological type in other cerebral and spinal CNS locations. As far as tumor grading is concerned, the majority of supratentorial PNETs can be considered as grade III or grade IV neoplasms.

In summary, all participants in this podium discussion agreed that the PNET discussion must be continued from the molecular, neuropathological, and clinical point of view.

References

1. Fields WS (1989) Primary brain tumors. A review of histologic classification. Springer, New York Berlin Heidelberg London Paris Tokyo Hong Kong
2. Gould VE, Rorke LC, Jansson DS, Molenaar WM, Trojanowski JQ, Lee VMY, Packer RJ, Franke WW (1990) Primitive neuroectodermal tumors of the central nervous system express neuroendocrine markers and may express all classes of intermediate filaments. Human Pathology, 21:245–252
3. Gould VE, Jansson DS, Molenaar WM, Rorke LB, Trojanowski JQ, Lee VMY, Packer RJ, Franke WW (1990) Primitive neuroectodermal tumors of the central nervous system. Laboratory Investigation, 62:1–11
4. Rorke LB (1983) The cerebellar medulloblastoma and its relationship to primitive neuroectodermal tumors. J Neuropathol Exp Neurol 42:1
5. Rorke LB, Gilles FH, Davis RL, Becker LE (1985) Revision of the World Health Organization Classification of brain tumors for childhood brain tumors. Cancer 56:1887
6. Zülch KJ (1979) Histological typing of tumors of the central nervous system. WHO, Geneva

Prognosis of Supratentorial Gliomas in Children

J. Pospiech, R. Kalff, W. Kocks, and W. Grote[1]

Introduction

Comparing brain tumors of children and adults, a few distinguishing clinical features can be found:

1. Epileptic seizures are the initial symptom in 20%–30% of brain tumors in adults, whereas in children nonspecific symptoms such as headache, vomiting, and lethargy predominate [1].
2. Especially during the 1st decade of life, brain tumors are frequently located in the posterior fossa. Later on most neoplasms occur in the cerebral hemispheres.
3. Postoperative radiotherapy, which is generally acceptable in adults, can lead to cognitive and emotional impairment in children [2, 6].
4. The significance of brain tumors in childhood is underlined by their incidence. They account for 20% of all malignant neoplasms in children [2].

Between 10% and 20% of brain tumors in children are located in the cerebral hemispheres [5] and are of special interest because they constitute a small group of brain tumors of great histological variability. We wanted to evaluate the usefulness of an established tumor grading scheme as a prognostic indicator in clinical routine.

Patients and Methods

In this series there were 21 patients with supratentorial gliomas, representing 25% of all children with brain tumors treated at our institution since 1971. Patients with gliomas of the optic pathways, craniopharyngiomas, tumors of the pineal region, and all nonneuroepithelial neoplasms were excluded because they may not share the same oncological prognosis and present different surgical problems.

The patients were under 16 years of age at the time of operation (average 7 years 10 months, youngest 2 years 1 month, oldest 15 years 10 months). There were 10 boys and 11 girls. The duration of symptoms varied between some days (in a few cases) and a few months (in almost all cases). Headache, vomiting, lethargy, and behavioral disturbances were the most frequent symptoms. Nine children were admitted because of epileptic seizures. Neurological examination gave unremarkable

---

1 Neurochirurgische Klinik, Universitätsklinikum Essen, Hufelandstr. 55, D-4300 Essen, FRG

Advances in Neurosurgery, Vol. 19
W. J. Bock, Ch. Lumenta, M. Brock, M. Klinger (Eds.)

Table 1. Neurological grading on admission ($n = 21$)

Grade	Description	No. of patients
I	No neurological deficit	9
II	Mild neurological deficit	6
III	Severe neurological deficit	6

results in nine cases; six children had only mild neurological defitics (e.g., papilledema, sensory disorders, reflex differente; Table 1). There were six midline and 15 hemispheric tumors.

Total removal was achieved in six patients, five of them with low grade gliomas. Partial removal was carried out in 11 cases (six low grade gliomas, five high grade gliomas). Biopsy only was carried out in cases of diffuse tumor growth (four children). Two children suffered from postoperative complications: one bone flap osteomyelitis and one CSF fistula. No patient died in the immediate postoperative period.

Histological examination revealed low grade gliomas in 13 (62%) cases and high grade gliomas in eight cases (Table 2). Pilocytic and fibrillary astrocytomas constituted nearly 50%.

Patients who had undergone total tumor removal received no further therapy. In almost all others surgery was combined with local radiotherapy, depending on histology: no adjuvant therapy was given to eight out of 13 patients with low grade gliomas, whereas six out of eight children with high grade gliomas received postoperative radiotherapy, three of them in combination with systemic chemotherapy.

Table 2. Histological diagnoses in 21 patients, using Kernohan's tumor classification[a]

	Diagnosis	No.
Grade I	Pilocytic astrocytoma	3
	Gangliocytoma	1
Grade II	Astrocytoma	6
	Oligodendroglioma	2
	Ependymoma	1
Grade II–III	Astrocytoma	2
	Oligodendroglioma	1
Grade III + IV	Astrocytoma	1
	Oligodendroglioma	2
	Ependymoma	1
	Anaplastic glioma	1

[a] Low grade tumors: grades I and II
High grade tumors: grades III and IV

Results

Two patients were excluded from further analysis because the follow-up period was less than 2 years. Six children (two low grade gliomas, four high grade) died due to progressive tumor growth; their mean survival was 8.5 months.

Thirteen patients are still alive, with follow-up period varying between 38 and 211 months (average 107 months). In three cases of low grade glioma there was a tumor recurrence after total removal (average 63 months postoperatively). In all cases a second operation was carried out successfully.

At the end of the follow-up period 12 children showed only mild neurological deficit or none. No significant neurological deterioration occurred due to the operation. In relation to extent of surgical tumor removal, all children who underwent total removal are without any neurological deficit (mean survival 79 months), whereas both children who underwent only biopsy died due to tumor progression

Table 3. Neurological grades[a] before and after treatment, related to extent of tumor removal ($n = 19$)

Total removal			Partial removal			Biopsy		
Before	After	No.	Before	After	No.	Before	After	No.
I	I	3	I	II	2	I	†	2
				†	1			
II	I	2	II	I	2			
				†	1			
III	I	1	III	II	2			
				III	I			
				†	2			

[a] Classification as in Table 1

Table 4. Neurological grades[a] before and after treatment, related to histological diagnosis ($n = 19$)

Low grade tumor			High grade tumor		
Before	After	No.	Before	After	No.
I	I	3	I	II	1
	II	1		†	2
	†	1			
II	I	2	II	I	2
				†	1
III	I	1	III	†	1
	II	2			
	III	1			
	†	1			

[a] Classification as in Table 1.

(mean survival 7.5 months; Table 3). In relation to tumor grading, two out of 13 patients with low grade gliomas and four out of seven children with high grade gliomas died (mean survival 9 months and 8 months respectively; Table 4).

Discussion

Before comparing our own results with those from the literature we must draw attention to the inhomogeneity of our material, especially, as far as histology is concerned. It is obvious that, for example, an ependymoma II of the lateral ventricle will not have the same oncological prognosis as a temporal astrocytoma II [1]. This must always be borne in mind when brain tumors are being categorized only as low and high grade.

Nevertheless, it appears that low grade gliomas do have a far better prognosis than high grade tumors. According to the literature, they are often much more accessible to total surgical removal [1]. So extent of tumor removal and histological grading are the criteria with the best prognosis value in supratentorial gliomas of childhood (1, 3, 5]. It would appear that, despite the histological variability among supratentorial brain tumors in children, grading schemes based mainly on histological features, such as the classification by Kernohan, remain useful prognostic indicators [4].

Tumors in the midline have a worse prognosis, since it is frequently impossible to remove enough tumor.

We agree with the literature [3, 5] in failing to find any advantage from postoperative radiotherapy. We therefore recommend that this mode of therapy should be employed only in cases of tumor recurrence, in combination with surgery.

Conclusions

1. Surgery is the only effective treatment for supratentorial gliomas in children.
2. A low histological grading and location in the cerebral hemispheres are associated with a generally good prognosis.
3. Adjuvant therapies such as radiation and chemotherapy seem to be of very little value.

References

1. Hirsch JF, Sainte Rose C, Pierre-Kahn A, Pfister A, Hoppe Hirsch E (1989) Benign astrocytic and oligodendrocytic tumors of the cerebral hemisphere in children. J Neurosurg 70:568–572
2. Kun LE, Mulhern RK, Crisco JJ (1983) Quality of life in children treated for brain tumors. J Neurosurg 58:1–6
3. Mercuri S, Russo A, Palma L (1981) Hemispheric supratentorial astrocytomas in children. J Neurosurg 55:170–173

4. Nazar GB, Hoffman HJ, Becker LE, Jenkin D, Humphreys RP, Hendrick EB (1990) Infratentorial ependymomas in childhood, prognostic factors and treatment. J Neurosurg 72:408–417
5. Nishio S, Takeshita I, Fujii K, Fukui M (1989) Supratentorial astrocytic tumors of childhood, a clinicopathological study of 41 cases. Acta Neurochir (Wien) 101:3–8
6. Packer RJ, Sutton LN, Atkins TE, Radcliffe J, Bunin GR, D'Angio G, Siegel KR, Scut L (1989) A prospective study of cognitive function in children receiving whole-brain radiotherapy and chemotherapy. J Neurosurg 70:707–713

Proliferative Activity of Pilocytic Astrocytomas: Examination Using Monoclonal Antibody Ki-67*

R. Schröder and K. Bien[1]

Pilocytic astrocytomas occupy an exceptional position among the tumors of astrocytic differentiation because of the characteristically very low age of patients and the predilection of the tumors for the midline and infratentorial regions. As a rule these tumors grow very slowly and patients have a relatively good prognosis [1, 5, 7]. The question then arises whether this slow growth in comparison to other glioma types can be quantified in biopsy material, and whether it will be possible to define subtypes of pilocytic astrocytoma on this basis.

In this type of tumor mitoses are so extremely rare in histological sections, or sometimes completely absent, that determining a mitotic index is impossible. Compared to other more complicated methods for labeling DNA synthesizing cells today, it is simple to measure the part of proliferating cells within the total tumor cell population, the growth fraction, by immunohistochemistry using the monoclonal antibody Ki-67 on frozen sections.

We used this technique to examine 21 pilocytic astrocytomas of various locations. The age of the patients varied from 9 months to 57 years; 15 were male and 6 female. The labeling index, i.e., the growth fraction, was determined in regions of frequently labeled cells.

Table 1. Percentage of Ki-67-positive cells in pilocytic astrocytomas

Authors	%	*n*
Burger et al. [3]	0.6–1.4	3
Giangasparo et al [6]	1	1
Shibata and Burger [12]	0.4–1.4	5
Böker and Stark [2]	1	1
Kleihues et al. [12]	0.3–1.6 (X = 0.9)	13
Zuber et al. [13]	0.1	4
Deckert et al. [4]	0–< 1	4
Personal data	0.001–7.5 (X = 0.6)	21

* Supported by the Verein der Freunde und Förderer der Universität Köln

1 Neuropathologisches Labor, Institut für Pathologie der Universität Köln, Joseph-Stelzmann-Str. 9, W-5000 Köln 41, FRG

Advances in Neurosurgery, Vol. 19
W. J. Bock, Ch. Lumenta, M. Brock, M. Klinger (Eds.)

Table 2. Percentage of Ki-67-positive cells in different gliomas

	Median	Range	*n*
Glioblastomas	13.9	5.8 – 39.5	32
Astrocytomas III	9.7	4.0 – 15.5	20
Astrocytomas II	4.8	2.4 – 9.0	16
Pilocytic astrocytomas	0.16	0.001 – 7.5	21

Our results in this fairly larger number of cases agree very well with those of other authors (Table 1). The mean growth fraction was lower than 1%. The median values of such measurements are generally somewhat lower because of skewed distribution.

Table 2 compares our data with those for grade II and grade III astrocytomas and glioblastomas [11]. In the latter two types of tumor, the values of neighboring grades of malignancy differ by a factor of two at the most. Against that, pilocytic astrocytomas have a 40-fold smaller growth fraction than grade II astrocytomas.

Furthermore the extraordinary wide variation between the individual values is remarkable, as shown in Fig. 1. It should be noted that the abscissa is logarithmic in this graph, which leads to symmetrical distributions of similar width appearing for grade II astrocytomas and glioblastomas (grade III astrocytomas have been excluded for the sake of clarity). The range among pilocytic astrocytomas is much wider, covering several orders of magnitude, and may include several different peaks.

For this reason, we have divided up our data according to several different variables in order to find any correlations with differing proliferative activity. Statistical calculations are based upon the nonparametric Mann-Whitney U test. The results are shown in Table 3.

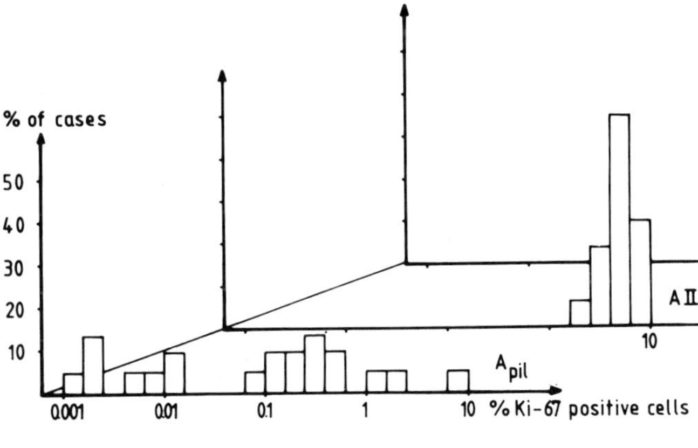

Fig. 1. Distribution of Ki-67 labeling indices over a logarithmic scale in pilocytic astrocytomas *(A_{pil})* compared to grade II astrocytomas *(A II)* and glioblastomas *(Gbl)*

Table 3. Percent Ki-67-positive cells in relation to patient age, location, and histopathologic characteristics

	Median	Range	*n*	
Patients age				
≤ 16 years	0.24	0.001–1.9	11	n. s
> 16 years	0.14	0.007–7.5	7	
Optic nerve	1.9	0.3–7.5	3	$p < 0.05$
Other	0.11	0.001–1.3	18	
Supratentorial (without optic nerve)	0.01	0.001–0.52	9	n. s.
Infratentorial	0.16	0.003–1.3	9	
Juvenile type	0.02	0.001–1.3	12	n. s.
Adult type	0.15	0.01–0.31	6	

There is no demonstrable difference in the growth fraction of pilocytic astrocytomas in infancy and in adulthood. Regarding location, three optic gliomas are conspicuous for significantly elevated labeling indices, possibly indicating the existence of a special variant of pilocytic astrocytoma. To determine this, however, additional investigations would be needed. Despite very different medians, no statistically significant difference could be demonstrated between infra- and supratentorial tumors. Likewise, histological type – the so-called juvenile and adult type – apparently makes no difference, and the same can be said of the presence or absence of microcystic degeneration or of calcifications.

To summarize: the very low growth tendency of pilocytic astrocytomas is explained by their extremely small growth fraction, although other cell kinetic factors of course also play a part. The striking variability of the individual measurements is an unresolved problem. This has already been observed in in vivo labeling of DNA synthesizing cells in this tumor [9]. Optic gliomas, with their somewhat higher growth fraction, may form a separate group, but this has still to be confirmed. Particularly in adults, these tumors show a tendency to malignant transformation [8]. No other subtype has yet been detected among pilocytic astrocytomas in other locations. It is possible that the striking variability of the labeling index is due to inherent inhomogeneity of proliferation within a given tumor, as is known in cell-rich tumors of other kinds [11]. However, because of the paucity of cells and the large distances between proliferative clusters, it is difficult to observe this in pilocytic astrocytomas.

References

1. Afra D, Müller W, Slowik F, Firsching R (1986) Supratentorial lobar pilocytic astrocytomas: report of 45 cases, including 9 recurrences. Acta Neurochir (Wien) 81:90–93
2. Böker D-K, Stark H-J (1988) The proliferation rate of intracranial tumors as defined by the monoclonal antibody Ki 67. Application of the method to paraffin embedded specimens. Neurosurg Rev 11:267 272
3. Burger PC, Shibata D, Kleihues P (1986) The use of the monoclonal antibody Ki-67 in the identification of proliferating cells: Application to surgical neuropathology. Amer J Surg Pathol 10:611-617
4. Deckert M, Reifenberger G, Wechsler W (1989) Determination of the proliferative potential of human brain tumors using the monoclonal antibody Ki-67. J Cancer Res Clin Oncol 115:179–188
5. Febert A, Gullota F (1985) Remarks on the follow-up of cerebellar astrocytomas. J Neurol 232:134–136
6. Giangasparo F, Doglioni C, Rivano MT, Pileri S, Gerdes J, Stein H (1987) Growth fraction in human brain tumors defined by the monoclonal antibody Ki-67. Acta Neuropathol 74:179–182
7. Gjerris F, Klinken L (1978) Long-term prognosis in children with benign cerebellar astrocytoma. J Neurosurg 49:179–184
8. Harper CG, Stewart-Wynne EG (1978) Malignant optic gliomas in adults. Arch Neurol 35:731–735
9. Hoshino T, Nagashima T, Murovic JA, Wilson CB, Edwards MSB, Gutin PH, Davis RL, De Armond SJ (1986) In situ cell kinetics studies on human neuroectodermal tumors with bromodeoxyuridine labeling. J Neurosurg 64:453–459
10. Kleihues P, Meer L, Shibata T, Bamberg M (1988) DNA-Reparatur und DNA-Replikation als Kriterien für therapeutische Effizienz. In: Bamberg M, Sack H (eds) Therapie primärer Hirntumoren. Zuckschwerdt, München, pp 1–8
11. Schröder R, Bien K, Kott R, Meyers I, Vössing R (in press) The relationship between Ki-67 labeling and mitotic index in gliomas and meningiomas. Acta Neuropathol
12. Shibata T, Burger PC (1987) The use of the monoclonal antibody Ki-67 in determination of the growth fraction in pediatric brain tumors. Child's Nerv Syst 3:364–367
13. Zuber P, Hamou M-F, de Tribolet N (1988) Identification of proliferating cells in human gliomas using the monoclonal antibody Ki-67. Neurosurgery 22: 364–368

Immunohistochemical Investigations with a Monoclonal Anti-Epidermal Growth Factor Receptor Antibody in Supratentorial Tumors in Children

J. Behnke, H. Ludwig, G.A. Luckenbach, B. Rama, and E. Markakis[1]

Introduction

In the search for more specific tumor antigens, epidermal growth factor (EGF) receptor-mediated mechanisms have been found to play an important role in the growth of malignancies. The EGF receptor is a transmembrane mitogenic glycoprotein of 170 kDa. In addition to increased expression in human cervical, ovarian, and vulval carcinomas [1] and human sarcomas [2], expression of EGF receptor has been found to be increased in human brain tumors [5].

In a previous investigation of more than 200 tumors of adults and children obtained after resection in our neurosurgical department (publication in preparation), nearly 80% of the glioblastomas and anaplastic astrocytomas tested and more than 90% of the oligodendrogliomas tested bound the monoclonal antibody (Mab) 425, a murine IgG2a which specifically detects EGF receptor [7]. Forty percent of all resected tumors, but 50% of supratentorial tumors, bound Mab 425.

In the present study, supratentorial tumors in children were examined for expression of EGF receptor by means of binding Mab 425.

Methods

The study covered tumors of children aged up to 20 years and treated during the last 3 years.

Of the 42 tumors examined, 25 were located supratentorially; one was located both supra- and infratentorially. From the clinical point of view, five main localizations of supratentorial tumors can be distinguished according to Jacobi and Kornhuber [4]:

1. Tumors of the cerebral hemispheres and within the ventricles ($n = 10$, including one tumor with local recurrence, one metastasis of a group IV tumor and one tumor of imflammatory origin)
2. Tumors of the basal ganglia and thalamus ($n = 1$)
3. Tumors within the third ventricle, anterior visual pathway, and anterior hypothalamus ($n = 2$, including one tumor of inflammatory origin)
4. Tumors in the pineal region, posterior part of the third ventricle, hypothalamus, and quadrigeminal plate ($n = 4$)

1 Neurochirurgische Klinik, Universität Göttingen, Robert-Koch-Str. 40, W-3400 Göttingen, FRG

Advances in Neurosurgery, Vol. 19
W. J. Bock, Ch. Lumenta, M. Brock, M. Klinger (Eds.)

5. Extrinsic tumors of the suprasellar region and within the sella ($n = 8$, including one tumor together with a part of it which remained and was operated upon as a secondary procedure).

The tumor material was frozen immediately after resection in isopentane, cooled in liquid nitrogen, and then kept at –80°C until the tissues were cut into 10–µm-thick sections at –20°C on a cryostat. The sections were fixed in 4°C cold acetone for 5 min and were kept at –20°C overnight or for up to 5 days. For immunohistochemistry with Mab 425 the three-stage avidin-biotin immunoperoxidase method was used. 3-Amino-9-ethylcarbazole was used as chromogen and counterstaining was done with Gill's hematoxylin. The slides were mounted in Mowiol. The slides were checked for Mab 425-binding cells and the "EGF receptor-positive" (Epidermal Growth Factor) tumors defined in this way examined with regard to ultrastructure, histopathology, and the clinical course of the patient.

Results

Tumors which bound Mab 425 to the EGF receptor were found only in group I, tumors of the cerebral hemispheres and within the lateral centricle. All tumors in groups II, III, IV, and V and the tumor which situated supra- and infratentorially were negative for binding of Mab 425.

In group I, one occipital metastasis of an epithelial tumor and two primitive neuroectodermal tumors, one with a local recurrence, were positive. In the same group, one anaplastic astrocytoma, one inflammatory process, one cavernous angioma, one fibrosarcoma, one ganglioglioma, and a bifrontal metastasis of a tumor whose primary manifestation was in group IV were negative for expression of EGF receptor as shown by binding of Mab 425. Tumors which express EGF receptor at a high rate in adults did not bind Mab 425 in our study; in these cases the disease did not take a malignant course clinically. The two primitive neuroectodermal tumors appear particularly interesting, because expression of EGF receptor by epithelial metastases is not a speciality of tumors in childhood (publication in preparation).

Not all of the primitive neuroectodermal tumors tested expressed EGF receptor: the bifrontal metastasis of an ependymoblastoma of group IV, histopathologically estimated as a primitive neuroectodermal tumor, one further primary germinoma of group IV together with its local recurrence were negative for binding the EGF receptor antibody. Only the two primary hemispheric neuroectodermal tumors were positive for binding Mab 425, as was the local recurrence of one of them. Both positive primitive neuroectodermal tumors took a malignant course. In case 1 of these, a 9-year-old girl suffered from a right paraventricular primitive neuroectodermal tumor. She had local recurrence 5 months after operation and died 11 months after first diagnosis. In case 2, a 7-year-old boy had a sudden fit and was admitted with the clinical signs of encephalitis. Computed tomography showed a left temporal mass without contrast enhancement. With virostatic and antiedema therapy, the mass was reduced. Four months later the mass had the appearance of a brain tumor on multiple contrast enhancements and subtotal temporal lobe extirpation was performed. Three months later the whole temporal space was again filled by tumor masses and the boy was reoperated upon, but died 1 year after the onset of his illness.

The two positive primitive neuroectodermal supratentorial hemispheric tumors had similar histopathological and ultrastructural features. They were composed of sheets and clumps of small undifferentiated cells with little cytoplasma. Electron microscopy showed the tumors to be composed of small undifferentiated cells with prominent nuclei and thin rims of cytoplasm containing few mitochondria, occasionally a tiny granular endoplasmic reticulum, rare Golgi complexes, and many free ribosomes and polysomes. These primitive cells "float" in the cytoplasm, containing broad filaments, of cells with processes – astrocytes. Some capillaries have a thickened basement membrane and endothelial padding without endothelial proliferation.

Discussion

Apart from an epithelial metastasis, the only supratentorial tumors of childhood which bound Mab 425 were two tumors which arose out of the cerebral hemispheres and whose biological behavior was malignant.

Histological examination and electron microscopy showed these tumors to be composed of small undifferentiated cells without significant cytoplasmic differentiation or junctional complexes, suggesting that the predominant cell is a primitive, undifferentiated neuroectodermal cell of the cerebrum. Other primitive neuroectodermal tumors of the pineal region did not express the EGF receptor; neither did cerebellar medulloblastomas (publication in preparation).

Rubinstein [8] has pointed out that specific types of primitive neuroectodermal tumors, such as medulloephitheliomas, cerebral neuroblastomas, polar spongioblastomas, ependymoblastomas, pineal parenchymal tumors and cerebellar medulloblastomas, deserve special designations because of their location and histologic appearance. Hart and Early [3] have pointed out that there remains a group of largely undifferentiated neoplasms in children which are uncommon, are sometimes mistaken for metastatic tumors, have a hemispheric location, and whose biological behavior is malignant. Unlike these authors, but like Markesbery and Challa [6], we saw no mesenchymal tumor component in our two hemispheric primitive neuroectodermal tumors but nevertheless we did see EGF receptors as a marker of this subgroup of primitive neuroectodermal tumors.

References

1. Gullick WJ, Marsden JJ, Whittle N, Ward B, Babrow L, Waterfield MD (1986) Expression of epidermal growth factor receptors on human cervical, ovarian, and vulval carcinomas. Cancer Res 46:285–292

2. Gusterson B, Cowley G, McIlhinney J, Ozanne B, Fisher C, Reeves B (1985) Evidence for increased epidermal growth factor receptors on human sarcomas. Int J Cancer 36:689–693
3. Hart MN, Earle KM (1973) Primitive neuroectodermal tumors of the brain in children. Cancer 32:890–895
4. Jacobi G, Kornhuber B (1987) Malignant brain tumors in children. In: Jellinger K (ed) Therapy of malignant brain tumors. Springer, Vienna New York, pp 396–493
5. Libermann TA, Razon N, Bartal AD, Yarden Y, Schlessinger J, Soreq H (1984) Expression of epidermal growth factor receptors in human brain tumors. Cancer Res 44:753–760
6. Markesbery WR, Challa VR (1979) Electron microscopic findings in primitive neuroectodermal tumors of the cerebrum. Cancer 44:141–147
7. Murthy U, Basu A, Rodeck U, Herlyn M, Ross AH, Das M (1987) Binding of an antagonistic monoclonal antibody to an intact and fragmented EGF-receptor polypeptide. Arch Biochem Biophys 252:549–560
8. Rubinstein LJ (1972) Cytogenesis and differentiation of primitive central neuroepithelial tumors. J Neuropathol Exp Neurol 31:7–26

Neurosurgical Intensive Care

Neurosurgical Intensive Care – An Interdisciplinary Field

A. Encke[1]

Greeting of the General Secretary of the Deutsche Interdisziplinäre Vereinigung für Intensiv- und Notfallmedizin.

DIVI was founded in June 1977 as a corporative association of medical societies and professional associations of those medical specialties closely involved with intensive care. Meanwhile DIVI has among its members representatives of the specialties of anesthesiology, surgery including accident, thoracic and cardiovascular surgery, neurosurgery, medicine, gynecology and obstetrics, neurology and pediatrics.

The foundation intentionally took the form of an interdisciplinary association rather than a German society for intensive care medicine to prevent the development of a separate specialty "intensive care medicine" and a "specialist in intensive care medicine". Regulations therefore do not include personal membership or exclusively admit scientific societies and professional associations.

Member societies of DIVI invariably represent the principle that intensive care is an integral part of many specialties and in its broad spectrum cannot competently be mastered and represented by any one individual physician.

Neurosurgery is an excellent example for optimal intensive care, monitoring and general therapy with their specific aspects overlap and specialist knowledge and experience are of vital importance for the success of therapy. Central nervous system disorders or injury with their influence on vital functions require competent cooperation with the neurosurgeon. Another aspect closely linking neurosurgeons to general surgeons is the fact that responsibilities especially in the critical postoperative period cannot be delegated and that the exact intraoperative finding in the individual case along with the possible complications there, are only known to the individual surgeon.

On the other hand modern intensive care medicine on which alone our operative success is founded is quite unthinkable without the cooperation and activities of anesthesiology. This again emphasizes the integral specific and interdisciplinary character of surgical intensive care medicine. Last but not least, intensive care medicine is a cornerstone of our clinical research.

During the past 10 years DIVI has succeeded in building up a modern interdisciplinary intensive care medicine through reliable cooperation. However, we have to

---

1 Zentrum der Chirurgie, Abteilung für Allg. und Abdominalchirurgie, Theodor-Stern-Kai 7, W-6000 Frankfurt/Main 70

Advances in Neurosurgery, Vol. 19
W. J. Bock, Ch. Lumenta, M. Brock, M. Klinger (Eds.)

accept that this view is not necessarily shared by other countries. A number of neighboring countries aim at an “independent intensive care physician” who is to guarantee agreement, continuity and competence. To follow our own concept, we are therefore obliged to be particularly dedicated to high demands in clinical intensive care medicine and related scientific research. Intensive care medicine is quite unsuitable as a mere battlefield.

An obvious measure of the constructive work done on the part of DIVI is the number of publications on problems of organizational problems of critical care medicine. Special sections were founded to look after a variety of topics. The section on rescue medicine, founded in 1980, has sent out important impulses concerning problems of emergency medicine and rescue. In addition, in 1988, the section on disaster medicine was founded.

In recent years DIVI has established principles for hospital hygiene, as well as spatial and technical equipment standards for intensive care units. A special aim has been to adjust the highly inadequate staffing figures produced by the Deutsche Krankenhausgesellschaft (German Hospital Society) for intensive care units, especially for the nursing staff, to modern developments of critical care medicine. Of the problems in this field you will be very well aware but, unfortunately neither the general public nor politicians involved. Following years of fruitless discussions between representatives of the hospitals and national sociel insurance companies the Bundesminister für Arbeit und Soziales (Federal Department of Work and Social Affairs) will have to lay down new figures as a statutory order for 1st July, 1980.

Based on their own investigations in analogy to the injury severity score (TISS scale) DIVI has produced their own figures now accepted by the German Hospital Society (Deutsche Krankenhausgesellschaft).

Here as well as in other areas special credit goes to Professors Bock, Karimi and Lorenz for their dedicated cooperation.

These activities emphasize another aspect of DIVI, which is the representation of common efforts, and principles in the field of health politics. Next to improving the cooperation between various scientific societies there is increasing importance in the representation of common interest of intensive care and emergency medicine confronting authorities, medical professional societies and other groups. The dedicated activities of the Deutsche Gesellschaft für Neurochirurgie in this area are greatly appreciated.

Neurosurgical Intensive Care: General Considerations

W.J. Bock, J. Piek, and C. Sprick[1]

It is 19 years since we last looked at the topic of neurosurgery on the occasion of an annual meeting, that time also in Düsseldorf. This local coincidence is by no means accidental, because in the early 1960s neurosurgical intensive care was instituted in the Düsseldorf University Hospital in a ward specially equipped for this purpose by Hans Kuhlendahl. The controversy as to whose responsibility it is has never ended, with expert advice from both neurosurgeon and anesthesist being required.

I therefore consider it a successful development to see the specialties participating in intensive care meet in the German Interdisciplinary Association of Intensive Care and Emergency Medicine (DIVI), whose General Secretary I welcome on this occasion. All those sent by their societies to be active in this association will rapidly find out that cooperation rather than controversy is the only option. Thus, as early as 1970 the German Societies of Anesthesiology and Neurosurgery decided that neurosurgical intensive care was to be supervised by a neurosurgeon with specialist advice from an anesthesiologist. Multidisciplinary intensive care wards, however, were to be supervised by an anesthesiologist, with the neurosurgeon responsible for specific neurosurgical care. Everything depends on a high degree of cooperation of both specialties to achieve a satisfactory result for the patient.

Looking at a course of treatment in general, you will quickly see that intensive care is at one extreme and, for example, rehabilitation at the other, but all treatment modalities merge into one another, so that separatist activities on behalf of one specialty appear to me to be disadvantageous.

What, then, are the main tasks of a neurosurgical intensive care ward?

1. Postoperative care of patients following elective surgery of the brain and upper cervical cord
2. Care of patients with spontaneous intracranial hemorrhage requiring either conservative or operative treatment
3. Care of head-injured patients and those with traumatic spinal lesions
4. Emergency care of patients with other forms of impaired consciousness, e.g., those in metabolic coma requiring further investigation

Looking at patients in Düsseldorf over the last 3 years (1987–1989), postoperative cases have increased from 42.6% to 45.8% to 49.0%. The percentage of head injuries has decreased from 26.6% in 1987 and 26.3% in 1988 to 21.8% in 1989, the absolute figures being from 201 to 166. This may be due to a reduction of beds caused by the present shortage of nursing staff in all neurosurgical intensive care

[1] Neurochirurgische Klinik, Universität Düsseldorf, Moorenstr. 5. W-4000 Düsseldorf, FRG

Advances in Neurosurgery, Vol. 19
W. J. Bock, Ch. Lumenta, M. Brock, M. Klinger (Eds.)

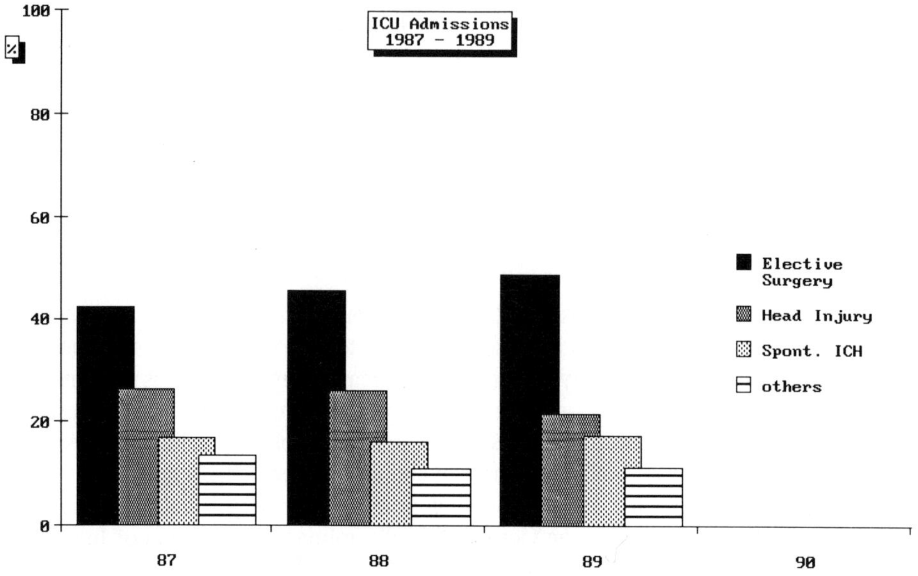

Fig. 1. Admission to the Düsseldorf neurosurgical intensive care unit from 1987 to 1989

units in Germany, one consequence of which is inadequate care of patients with severe head injuries – a situation likely to deterior further in the future. The percentage of cases of spontaneous hemorrhage has remained at 17.2%, whereas that of other conditions requiring intensive care has come down from 13.6% to 11.4%. These include extensive spinal injuries, of the cervical region in particular, but also cardiovascular and pulmonary problems requiring intensive rather than ordinary ward care. The total numbers of patients and the length of their stay in intensive care have remained stable (Fig. 1).

Postoperative or post-traumatic conditions tend to present as one of three major patterns of damage, i.e., either with loss of autonomic functions, or with neurologic damage, or with excessive activity and psychopathic syndromes. Autonomic symptoms will disappear in relation to the degree of damage. Neurologic deficits will resolve in relation to the site of the lesion. Psychopathic defects have the worst prognosis. In the acute phase there will be general autonomic abnormalities such as circulatory dysregulation, headache, fatigue, sweating, tachycardia, instability, and sleep disorders. Second only to impairment of consciousness, these patterns are the most important parameters for neurosurgical intensive care.

Neurologic deficits include dysphasia, apraxia, agnosia, and motor weakness, whereas sensory impairment matters less to the patient. In addition there are disturbances of coordination and cranial nerve palsies. Which of these symptoms predominate again depends on the site of the lesion.

Psychopathic lesions may be psychomotor in the form of a transistory syndrome, and later the organic psychosyndrome, which may be reversible. In addition, there are impairment of memory and affective changes compared to the situation before trauma or surgery. Frequently there is an impairment of critical judgement. Some of these are late sequelae which may establish themselves only after termination of therapy, i.e., after rehabilitation. If we want to keep the incidence of these late sequelae down in our patients, we have to insist that acute and, especially, intensive care must be oriented towards later rehabilitation. For this reason, in the early 1980s integration of acute care and early rehabilitation was suggested. Today we can be proud to show that these efforts have been successful, and that the persistent vegetative state has become a rarity thanks to intensive neurosurgical care and early rehabilitation beginning in the intensive care ward. It must, however, not be concealed that the results of intensive care and later rehabilitation procedures depend on age, in head injuries on the severity of trauma, on accompanying diseases, and on biological age, but above all the quality of acute care. Jennett [1–3] subdivided Glasgow results into "poor" and "good" outcome categories. "Poor" outcomes are death, the persistent vegetative state, and severe disability. "Good" outcomes are no or minor disability and moderate disability. The neurosurgeon may not withdraw from this task of early rehabilitation beginning in the intensive care unit and confine himself to operative procedures.

With the considerable expense in terms of equipment, staff, and financial resources, I have to face the question of whether measuring the efficacy of this therapy in these complex patients is at all feasible. One way is to look at mortality and to analyze this over the years with changes of management. We have analyzed our data for mortality in intensive care over the years 1982–1989 and found a reduction of almost half from 22.3% to 14.6% (Fig. 2). The slight increase in 1987 has not

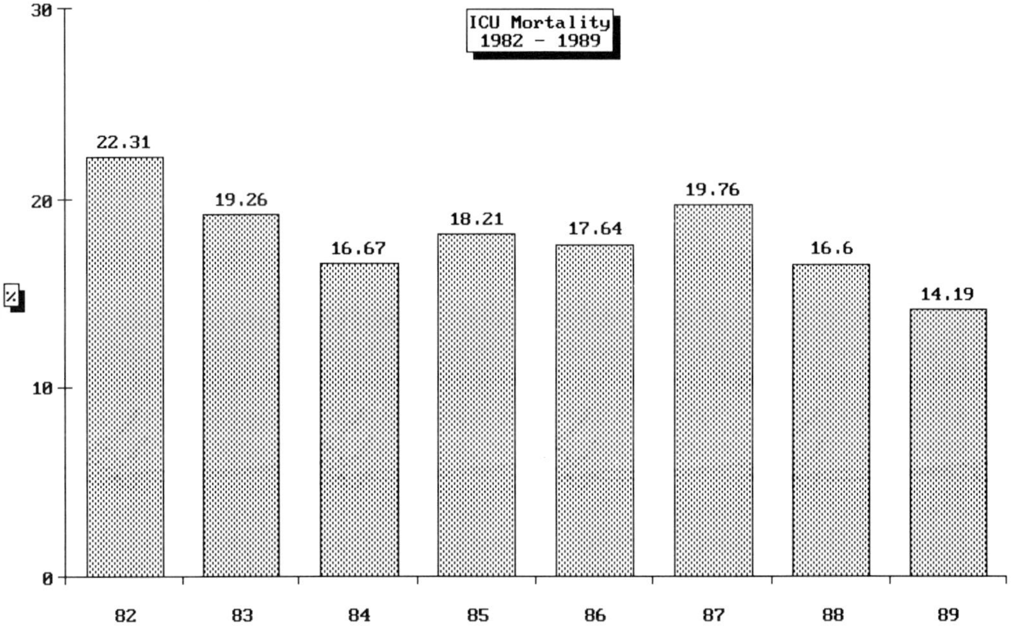

Fig. 2. Mortality in the Düsseldorf neurosurgical intensive care unit from 1982 to 1989

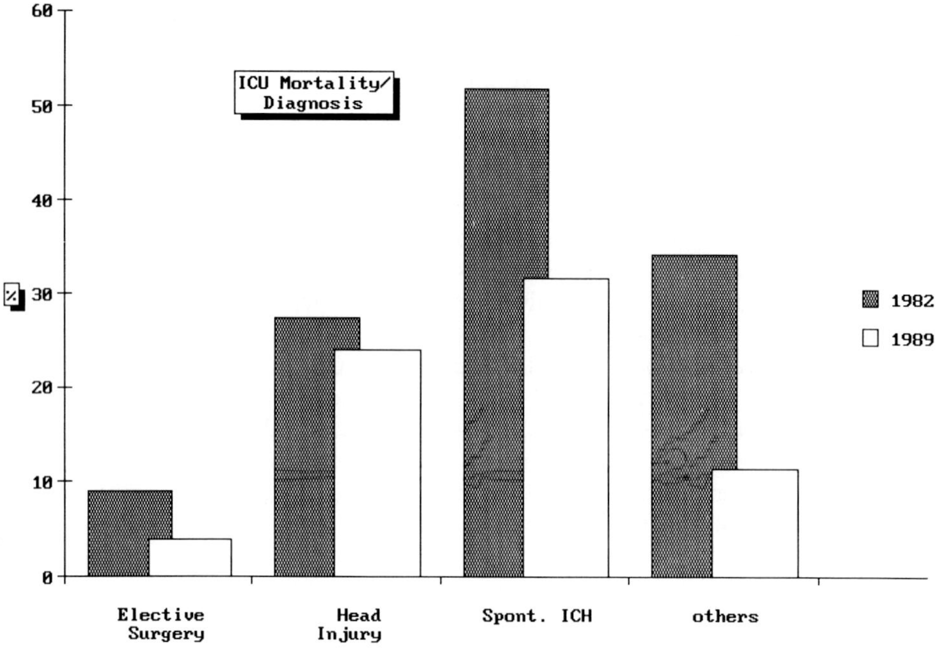

Fig. 3. Reduction in mortality in the intensive care unit according to a variety of diagnoses on admission. *Spont. ICH,* spontaneous intracranial hemorrhage

yet been analyzed and accounted for. Subdividing these figures by diagnosis, we find a reduction of mortality in all groups (Fig. 3). Thus, spontaneous intracranial hemorrhages were the major group in 1982 with a mortality of 52%; fortunately, a reduction to less than 32% has been possible in these 8 years. A similar reduction is seen elsewhere, with a drop to 4% in elective surgery, 24% head injuries, and from 34% to 11% in other conditions.

The high proportion of intracranial hematomas may be specific to Düsseldorf, because here the neurosurgical department alone is responsible for treatment, except in less severe cases which may be looked after in neurological or medical wards.

Looking at causes of death, cerebral causes outnumber extracerebral causes (Fig. 4). This plain statement is necessary because straightforward surgical complications both in the early and late periods and dysfunction of other organ systems dominate in general surgical intensive care wards. Central dysregulation due to raised intracranial pressure or postoperative hematomas are frequent causes of death in the early phase. Safe treatment requires special monitoring, which belongs to neurosurgery. In addition to clinical monitoring, this includes computed tomography, EEG, monitoring of evoked potentials, and intracranial pressure (ICP) monitoring, and also ICP therapy and neurosurgical operative procedures.

I should like to dwell for a moment on some necessities of treatment with organizational consequences. The majority of patients in neurosurgical intensive care

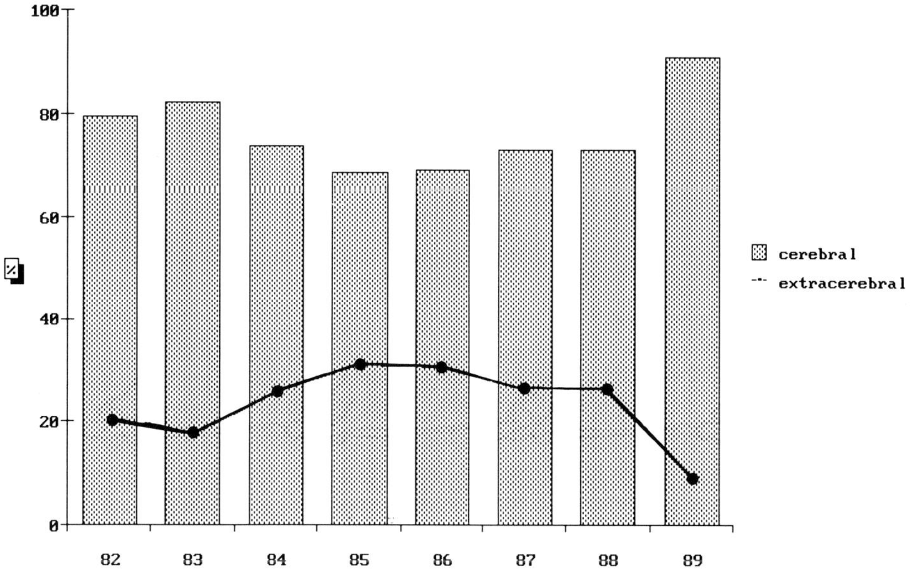

Fig. 4. Causes of death on the Düsseldorf neurosurgical intensive care unit from 1982 to 1989

units are emergency admissions, in Düsseldorf they constitute 48.6%. Most of these patients are admitted outside of normal working hours. To safeguard admission of these patients into the intensive care unit – running at almost 100% capacity in Düsseldorf – other patients have to be prematurely transferred to the general wards or to intensive care units in other hospitals. The decision for transferral under these circumstances can only be made by the neurosurgeon as the doctor in charge. He or she is the only person to decide which patients may safely be transferred and to recommend further treatment. This again illustrates that a neurosurgeon is required to be the doctor in charge of such patients. These emergency admissions into intensive care therefore have far-reaching consequences for the organization of the whole department, theatre, radiology, and also the ordinary neurosurgical wards.

To conclude: neurosurgical treatment is impossible without competent neurosurgical intensive care, i.e., specialist diagnostic and therapeutic advice by the neurosurgeon in critical care. In addition, neurosurgical intensive care is only a part of the overall treatment. For this reason, instruction in neurosurgical intensive care within the context of specialist training is necessary, as laid down in the specialist training scheme.

References

1. Jennett (1972) Lancet i:734–737
2. Jennett (1975) Lancet i:480
3. Jennett (1978) NY Acad Sci 35:293–306

Prognostic Value of Motor Evoked Potentials in Traumatic and Nontraumatic Coma

V. Rohde and J. Zentner[1]

Introduction

With the recently introduced method of transcranial electrical and magnetoelectric stimulation of the motor cortex and recording of the electromyographic (EMG) response (motor evoked potential, MEP), noninvasive assessment of the descending pathways has become possible for the first time [1, 4]. Up to the present, however, no data have been available on the prognostic value of MEP in patients in severe traumatic or nontraumatic coma. Therefore, in this study MEP were elicited by electrical and magnetoelectric stimulation in 201 comatose patients. Our aim was to test the prognostic value of MEP and to compare the recordings obtained by electrical and by magnetoelectric stimulations.

Patients and Methods

A total of 201 patients (131 male, 70 female) aged between 3 and 89 years (average age 32 years) were studied. All patients were comatose with a Glasgow Coma Score ranging between 3 and 8 [5]. They were intubated and artificially respirated. Most were receiving midazolam and fentanyl. In 132 patients coma had been caused by a severe head injury and in 69 by either subarachnoid or intracerebral hemorrhage or by cerebral ischemia and hypoxia. MEP were elicited by electrical stimulation in all patients, and in 26 additionally by magnetoelectric excitation of the motor cortex. Stimulation of the lower cervical spine was performed in every case using the electrical technique. MEP recordings were performed on the 1st–3rd day of coma. In 34 patients serial recordings were done at 2- to 5-day intervals, but for prediction of outcome only the results of the first examination, between day 1 and day 3 after onset of coma, were used. The outcome was evaluated according to the Glasgow Outcome Scale [3], in which a score of 1 means good recovery and a score of 5 death. Observation time ranged from 2 months to 4 years.

Transcranial electrical stimulation of the motor cortex was performed with constant-voltage condenser discharges using a Digitimer D 180, which delivers a maximum output of 750 V with a time constant of 100 μs. In each patient stimulation of both the motor cortex (transcranially; anode over the motor hand area, cathode

---

[1] Neurochirurgische Klinik, Universität Tübingen, Hoppe-Seyler-Str. 3, W-7400 Tübingen, FRG

Advances in Neurosurgery, Vol. 19
W. J. Bock, Ch. Lumenta, M. Brock, M. Klinger (Eds.)

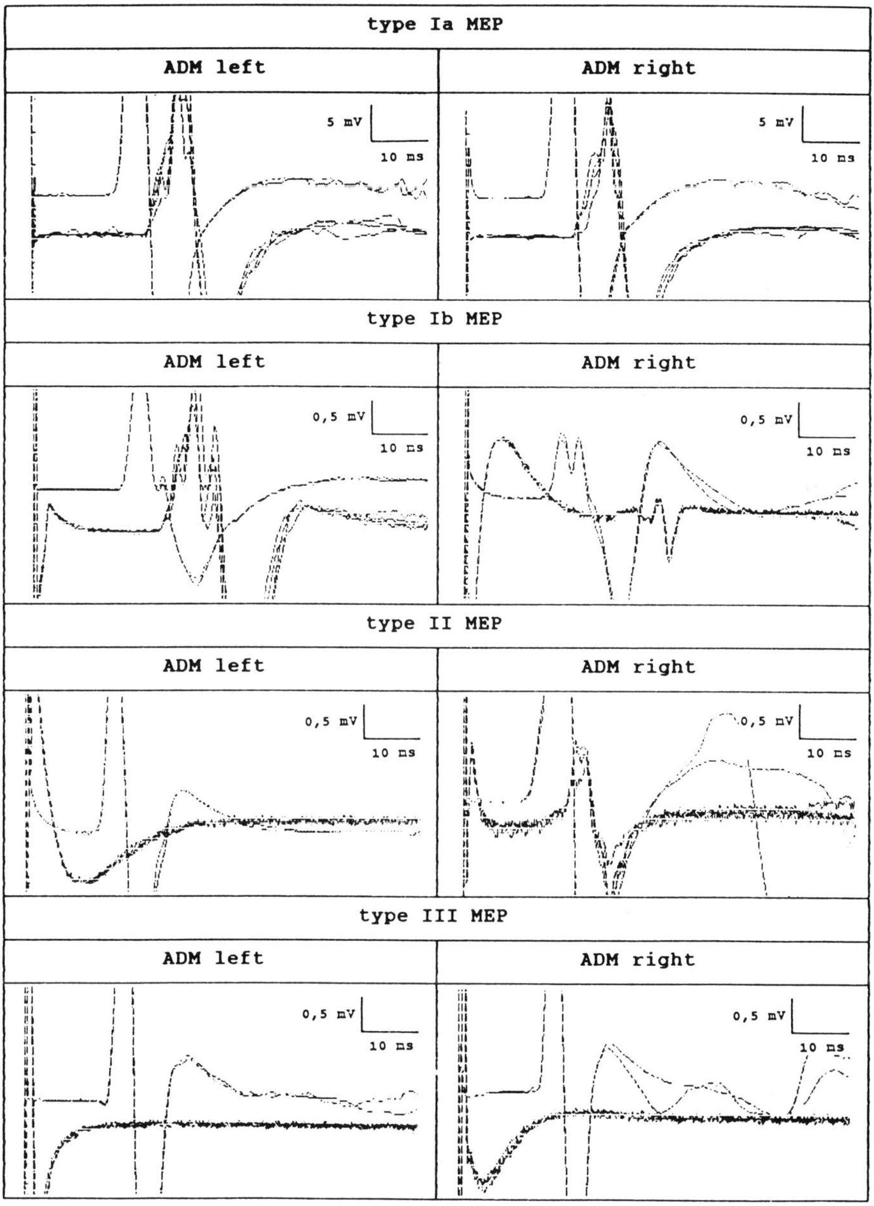

Fig. 1. MEP patterns (two recordings superimposed). Type Ia: bilaterally preserved EMG response following cortical and lower cervical stimulation. Type Ib: bilaterally preserved response following cortical and cervical stimulation; CμCT > 6 ms at least one side. Type II: unilateral loss of EMG response following cortical stimulation; bilaterally preserved response following lower cervical stimulation. Type III: bilateral loss of EMG response following cortical stimulation, bilaterally preserved response following lower cervical stimulation. *ADM*, abductor digiti minimi

over the vertex) and subsequently the lower cervical spine (cathode over the intervertebral space C6-7 and anode 6 cm from the midline homolateral to the recording side) was performed using ECG electrodes 1 cm in diameter.

Transcranial magnetoelectric stimulation was performed using a Magstim 200 (Novametrix, 1.5 T). The stimulation coil was placed over the vertex with the center at C_z. For recordings from the right side the direction of current was clockwise and for recordings from the left side it was counterclockwise.

MEP were recorded from the contralateral hypothenar muscle using EMG electrodes (abdomen/tendon fashion). Stimulus strength was gradually increased until a clear EMG response was obtained or absence of any response even at maximum stimulus strength was documented. The time base was 100 μs with a gain ranging from 100 μV per division. Filter settings were restricted to 20 Hz (low) and 3 Hz (high). Central motor conduction time (CMCT) was calculated by subtracting the latency of the hypothenar potential obtained by lower cervical stimulation from that obtained by transcranial stimulation. We decided upon acceptable limits for CMCT of 5.3 ± 0.6 ms following electrical stimulation (our own normative data) and 9.4 ± 1.0 ms in response to magnetoelectric stimulation [2]. Depending on the presence or absence of EMG responses and CMCT, potential findings were categorized into four types (Fig. 1).

Results

An EMG response from the hypothenar muscle following electrical stimulation of the lower cervical spine was obtained in all patients. Depending on the transcranial stimulation technique used (electrical vs. magnetoelectric), our findings were as described below.

Electrical Stimulation

Fourteen of 48 patients (29.2%) with type Ia and 11 of 87 patients (12.6%) of type Ib patterns died. The remainder survived with Glasgow Outcome Scores ranging from 1 to 4. Of the 31 patients with type II, only 9 (29%) had outcome scores from 1 to 3, while the others either survived in a vegetative state (25.8%) or died (45.2%). All patients with type III patterns died (Fig. 2). Figure 3 shows the MEP findings in 2 patients.

Magnetoelectric Stimulation

There were approximately equal numbers of favorable and unfavorable outcomes in patients with type Ia patterns. Four of 5 patients (80%) with type Ib survived with outcome scores of 2 or 3, and 1 patient (20%) died. One patient (20%) with a type II pattern survived with an outcome score of 2, while 3 (60%) remained in a

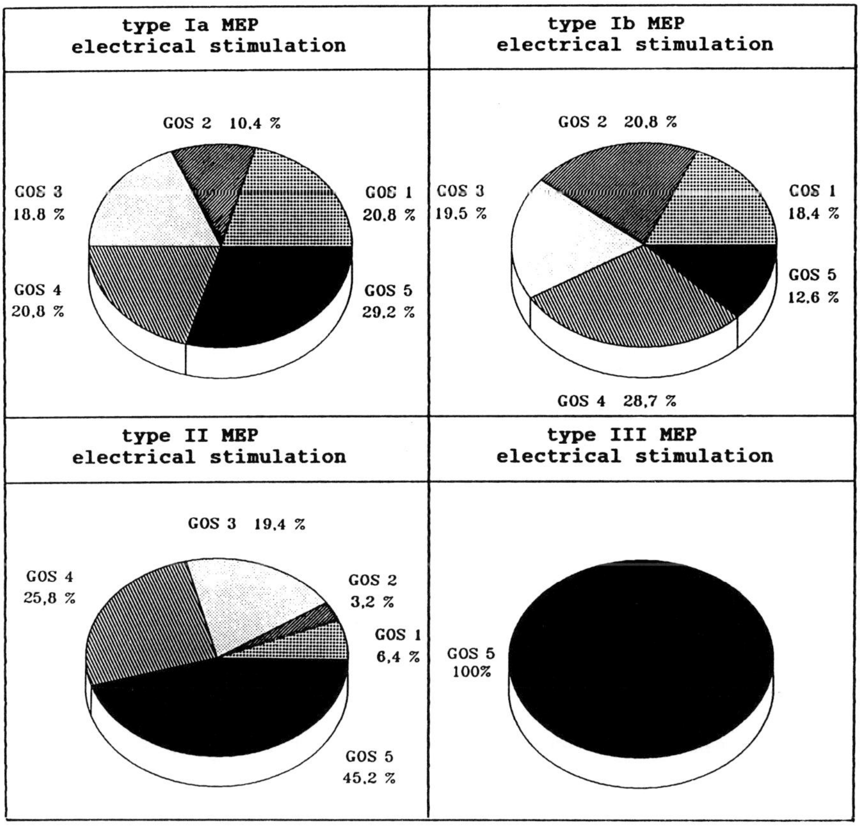

Fig. 2. MEP findings in response to electrical excitation of the motor cortex and Glasgow Outcome Score. Results for 201 patients are shown

vegetative state, and 1 (20%) died. Seven of the 11 (63.6%) type III patients died, 3 (27.3%) survived in a vegetative state, and 1 (9.1%) survived with an outcome score of 2 (Fig. 4).

Discussion

The aim of the present study was to assess the prognostic value of MEP in comatose patients by comparing the results of electrical and magnetoelectric stimulation. Our results clearly indicate that bilateral presence of both electrically and magnetoelectrically evoked potentials with a normal (type Ia) or prolonged (type Ib) CMCT has no prognostic value, since approximately as many patients with these patterns had a favorable outcome as an unfavorable one. Although the majority of patients with unilaterally absent responses (type II) had an unfavorable outcome, there were

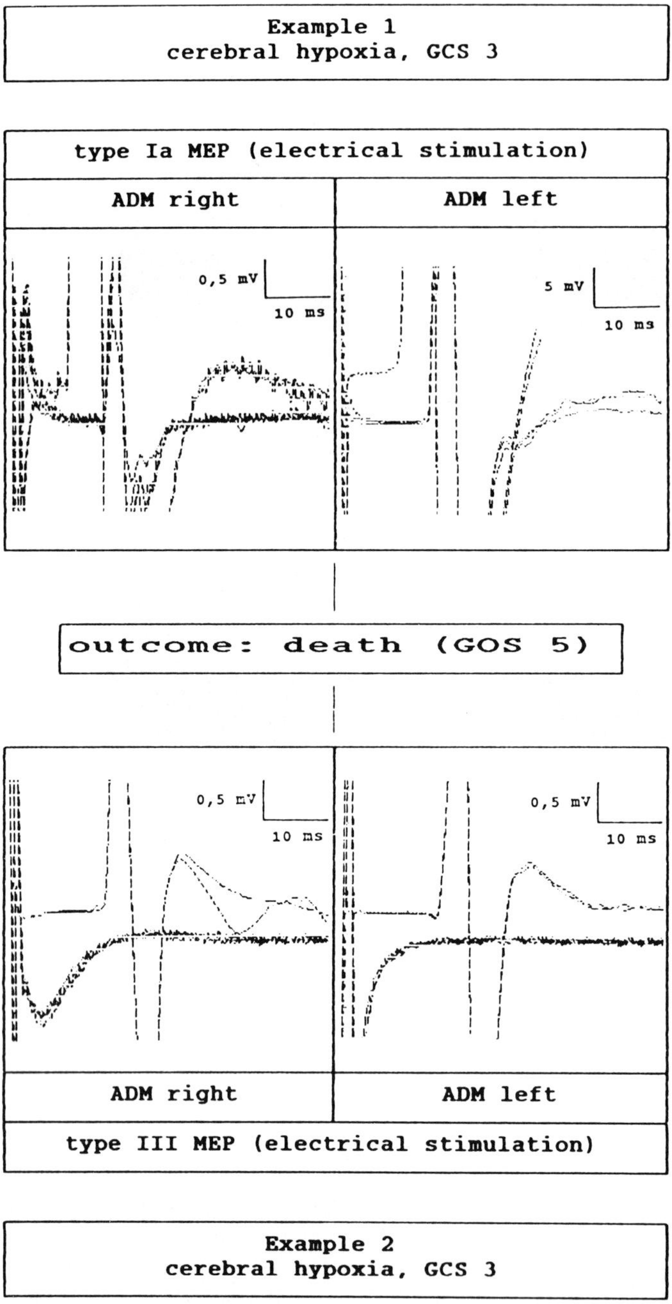

Fig. 3. MEP findings in response to electrical stimulation in two patients, and outcome. One patient had normal MEP (type Ia), the other bilaterally absent responses (type III). Both died. *GCS*, Glasgow coma score; *GOS*, Glasgow Outcome Score; *ADM*, abductor digiti minimi

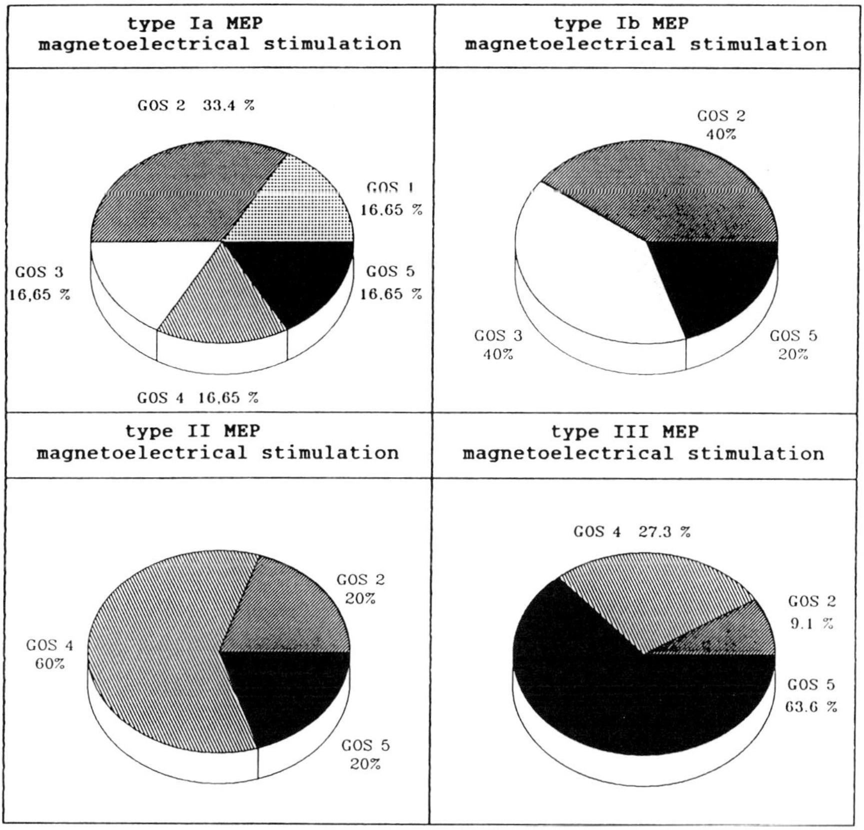

Fig. 4. MEP types obtained in response to magnetoelectrical stimulation of the motor cortex and Glasgow Outcome Score. Results for 26 patients are shown

several who survived in good condition. Only an absence of MEP (type III) following electrical stimulation had high prognostic value, as all patients with this pattern type died. However, the same is not true for magnetoelectric stimulation, since here some patients with no responses survived. Thus, there is no type of magnetoelectrically elicited MEP that can be used as a basis for definite prognostic conclusions.

In our opinion, the varying prognostic value of electrically and magnetoelectrically evoked potentials in regard to absence of responses is the result of the different action sites of the two stimulation techniques and the relatively weak impulse delivered by the 1.5-T machine as used for magnetoelectric stimulation.

To conclude, examination of descending pathways by magnetoelectric stimulation of the motor cortex cannot be recommended for prognostic evaluation of comatose patients. In regard to the electrical technique, absence of responses undoubtedly indicates an unfavorable outcome.

References

1. Barker AT, Jalinous R, Freeston IL (1985) Non-invasive magnetic stimulation of the human motor cortex. Lancet 1:1106–1107
2. Barker AT, Fresston IL, Jalinous R, Jarrett A (1986) Clinical evaluation of conduction time measurements in central motor pathways using magnetic stimulation of the human brain. Lancet 1:1325–1326
3. Jennett B, Bond M (1975) Assessment of outcome after severe brain damage: a practical scale. Lancet:480–484
4. Merton PA, Morton HB (1980) Stimulation of the cerebral cortex in the intact human subject. Nature 285:227
5. Teasdale G, Jennett B (1974) Assessment of coma and impaired consciousness. A practical scale. Lancet 2:81–84

The Temporal Structure of Information Processing in Patients Following Diffuse Head Injuries: Electrophysiological Studies

B.M. Reuter, D.B. Linke, and M. Kurthen[1]

Introduction

After cerebral trauma patients often suffer fundamental disturbances in selective attention. Consequently, other cognitive processes such as memory, language, learning etc. may be impaired as well. What fundamental physiological dysfunctions are responsible for these disturbances? There are many indications that disorganization of the temporal progression of the physiological processing plays an important part. The following disturbances seen in patients suffering head injuries support this theory: disturbed estimation of time, slowing of the flicker fusion threshold, decreased performance in the Tapping test, impaired order threshold, and slowed reaction times [3]. A cerebral rhythmic timer appears to be disturbed.

Is there an electrophysiological correlate to these cyclic processes of information processing? Since the beginning of scientific study of the EEG, the EEG oscillations have been suspected of representing a rhythm of excitability (or a scanning mechanism), describing alternating facilitation and inhibition of the afferent and efferent impulses. In a study published in 1987, Reuter and Linke [4] were able to show that the EEG α rhythm cannot be regarded as a rhythm of excitability for cognitive processes. The present study therefore deals with the EEG oscillations of the 40-Hz range. Focused arousal in man and higher mammals is especially associated with the occurrence of this particular frequency. During problem solving, depending on the nature of the task, the 40-Hz rhythm may also be lateralized [6, 7]. The 40-Hz rhythm appears in the EEG surface recordings at a low altitude, approximately 10 times smaller than the standard EEG. With deep recordings the rhythm can be demonstrated as prominent frequency of the power spectrum [2, 5].

Three questions were to be answered by this study. First, is the 40-Hz rhythm a rhythm of excitability for cognitive processes? That is, does the running 40-Hz EEG exhibit phases of greater and lesser excitability? Basar et al. [1], for example, states that excitability is greatest during the negative 40-Hz phase. It remains to be shown whether this in turn affects the latency of the endogenous components of the event-related potentials.

Second, is the excitability of the 40-Hz rhythm disturbed in patients with head injuries? Also, does the pathophysiology of the disturbed rhythm of excitability allow us to draw any conclusions about the temporal organization of the healthy brain? And third, is the 40-Hz rhythm, whose significance for cognitive processes

---

[1] Neurochirurgische Universitätsklinik, Sigmund-Freud-Str. 25, W-5300 Bonn 1, FRG

Advances in Neurosurgery, Vol. 19
W. J. Bock, Ch. Lumenta, M. Brock, M. Klinger (Eds.)

has been demonstrated, in any other way disturbed in patients with cerebral impairment?

Methods

Twelve right-handed controls and six right-handed patients with a history of diffuse head injury were studied using a classical event-related potential (ERP) selective attention paradigm.

Significant neurological deficits were no longer present. Patients showed no aphasia or other noticeable grave neuropsychological disturbances, but did suffer from impairment of attentiveness. The battery of neuropsychological tests used for more detailed examination included the Wechsler Adult Intelligence Scale (WAIS), the Benton test and Brickenkamp's attentiveness stress test D2.

The "omitted click" method was employed to evoke P300. Click sounds were given at constant intervals of 1.3 s. Participants were asked to silently count the random omissions in the sequence. Besides EEG recording, EOG and EMG of the chin and neck muscles were collected as control data.

The entire session was stored on FM or PCM tapes in order that the 40-Hz phase at the beginning of stimuli could be determined retrospectively. For this purpose, the EEG obtained during stimulation was filtered digitally, without artificial shiftings of phase, in the range of the 32- to 48-Hz band. The results were then examined by computer for the phase at the beginning of the stimulus. In other words, responses to single stimuli were selected which exhibited a specific 40-Hz phase at the beginning of stimulus: positive maximum, negative maximum, positive slope, and negative slope. Subsequently, the original event-related potentials were averaged for each phase category.

Using digital filtering, the responses to the frequent clicks, the information processing-associated peaks N100 and P200 of the ERP, could be analyzed in regard to their latency.

Results

The effects of the four selected phase conditions on the latency of the event-related potentials were small. When the ERPs from the different phase conditions were superimposed, intraindividual deviations in the latency of N100 and P200 of controls were found to be not greater than 8 ms. The grand average of the 12 controls showed deviations in latency of only approximately 5 ms. A relationship between the individual 40-Hz phases and the components of the ERPs could therefore not be demonstrated in test subjects without cerebral trauma. In patients with a history of diffuse head injury, superposition within the grand average also revealed no significant systematic deviations in relation to the 40-Hz phase. However, measurement of the absolute amplitude of the running 40-Hz EEG revealed a significant reduc-

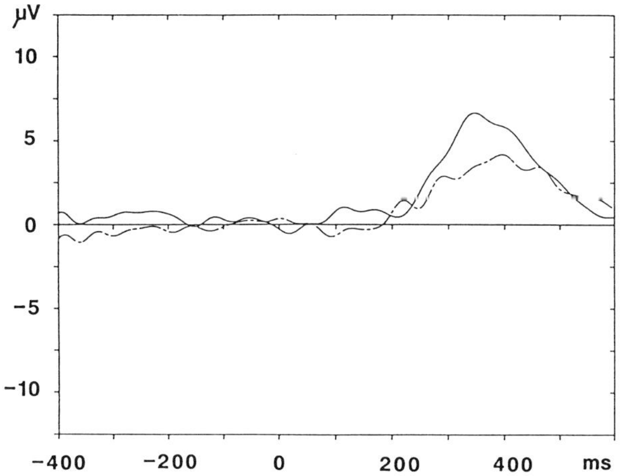

Fig. 1. Grand average of the P300 wave ("omitted click paradigm"). Patients who had suffered head trauma (*broken line*) showed a clear delay in the latency of P300 as compared with the control subjects (*solid line*)

tion in amplitude to an average ov 1.45 µV. The comparable value of the healthy controls was 4.3 µV (U test, $p < 0.05$).

Other ranges of frequency, such as the θ and δ rhythm, deviated slightly but not significantly from the control group.

Finally, in patients with a history of diffuse head injury, a significant deviation of 42 ms was found for the latency of P300 in the grand average (U test, $p < 0.05$, Fig. 1). No specific neuropsychological signs were demonstrable with the WAIS following the criteria of Wechsler. However, five of the six patients showed significant decreases in performance in the Brickenkamp's D2 attentiveness stress test following periods of stress and attentiveness. This may be related to the similarly significantly low amplitude of the 40-Hz EEG.

Discussion

A rhythm of excitability associated with the phases of the 40-Hz EEG could not be determined. Yet, rhythmical events appear to be necessary and possibly have a functional significance in the nervous system. Evidence for a correlation between focused cognitive arousal and coherent 40-Hz EEG activity can be found. Disturbances of attentiveness manifest themselves in a reduction of the central rhythms. The factor "time required for processing" appears to play an important role, as is also indicated by the delay of latency of P300 in patients. Our studies suggest that the computer-analyzed EEG scan serve as a simple diagnostic instrument for the demonstration of disturbances of attentiveness in patients following head injury.

References

1. Basar E, Rosen B, Basar-Eroglu C, Greitschus F (1987) The associations between 40 Hz-EEG and the middle latency response of the auditory evoked potential. Int J Neurosci 33:103–117
2. Bressler SL, Freeman WJ (1980) Frequency analysis of olfactory systems EEG in cat, rabbit, and rat. Electroencephalogy Clin Neurophysiol 50:19–24
3. Grüssler OJ (1983) Zeit und Gehirn. Zeitliche Aspekte der Signalverarbeitung in den Sinnesorganen und im Zentralnervensystem. In: Peisl A, Mohler A (eds) Die Zeit. Oldenbourg, Munich, pp 79–132
4. Reuter BM, Linke DB (1987) Stehen kognitive Prozesse in Beziehung zur EEG-Alpha-Phase? Eine experimentelle Studie zu P300.Z EEG EMG 18:58–60
5. Sheer DE (1984) Focused arousal, 40 Hz EEG, and dysfunction. In. Elbert T, Rockstroh B, Lutzenberger W, Birbaumer N (eds) Self-regulation and behavior. Springer, Berlin Heidelberg New York, pp 64–84
6. Spydell JD, Sheer DE (1982) Effect of problem solving on right and left hemisphere 40 Hertz EEG activity. Psychophysiology 19:420–4425
7. Spydell JD, Ford MR, Sheer DE (1979) Task dependent cerebral lateralisation of the 40 Hertz EEG Rhythm. Psychophysiology 16:347–350

TCD, SEPs and ICP: Comparative Analysis in Severe Head Injury

M. Lorenz, G. Dorfmüller, W.-P. Sollmann, and M.R. Gaab[1]

Introduction

Several methods are available for the assessment of brain damage and for planning of therapeutic strategy after severe head trauma:

- Clinical examination, which is of limited value in deeply sedated patients
- Anatomical imaging (computerized tomography), in which there sometimes discrepancies between images and clinical status, and which is only possible at intervals
- Monitoring of physiological parameters: EEG and somatosensory evoked potentials (SEP), transcranial Doppler sonography (TCD) to monitor blood flow, and continuous recording of intracranial pressure (ICP)

SEP, TCD, and ICP are influenced by several factors which can be therapeutically varied to a greater or lesser extent (morphological damage, elastance and resistance, systemic blood pressures, PO_2, PCO_2, hematocrit, drug interactions, etc.).

Patients and Methods

Eighty-four patients with a Glasgow Coma Scale (GCS) score of less than 9 were examined (brain death investigations excluded). Continuous ICP monitoring was carried out in 46. In 22, simultaneous registration of SEP, TCD, and ICP was performed. SEPs were recorded after median or ulnar nerve stimulation contralaterally over $C_{3,4}/F_z$ and above the neck (Nicolet CA1000 or Biologic Traveller). The central conduction time (CCT) and ratio of amplitudes from cortical and cervical responses were calculated [3]. In TCD, the pulsatile index and systolic, diastolic, and mean flow in both middle cerebral arteries were registered (EME/3D Transcranial Doppler Scanner, TCD 2-64B). In ICP monitoring, we used the Gaeltec system with epidurally applied sensors.

[1] Neurochirurgische Klinik, Medizinische Hochschule Hannover, Konstanty-Gutschow-Str. 8, W-3000 Hannover 61, FRG

Advances in Neurosurgery, Vol. 19
W. J. Bock, Ch. Lumenta, M. Brock, M. Klinger (Eds.)

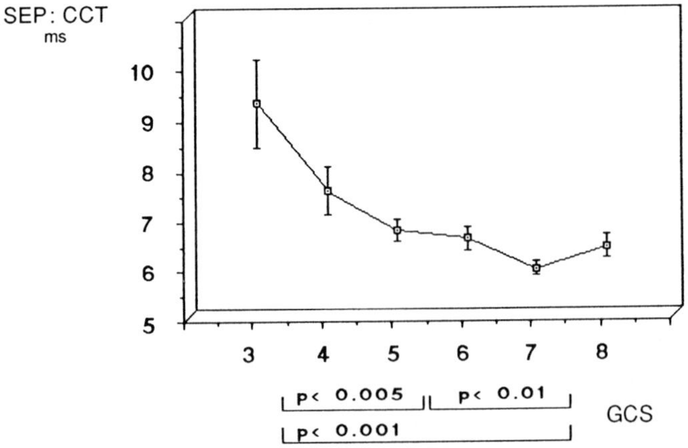

Fig. 1. SEP:CCT in relation to Glasgow Coma Scale score (GCS): CCT longer with lower GCS score

Results

Somatosensory Evoked Potentials

There was a significant correlation between CCT or amplitude ratio and coma grade. CCT increased as clinical condition deteriorated ($p < 0.001$; Fig. 1).

In patients fulfilling our inclusion criteria (GCS < 9), there was a higher incidence of poor outcome 6 months after injury: Glasgow Outcome Scale (GOS) score I: 7 patients, II: 23, III: 21, IV: 2, and V: 28 (follow up too short: 3 patients).

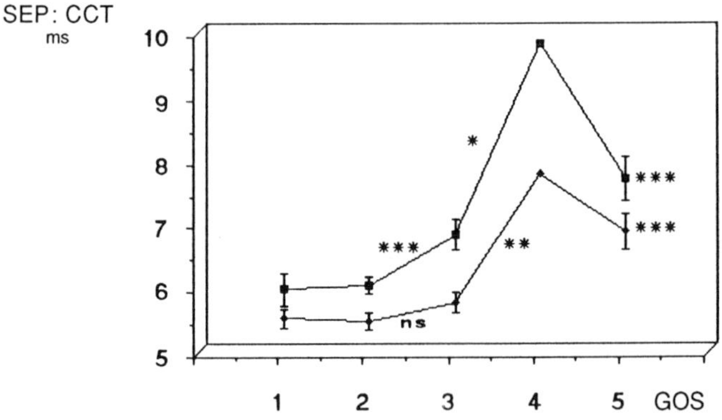

Fig. 2. SEP: mean CCT (± SEM) of the more (*upper trace*) and less (*lower trace*) affected hemisphere in relation to Glasgow Outcome Scale score; significant increase in CCT with worsening of outcome

A GOS scored I was only awarded for a patient working at his former job 6 months after trauma. SEPs predicted outcome reliably. CCT and amplitude ratio were in high correlation to outcome comparing the outcome groups I and II to IV and V. Patients of outcome group III also had a significant increase of the CCT of the more affected hemisphere compared to those of outcome groups I and II (Fig. 2). A striking difference between the SEP signals of both sides was a predictor of the development of hemisymptomatic disorders afterwards. Only two patients who showed bilateral electrical cortical silence survived, one in a vegetative state, the other severely disabled.

Transcranial Doppler Sonography

There seemed to be no interrelation between GCS score and blood-flow velocity or wave form of the TCD signal. The interrelation between flow-velocity and PCO_2, however, is well known and can lead to difficulties in signal interpretation in comatose and ventilated patients. In one case, a drop in PCO_2 from 32.6 to 25.5 mmHg only led to a decrease in ICP from 19 to 9 mmHg, but caused a reduction of systolic/diastolic flow velocity from 242/95 cm/s to 132/60 cm/s.

We had no evidence of a statistically clear correlation between TCD signals and outcome. However, those patients in whom a high systolic/diastolic flow velocity ratio coincided with elevated ICP had a poorer outcome. On the other hand, many patients with raised ICP did not have a greatly increased pulsatile index or systolic/diastolic flow ratio.

Intracranial Pressure

The ICP monitoring revealed ICP to be in highly significant correlation to coma grade and outcome.

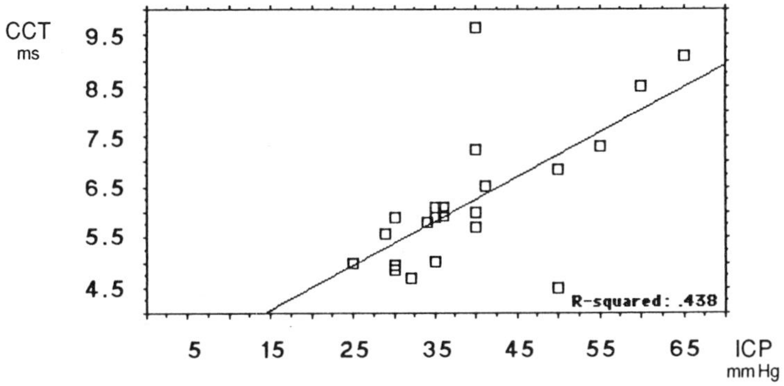

Fig. 3. SEP:CCT in relation to actual ICP: CCT increases with ICP in high pressure coma ($p < 0.05$). Patients without cortical response not included

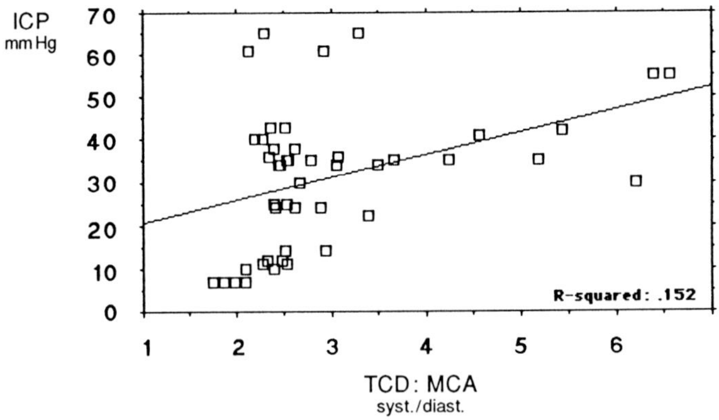

Fig. 4. TCD:ratio of systolic and diastolic flow velocity in the middle cerebral artery in relation to ICP

In low pressure coma there was no correlation between SEPs and pressure level. In the range above 25 mmHg, however, there was a clear trend for the CCT to lengthen as ICP rose ($r = 0.438$; $p < 0.05$; Fig. 3). However, we examined one patient who evinced no changes in CCT or amplitude with an ICP ranging from 60 to 22 mmHg during mannitol treatment of a pressure wave. Obviously this patient tolerated the elevated ICP well and showed no systemic pressure response.

Several single TCD recordings from different patients indicated that there was a trend towards increased systolic and decreased diastolic flow velocity as ICP rose. The pulsatile index and ratio of systolic/diastolic flow velocity showed variable correlation with higher levels of ICP (Fig. 4). These trends became more evident in multiple recordings from single patients at different levels of ICP.

Conclusion

In the examination of patients following severe head injury, deleterious signs can rarely be seen and are commonly indicators for developing brain death: complete disappearance of the primary cortical response in SEPs [6, 10], reverberating intracranial blood flow in TCD [4, 9], and, in ICP monitoring, an alignment of intracranial and systemic pressure during transtentorial herniation. Where the clinical course is less complicated, changes are incomplete, and if further deterioration sets in, efforts have to be made to prevent further substantial brain damage. Thresholds for normal values therefore need to be defined in order to help the physician in his assessment of the patient's clinical condition and progress.

SEPs have been shown to correlate well with coma grade and outcome and can be recorded even in deeply sedated patients [6, 10]. If the CCT is within the normal range or shows rapid normalization of slightly elevated values, a good recovery can be expected. However, if CCT remains increased, a poorer outcome is rather likely. Bilateral electrical silence is usually a sign of a bad prognosis and is in most cases

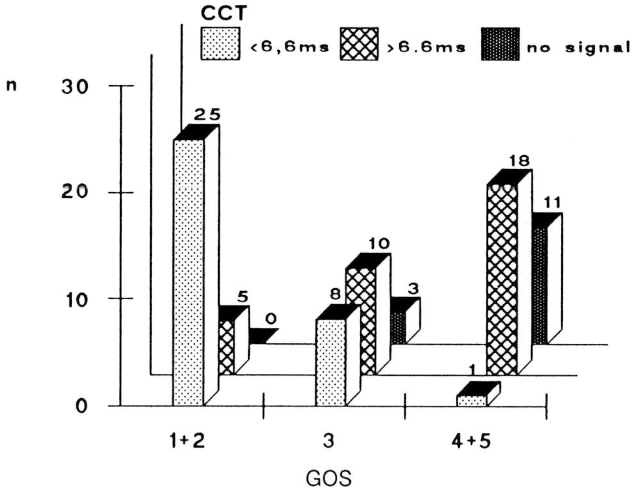

Fig. 5. SEP: Relation between outcome (GOS) and CCT of the more affected hemisphere

a predictor of death [10] (Fig. 5). There seems to be a relationship between a drop in cerebral perfusion pressure/cerebral blood flow and CCT [2, 5]. However, we found no correlation between SEPs and TCD.

The importance of TCD in severe head injuries remains to be defined. Since brain perfusion mainly takes place in the diastole, a marked decrease in flow velocity accompanied by an increase of the pulsatile index and a deformation of flow profile may indicate reduced cerebral blood flow and support the indication for ICP monitoring [7, 8, 11]. Major differences between the two hemispheres are sometimes recorded and suggest a significant metabolic influence. The PCO_2 should be kept constant between two recordings [8, 9].

The value of ICP monitoring in high-pressure coma is well accepted and needs no further comment [1]. In low-pressure coma, however, ICP supplies no information about the extent of brain damage. In these cases, SEPs correlate better with the functionality of the injured brain [6]. No reliable mathematical conclusion could be obtained from SEPs or TCD recordings to assess actual ICP; they cannot replace ICP monitoring.

References

1. Gaab MR, Heissler HE (1988) Monitoring intracranial pressure. Wiley, New York, pp 1961–1983 (Encyclopedia of medical devices and instrumentation, vol 3)
2. Handa Y, Hayashi M, Hirose S, Shirasaki N, Kobayashi H, Kawano H (1989) Changes of evoked potentials during pressure waves. In: Hoff JT, Betz AL (eds) Intracranial pressure VII, Springer, Berlin Heidelberg New York, pp 238–240
3. Hume AL, Cant BR (1978) Conduction time in central somatosensory pathways in man. Electroencephalogr Clin Neurophysiol 45:361–375

4. Kirkham FJ, Levin SD, Padayachee TS, Kyme MC, Neville BRG, Gosling RG (1987) Transcranial pulsed Doppler ultrasound findings in brain stem death. J Neurol Neurosurg Psychiatry 50:1504–1513
5. Koehler RC, Backofen JE, McPherson RW, Rogers MC, Traystman RJ (1986) Relationship of regional cerebral blood flow, evoked potential responses, and systemic hemodynamics during intracranial hypertension. In: Miller JD, Teasdale GM, Rowan JO, Galbraith SL, Mendelow AD (eds) Intracranial pressure IV. Springer, Berlin Heidelberg New York, pp 365–368
6. Lorenz M, Gaab MR Sollmann WP (1989) Somatosensory evoked potentials: diagnostic and prognostic value in head injuries. Adv Neurosurg 17:97–101
7. Lundar T, Lindegaard KF, Nornes H (1990) Continuous recording of middle cerebral arterial blood velocity in clinical neurosurgery. Acta Neurochir (Wien) 102:85–90
8. Nakatani S, Ozaki K, Hara K, Mogami H (1989) Simultaneous monitoring of ICP and transcranial Doppler sonogram on the middle cerebral artery. In: Hoff JT, Betz AL (eds) Intracranial pressure III. Springer, Berlin Heidelberg New York, pp 113–115
9. Ringelstein EB (1986) Transcranial Doppler monitoring. In: Aaslid R (ed) Transcranial Doppler sonography. Springer, Berlin Heidelberg New York, pp 147–163
10. Rumpl E, Prugger M. Gerstenbrand F, Hackl JM, Pallua A (1983) Central somatosensory conduction time and short latency somatosensory evoked potentials in post-traumatic coma. Electroencephalogr Clin Neurophysiol 56:583–596
11. Saunders FW, Cledgett P (1988) Intracranial blood velocity in head injury. A transcranial ultrasound Doppler study. Surg Neurol 29:401–409

Parenteral Nutrition in Patients with Spontaneous Intracranial Hemorrhages

J. Piek and W.J. Bock[1]

Introduction

The optimum food intake for neurosurgical patients has been a matter of controversy for the last 20 years. Nevertheless, since 1975 [10] it has been beyond doubt that the energy requirements of most neurosurgical patients rarely exceed 3000 kcal/day and are comparable to those of other patients under intensive care. However, in most studies in which indirect calorimetry was used to determine the energy consumption of neurosurgical patients, only patients with head injuries were studied, or indirect calorimetry was performed only for a short period of time. The aim of the present study was (a) to determine the energy requirements of patients with spontaneous intracranial hemorrhages by indirect calorimetry and (b) to use the values obtained as a basis for parenteral nutrition in such patients.

Patients and Methods

Indirect calorimetry was performed in 11 patients (group A) with spontaneous intracranial hemorrhages (7 men, 4 women; age 51 ± 13.4 years; coma score 3–6 points on the Glasgow Coma Scale [8]) during the first 5 days after their admission to the intensive care unit. In each patient a daily cycle of 8 h of indirect calorimetry was performed, using the MMC Horizon Metabolic Computer (Beckmann Instruments Inc., 1630 South State College Boulevard, Anaheim, California 92806, USA). Inspired and expired gas concentrations were measured via sample adapters in the inspiratory and expiratory limb of the ventilator circuit. Before each measuring period O_2 calibration was performed and possible leaks ruled out by an artificial test lung. This calorimetric system has been validated by comparison with gases and volumes of known composition [3, 9].

The effects of parenteral nutrition were studied in eight additional patients (group B) with either isolated ventricular hemorrhages ($n = 6$) or hemorrhages of the basal ganglia ($n = 2$). These patients had a median score of 5 points on the Glasgow Coma Scale.

The regimen for parenteral nutrition is shown in Fig. 1. It is to be noted that: only water and electrolytes were given on the 1st day; carbohydrates were given as

[1] Neurochirurgische Klinik, Medizinische Einrichtungen der Heinrich-Heine-Universität Düsseldorf, Moorenstr. 5, W-4000 Düsseldorf, FRG

Advances in Neurosurgery, Vol. 19
W. J. Bock, Ch. Lumenta, M. Brock, M. Klinger (Eds.)

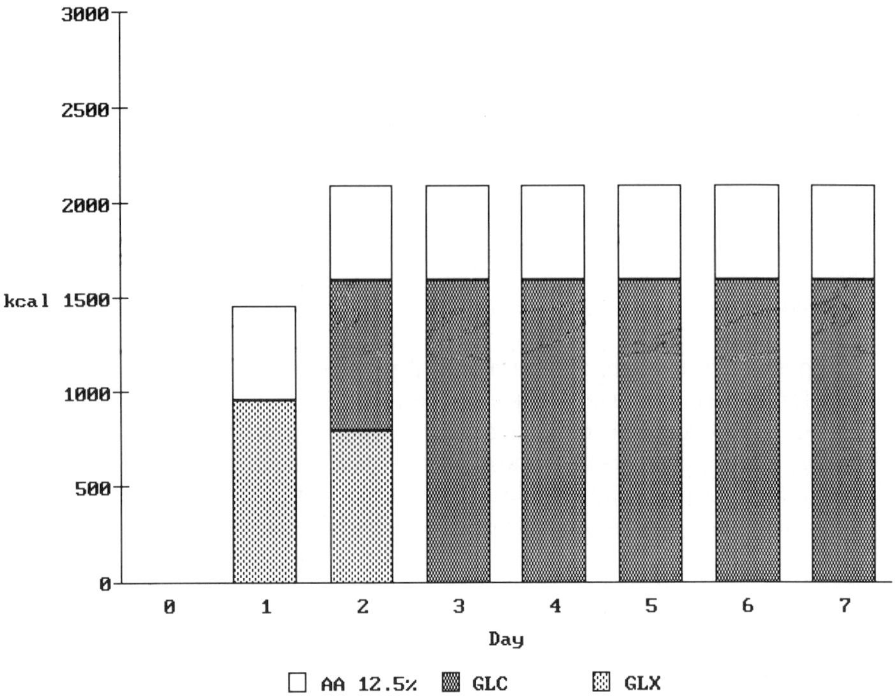

Fig. 1. Nutritional regimen in the study group. *AA 12.5%,* 12.5% amino acid solution; *GLC*, glucose solution; *GLX*, glucose-fructose-xylitol solution, ratio 2:1:1

glucose-fructose-xylitol (2:1:1 ratio) solutions on days 2 and 3 and as pure glucose solutions on the following days; amino acids were given at a mean dose of 1.67 g/kg body weight/day in a commercially available 12.5% solution (Neoaminomel 12.5%, Boehringer Mannheim GmbH, 6800 Mannheim 31, FRG).

Treatment in both patients groups included controlled hyperventilation under sedation (droperidol and fentanyl) during the study period. No patient required osmotherapy of barbiturates for treatment of raised intracranial pressure. Apart from implantation of ventricular catheters (six patients from group A, three patients from group B), no major surgical procedure was carried out. Steroids with a mean dose of 24 mg dexamethasone/day were administered in both groups.

Results

Energy Expenditure

The results of the study are summarized in Table 1. During the whole study period, resting energy expenditure remained fairly constant, varying from a minimum of

Table 1. Resting energy expenditure in patients with spontaneous intracranial hemorrhages

	Day 1	2	3	4	5
	kcal/m² per day				
Mean	1013	982	1047	945	1093
SD	234	193	167	254	239
	% of predicted basal metabolic rate				
Mean	116.2	113.5	121.3	119.4	132.8
SD	25.0	22.4	23.1	37.6	27.7

945 kcal/m^2 per day on day 4 to a maximum of 1093 kcal/m^2 per day on day 5, representing 113.5%–132.8% of the predicted basal metabolic rate (BMR) [2].

Parenteral Nutrition

Numerous standard laboratory tests were performed to measure the efficacy and tolerance of total parenteral nutrition in our patients (e.g., red and white blood cell count, blood glucose, liver enzymes, blood urea nitrogen, serum creatinine, various

Table 2. Laboratory test results (body proteins) in the study group

	Day 0	1	2	3	4	5	6	7
	Total serum protein (65–80 g/l)							
Mean	63.38	61.30	58.80	61.45	59.80	59.89	58.46	59.23
SD	4.22	4.54	5.36	6.88	6.26	5.14	4.62	6.21
	Albumin (35–50 g/l)							
Mean	39.15	44.66	41.23	41.04	41.85	38.91	39.86	38.67
SD	4.53	2.22	4.81	3.01	6.02	6.32	3.23	3.51
	Prealbumin (0.1–0.4 g/l)							
Mean	0.354	0.329	0.314	0.296	0.314	0.342	0.291	0.291
SD	0.049	0.069	0.121	0.067	0.123	0.105	0.112	0.130
	Retinol-binding protein (0.03–0.06 g/l)							
Mean	0.063	0.066	0.052	0.051	0.062	0.059	0.051	0.052
SD	0.026	0.013	0.019	0.017	0.019	0.018	0.022	0.032

Figures in parentheses refer to range of normal values.

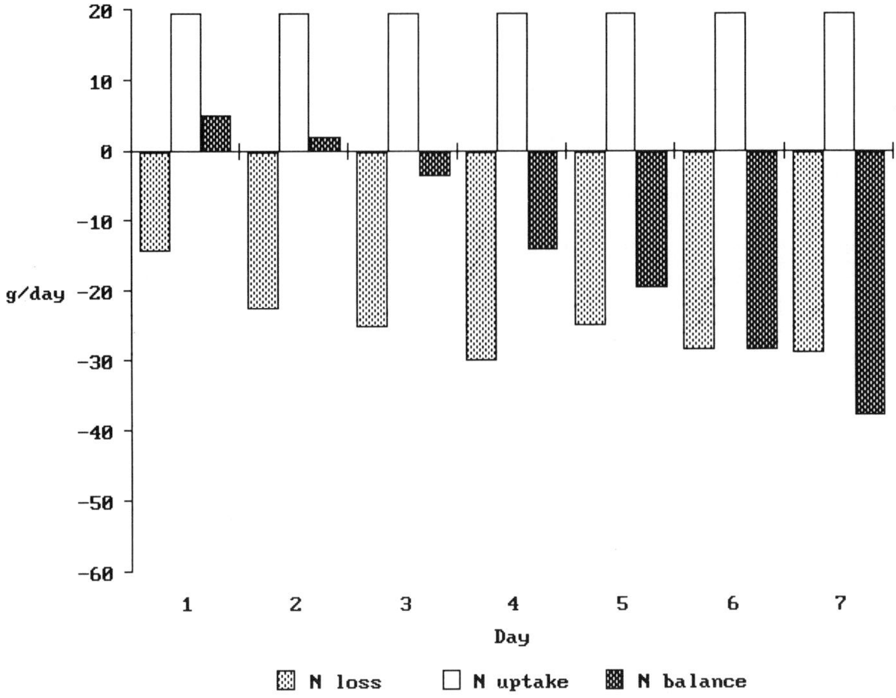

Fig. 2. Renal nitrogen loss and nitrogen balance (cumulative) in patients with spontaneous intracranial hemorrhage

indices of blood coagulation, blood gas analysis). Apart from a tendency to mild alkalosis and mild hyperglycemia (with blood glucose levels up to 242 mg/dl), all these tests showed normal results.

In regard to protein and amino acid metabolism, short-lived serum proteins (prealbumin and retinol-binding protein) were measured daily as well as total serum protein and albumin. Plasma levels of free amino acids were measured on days 1, 3, 5, and 7. Nitrogen balance was calculated from nitrogen uptake minus renal nitrogen loss minus 2 g/day (nitrogen loss via feces and perspiration). All results are shown in Table 2.

For short-lived serum proteins, albumin, and total serum protein, only normal values were observed. Free plasma amino acids remained within twice the normal range. Renal nitrogen loss increased steadily from –12.35 g/day on day 1 to –27.96 g/day on day 4, but remained as high as –25 g/day afterwards (Fig. 2). In patients receiving total parenteral nutrition, the cumulative nitrogen balance was reduced to –38 g nitrogen at the end of the study period.

Discussion

Before indirect calorimetry became available as a bedside method of measuring individual energy expenditure, neurosurgical patients were thought to have extremely high metabolic rates. Patients with severe head injuries especially were believed to require up to 6000 kcal/day [1, 4]. Although numerous studies have shown that energy requirements of patients with severe head injuries are much lower, to our knowledge rarely exceeding 150% of the basal metabolic rate, no comparable study has been performed in patients who have suffered spontaneous intracranial hemorrhages. The present study clearly shows that patients who have had spontaneous intracranial hemorrhages have an energy expenditure that is even lower than those who have suffered isolated head injury.

In order to prove the tolerance and the efficacy of such a low-calorie, high-protein nutritional regimen, a subsequent nutritional study was performed in another group of patients with spontaneous intracranial hemorrhages. The regimen consisted mainly of 1600 nonprotein kcal/day (given only as carbohydrates), together with 125 g amino acids/day (= 1.67 g/kg body weight).

Spontaneous intracranial hemorrhage results in typical hormonal changes causing changes in metabolism usually defined as "postaggression syndrome." In glucose metabolism this means low levels of circulating insulin, insulin resistance, and hyperglycemia [5, 6]. If high doses of glucose are infused during this time, hyperglycemia may be even more severe, as exogeneous insulin is not able to stimulate utilization of glucose [5, 6]. Mild hyperglycemia (maximum blood glucose levels up to 240 mg/dl) indicates that the energy intake of our patient group met its energy expenditure, avoiding the negative effects of high glucose loads. The normal results for most standard laboratory tests indicate that this nutritional regimen was well tolerated.

Catabolism usually results in protein loss and a negative nitrogen balance. Low levels of short-lived serum proteins may lead to suppression of imunological systems, increased infection rates, and impairment of wound healing. The pattern of free plasma amino acids is usually disturbed. In the present study both short-lived serum proteins and total serum protein and plasma albumin levels remained within the normal range. The pattern of free plasma amino acids was only slightly disturbed. This indicates that administration of amino acids up to 125 g/day was effective in the study group and was able to preserve normal levels of body proteins. Although renal nitrogen loss was high, negative nitrogen balance could be reduced to –38 g/7 days.

From the present studies we conclude that:

- In comatose patients with spontaneous intracranial hemorrhages, resting energy expenditure is usually low and rarely exceeds 130% of the predicted basal metabolic rate.
- Total parenteral nutrition with an energy intake that meets the requirements of this patient group is safe and avoids the negative effects [references in 7] of

"hyper" nutrition (e.g., hyperglycemia, increased CO_2 production, hyperosmolarity, fluid and electrolyte imbalance).
- Under these conditions, administration of high doses of amino acids is well tolerated, preserves body protein levels, and normalizes negative nitrogen balance.

References

1. Bauer BL, Pia HW (1966) Parenterale Ernährung in der Neurochirurgie. In: Lang K, Frey R (eds) Infusionstherapie, Anästhesie und Wiederbelebung, vol 13. Springer, Berlin Heidelberg New York, pp 124–133
2. Boothby WM, Berkson J, Dunn HL (1936) Studies of the energy metabolism of normal individuals: a standard for basal metabolism and with a nomogram for clinical application. Am J Physiol 116:468–484
3. Damask MC, Weissman C, Hyman I (1982) A systemic method for validation of gas exchange measurements. Anaesthesiology 218:213–218
4. Niedermeier B, Bock WJ (1973) Langzeit-Ernährung bei Schwerkranken und bewußtlosen Patienten. Dtsch Arztebl 38:2447–2449
5. Reinauer H (1983) Fettinfusion und Kohlehydratstoffwechsel. Infusionstherapie 10:134–141
6. Reinauer H (1987) Wechselwirkung zwischen Glukose und Fettstoffwechsel bei insulinresistenten Zuständen. In: Eckart J, Wolfram G (eds) Klinische Ernährung, vol 31. Zuckschwerdt, Munich, pp 89–103
7. Semsroth M (1985) Indirekte Kalorimetrie beim beatmeten polytraumatisierten Patienten. I. Untersuchungen beim Erwachsenen. Infusionstherapie 12:213–237
8. Teasdale G, Jennett B (1974) Assessment of coma and impaired consciousness. A practical scale. Lancet 2:81–84
9. Weissman C, Damask MC, Askanazi J (1982) Evaluation of the Beckman metabolic measurement chart. Crit Care Med 10:231
10. Wesemann W (1975) Dauerregistrierung des Leistungsumsatzes bei Patienten mit Schädel-Hirn-Trauma und Hirntumoren. Infusionstherapie 2:365–376

Susceptibility to Infection During Continuous Thiopentone Therapy

J. Nadstawek[1], D. Moskopp[2], M. Fischer[1], M. Födisch[1], and A. Bartsch[1]

Introduction

Several in vitro studies have confirmed an immunosuppressive effect of the barbiturate thiopentone [3–5, 7]. At present, high-dose thiopentone is given to patients with increased intracranial pressure (ICP) after cranial trauma if they show no response to other therapeutic measures, although no positive effect on outcome has been verified. Clinical experience shows that these thiopentone-treated patients are especially prone to infections. Furthermore, the few existing prospective studies designed to improve outcome in patients with high and therapy-resistant ICP by continuous thiopentone treatment suggest a slight but insignificant increase in the incidence of pneumonia [2, 9]. The goal of this retrospective study, therefore, was to document in vivo immunosuppression by continuous thiopentone treatment through biochemical tests and monitoring of clinical condition.

Patients and Methods

Fifty-three patients (32 male, 21 female) between 8 and 80 years of age (mean 39.4 years) with severe cranial trauma underwent continuous thiopentone treatment for therapy-resistant raised ICP, receiving 3 mg/kg body weight per hour for an average of 6 ± 3.2 days. The control group consisted of 53 patients (31 male, 22 female) between 7 and 75 years of age (mean 38.7 years), suffering from equally severe cranial injury but not receiving thiopentone. Criteria for the inclusion in the control group were: (1) cranial trauma matching that of the thiopentone group (Glasgow Coma Scale < 7), (2) acute midbrain syndrome on arrival and (3) unconciousness with consecutive ventilatory support for at least 10 days. The following were monitored in both groups: body temperature > 38.5°C, white blood cells (WBC), lymphocyte count, pathogenic colonization of pharynx, trachea, and urine, positive blood cultures, manifestation of sepsis (temperature above 40°C, catecholamines required, and roentgenological and clinical signs.

Statistic significance (level set at $p < 0.05$) was calculated using the Wilcoxon, Mann, and Whitney U test.

---

[1] Institut für Anästhesiologie der Rheinischen Friedrich-Wilhelms-Universität Bonn, Sigmund-Freud-Str. 25, W-5300 Bonn 1, FRG

[2] Neurochirurgische Klinik der Rheinischen Friedrich-Wilhelms-Universität, Sigmund-Freud-Str. 25, W-5300 Bonn 1, FRG

Advances in Neurosurgery, Vol. 19
W. J. Bock, Ch. Lumenta, M. Brock, M. Klinger (Eds.)

Results

While pathogenic colonization of the pharynx was found in 26 patients in the control group, the thiopentone group showed a significantly higher incidence, with pharyngeal colonization in 46 patients (Table 1). Pathogenic colonization of the trachea was nearly identical in both groups, that in the control group being slightly higher (Table 1). Urinary cultures gave positive results in a significantly higher number of patients of the control group (Table 1).

However, 43 patients of the thiopentone group, as against 27 patients of the control group, developed temperatures above 38.5°C ($p < 0.05$, Fig. 1). Temperature above 40°C due to sepsis were observed in 22 patients of the thiopentone group compared to 8 patients of the control group ($p < 0.05$, Fig. 1). Blood cultures from 12 thiopentone-treated patients gave positive results, against only 3 patients of the control group ($p < 0.05$, Table 1). Lymphopenia was detected more frequently in the thiopentone group (20 patients) than in the control group (13 patients; $p < 0.05$, Fig. 2). A raised WBC count was found more often in the thiopentone group, although this did not prove significant. Manifest sepsis with consequent changes in hemodynamic indices was seen in 26 patients of the thiopentone group, while only

Table 1. Pathogenic colonization of blood, urine, trachea, and pharynx in patients with severe head injury treated with and without thiopentone

	Control group +/–	Thiopentone +/–
Blood	3/50*	12/41*
Urine	15/38*	4/49*
Trachea	42/11	37/16
Pharynx	26/27*	46/7*

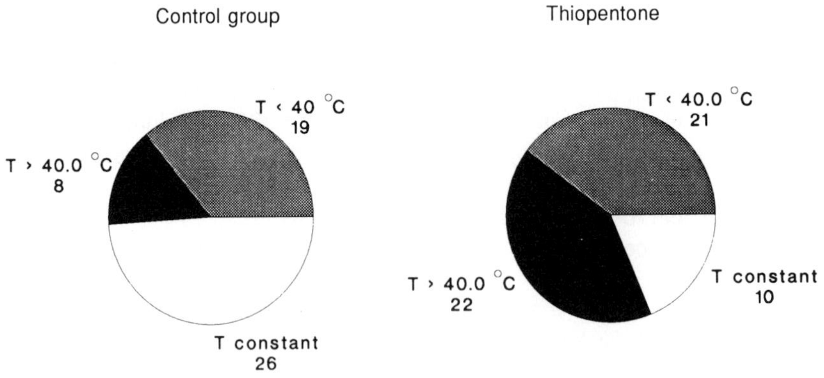

Fig. 1. Body temperature in neurotraumatized patients treated with and without thiopentone

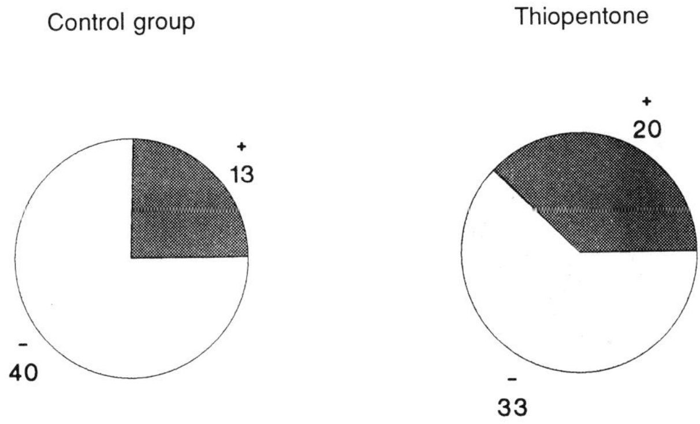

Fig. 2. Lymphopenia of patients treated with and without thiopentone

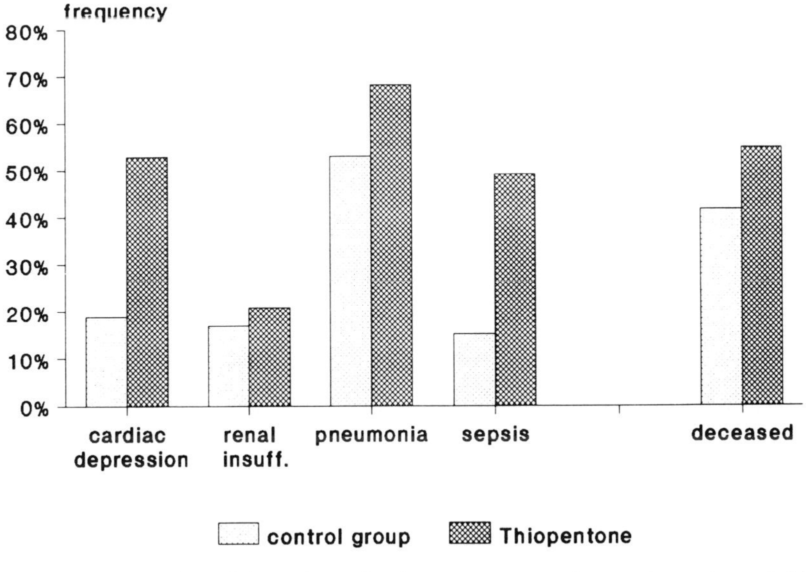

Fig. 3. Manifestation of hemodynamic changes, pneumonia, sepsis, and renal failure in patients treated with and without thiopentone

16 patients of the control group displayed similar signs ($p < 0.05$, Fig. 3); thus, more thiopentone patients were catecholamine-dependent. The incidence of pneumonia was 68% in the thiopentone group and 52% in the control group (difference not significant). Renal failure was noticed in both groups with no difference in relation to whether or not thiopentone had been received.

Discussion

Recent studies using different immunological systems have shown significant in vitro immune depression following high doses of the barbiturate thiopentone [3–5, 7]. Although no definite positive effect of high-dose thiopentone treatment on the outcome of severe, therapy-resistant raised ICP has yet been confirmed, and this stratagem is the subject of controversy in the literature [1, 2, 6, 8, 9], it is considered the last resort of treatment for raised ICP. The few existing prospective studies of the use of continuous administration of barbiturates to bring down raised ICP after cranial trauma report an increase in the incidence of infection. The present study was designed to verify these findings and own clinical experience. Although it is a retrospective study, our results clearly demonstrate a remarkable increase in susceptibility to infection in patients being treated with continuous high-dose thiopentone over several days for therapy-resistant increased ICP. Thus, we postulate that thiopentone too causes in vivo immunosuppression. Owing to this, the pathogenicity of bacterial colonies rises, resulting in a significant increase of septicemia in thiopentone-treated patients, although in our study pathogenic colonization of the trachea was identical in both groups, and even significantly higher in the control group in regard to urinary cultures.

Thiopentone treatment of patients with therapy-resistant increased ICP should therefore be reconsidered. Isolation of these patients in the intensive care unit, aseptic care comparable to that given to immunosuppressed patients, and intensive microbiological monitoring should be mandatory, as they contribute to patient safety. It would appear logical to extend immunological monitoring beyond the parameters studied here.

References

1. Abramson NS, Safar P, Detre K, Kelsey S, et al.(1983) Result of a randomized clinical trial of brain resuscitation with thiopentone. Anesthesiology 59(3):A101
2. Eisenberg HM, Frankowski RF, Contant CF, Marshall LF, Walker MD (1988) High-dose barbiturate control of elevated intracranial persure in patients with severe head injury. J Neurosurg 69:15–23
3. Kress HG, Segmüller R (1987) Intravenöse Anästhetika und Motilität humaner neutrophiler Granulozyten. Anasthesist 36:356–361
4. Krumholz W, Jorgall H, Käbisch S, Hempelmann G (1988) Narkoseeinleitungsmittel und Granulozytenadhärenz. Anasth Intensivther Notfallmed 23:69–72
5. Neuwelt EA, Kikuch K, Hill SA, Lipsky P, Frenkel E (1982) Barbiturate inhibition of lymphocyte function. Differing effects of various barbiturates used to induce coma. J Neurosurg 56:254–259
6. Nussmeier NA, Arlund C, Slogoff S (1986) Neuropsychiatric complications after cardiopulmonary bypass: cerebral protection by a barbiturate. Anesthesiology 64:165–170
7. Salo M, Perttilä J (1989) Effects of thiopentone on granulocyte oxidative microbicidal capacity. Acta Anaesthesiol Scand 33:339–342
8. Schwartz ML, Tator CH, Rowed DW, Reid SR, Meguro K, Andrews DF (1984) The University of Toronto head injury treatment study: a prospective, randomized comparison of pentobarbital and mannitol. Can J Neurol Sci 11:434–440

9. Ward JD, Becker DP, Miller JD, Choi SC, Marmarou A, Wood C, Newlon PG, Kenan R (1985) Failure of prophylactic barbiturate coma in the treatment of severe head injury. J Neurosurg 62:383–388

Infection Rate and Bacterial Spectrum in 413 Patients of a Neurosurgical Intensive Care Unit: Results of a 2-Year Prospective Study

A. Feldges[1], R. Kalff[1], E. Rosenthal[2], and W. Grote[1]

Introduction

The high incidence of unit-acquired infections in general intensive care units (ICUs) has reached critical importance in the past years. Advances in both surgery and drug treatment and the progress in invasive diagnostics and monitoring have also brought a higher risk of infections to the long-term patients of an ICU. Additionally trauma patients and long-stay patients are both groups in which the risk of infection with aerobic gram-negative bacteria is particularly well documented and is thought to influence mortality [6]. Should antibiotic therapy therefore be initiated at the first finding of bacteria? This question especially arises in a neurosurgical ICU, when bacteria are isolated from patients weakened by high doses of cortisone but as yet without a definite infection.

Patients and Methods

Over two years 3772 microbiological samples from 413 patients (238 males and 175 females) admitted to our neurosurgical ICU were examined. The distribution of the different age groups can be seen in Fig. 1. The most common diagnosis was severe head injury (36%). Intracranial hemorrhage was diagnosed in 32% and tumors in 18%. Three percent of all patients were admitted because of a primary cerebral infection, in most cases a cerebral abscess.

The duration of stay in the ICU reflected the severity of disease or injury. Thirty percent of all patients stayed for 15 days or longer, 55% of all patients had to be ventilated over 3 days or more, and 34% of all patients did not survive. Microbiological samples of gastric aspirate, tracheal aspirate, cerebrospinal fluid (CSF), and urine were taken twice a week. Additional samples for aerobic and anaerobic blood culture were taken, if body temperature exceeded 38.5°C. Intravascular catheters were always examined microbiologically when removed. If organisms were detected, experienced investigators verified whether a definite infection was present at the same time; otherwise bacterial findings were interpreted as colonization of a particular organ system.

[1] Neurochirurgische Klinik, Universitätsklinikum Essen, Hufelandstr. 55, W-4300 Essen, FRG

[2] Institut für Mikrobiologie, Universitätsklinikum Essen, Hufelandstr. 55, W-4300 Essen, FRG

Advances in Neurosurgery, Vol. 19
W. J. Bock, Ch. Lumenta, M. Brock, M. Klinger (Eds.)

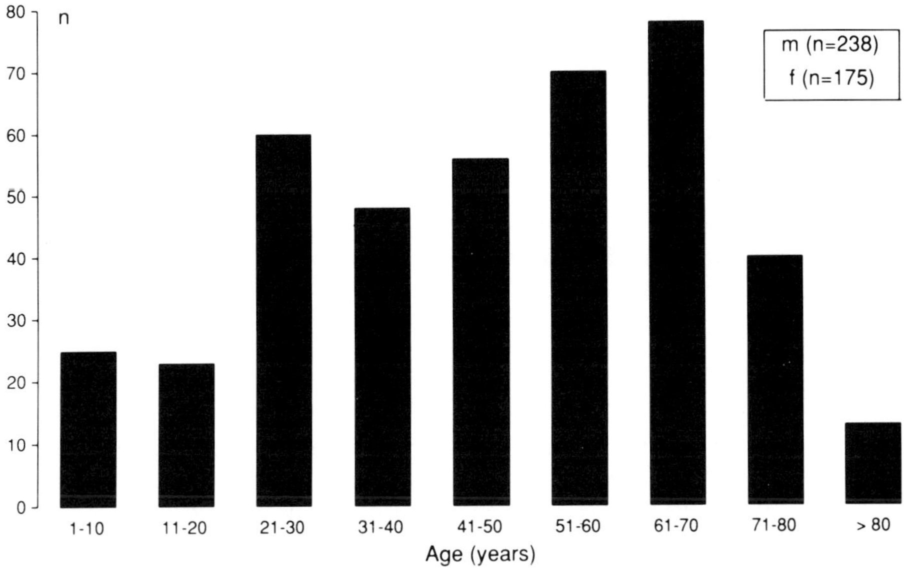

Fig. 1. Distribution of the various age groups. Most patients aged 21–30 years were victims of head trauma, while the majority of older patients (51–70 years) had suffered intracranial hemorrhage

All long-term ventilated patients (3 days or more controlled ventilation) received systemic antiobiotic prophylaxis consisting of 3 x 150 mg netilmicin and 3 x 2 g oxacillin. In the 2nd week of stay 4 x 500 mg amphotericin B was given additionally via the gastric tube. Antibiotic treatment was subsequently modified in accordance with continuous sensitivity tests.

Pneumonia was defined by the presence of at least three of the following:

1. White cell count > 12000/mm^3 and temperature spike > 38.5°
2. Purulent tracheal secretion
3. Pulmonary infiltrates visible on X-ray
4. Increase of 0.15 in inspired O_2 fraction to maintain oxygenation
5. Organisms detected in the tracheal aspirate

Septicemia was defined by the presence of all the following:

1. White cell count > 12000/mm^3 or < 4000/mm^3 starting from normal values and temperature spike > 38.5°C
2. Rise in of blood pressure amplitude to more than 50% of the original value accompanied by drop in diastolic blood pressure
3. Organisms detected in blood culture

The criteria for *urinary infections* were:

1. White cell count > 12000/mm^3 and temperature spike > 38.5°C
2. More then 5 white cells/mm^3 urine
3. Organisms detected in the urine

The criteria for *meningitis* were:

1. White cell count > 12000/mm^3 and temperature spike >38.5°C
2. More than 50 white cells/mm^3 in the CSF
3. Organisms detected in the CSF

Results

Over the 2 years there were 132 unit-acquired infections among the 413 ICU patients (32.5%). The most frequent was pneumonia, which occurred in 71 patients (17%) and accounted for 52.3% of all infections, followed by 36 cases of septicemia and 23 of urinary infections. We saw only two cases of meningitis. During the 1st week gram-positive bacteria predominated in the tracheal aspirate; especially *Staphylococcus aureus*, which was present in up to 11% of all patients. The general prophylactic antibiotic treatment given to long-term-ventilated patients reduced most of the *Staphylococci*. *Staphylococci* found between the 19th and 24th day in up to 5% of all tracheal samples were problematic organisms due to selection, but were well controlled by high potency antibiotics in all cases. A multiresistant

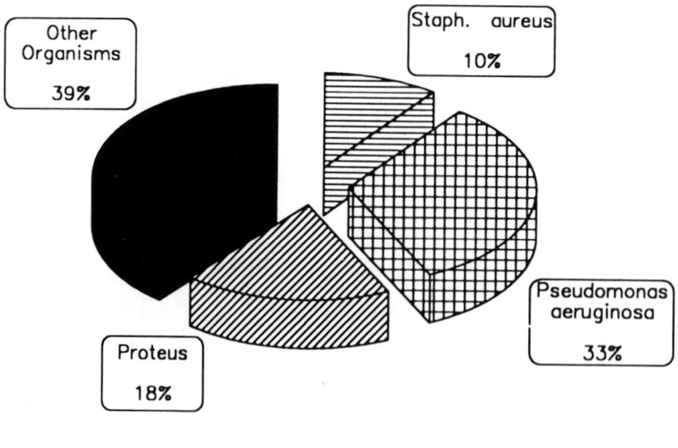

Fig. 2. Organisms isolated in episodes of pneumonia. *Pseudomonas aeruginosa* constituted one third of all organisms found as the main causative germ in pneumonia. Important bacteria subsumed in the group "other organisms" were *Escherichia coli* (12%), *Klebsiella* (6%), and *Streptococcus* (6%)

gram-positive bacteria didn't occur. Gram-negative bacteria were found in tracheal aspirate later. *Pseudomonas aeruginosa* was isolated in more than 18% of all tracheal samples after the 2nd week. Significant amounts of *Pseudomonas* during the first days in intensive care were seen only in patients who had acquired pneumonia before admission to the unit. Seventy five percent of cases of pneumonia were caused by one specific organism.

Pseudomonas aeruginosa was the most frequent causative bacteria (33%) (Fig. 2). Patients suffering from pneumonia had a significantly longer ICU stay (23 days, median) and spent longer under ventilation (16 days, median) than the other (2 days and 6 days respectively). Mortality in patients with pneumonia and/or septicemia was higher (43%) than in patients without these complications (36%). This difference was not statistically significant (CHi^2 test), $P < 0.05$), but suggested that pneumonia and septicemia might be contributory factors in a fatal outcome. Neoplasm or metabolic disturbances like diabetes mellitus did not significantly affect the incidence of pneumonia.

We differentiated between detection of bacteria in association with a definite infection and simply finding bacteria without any accompanying infection, called colonization. Thirty-seven percent of all *Streptococcus* findings in tracheal aspirate were associated with pneumonia, while only 12% of all *Candida* findings were.

Microbiological examination of gastric aspirate included additional investigation of pH value. An impressive example of an endogenous infection ascending from the gastric reservoir of the respiratory tract was the chronological tracking of *Klebsiella* in stomach and lung (Fig. 3). Minimum and maximum findings in gastric aspirate preceded the corresponding findings in tracheal secretion by 24–48 hours. In 90 cases the bacterial spectrum of the gastric and tracheal aspirate was the same.

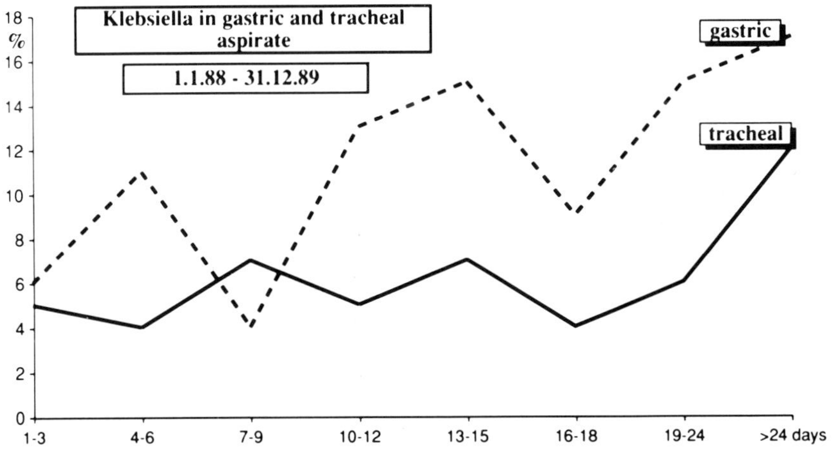

Fig. 3. Detection of *Klebsiella* in gastric and tracheal aspirate related to duration of stay. During the first 2 weeks the detection rates in the stomach anticipated the corresponding findings in the lung by 24–48 h. Later the findings ran parallel to each other

In 26% of all cases of pneumonia the same causative organism was found in the gastric aspirate a short time before onset of the symptoms of infection.

The organism most frequently found in the 1085 urine samples was *Candida albicans*. However, a definite urinary infection was seen in association with only 7% of all *Candida* findings. The other 93% could be interpreted as a result of secondary colonization of the urinary tract.

After 1 week *Staphylococcus epidermidis* was already detected in 18% of all blood cultures. Because of forming colonies on catheter surfaces hampering successful antibiotic therapy *Staphyloccus epidermidis* remained at this level of 18%. This bacteria was found in up to 47% of all cases of septicemia. Despite this high rate of detection however, its clinical significance had to be rated lower, as only 24% of all patients in whom *Staphylococcus epidermidis* was found developed a septicemia. Against this 71% of all *Staphylococcus aureus* findings were associated with septicemia.

Most of the 182 CSF samples were taken during the 1st week. Because of the relatively short time, external drainage of ventricles was usually performed. In accordance with its affinity for catheters *Staphylococcus epidermidis* was the most usual organism found in drainages in place for any length of time, but caused no case of meningitis.

Dexamethasone at doses of 16 mg or more consistent gastric protection by H_2-antagonists were given for 80% and 90%, respectively, of the patients' stay in the ICU. Despite this impairment of the immune systeme and the possible promotion of an ascending endogenous infection, only 17% of all ICU patients suffered from pneumonia. An important precondition for this low infection rate was the early institution of antibiotic prophylaxis in all long-term ventilated patients. Highly resistant gram-positive bacteria, which would be expected as a consequence of selection, were not seen with this prophylactic antibiotic regimen.

Discussion

To date few prospective studies evaluating infection rate and bacterial spectrum in ICUs have been published. Moreover interpretation of the various studies is impeded by the diversity of the patient populations. The overfall infection rate in our patients (32.5%) agrees with those in other studies. Hartenauer et al. [2] have reported 32.8%, Ledingham et al. [5] 39.4%, and Lackner et al. [4] 33%. Differences can be seen in the incidence of pneumonia; while we have diagnosed pneumonia in 17% of our patients, other studies have reported incidences between 42% [3) and 19% [4]. Further evidence of the diversity of the various studies is the mortality rate, which in our ICU was 34%, but in other patients populations has been between 13.2% [2] and 24% [5]. The isolates of organisms in episodes of pneumonia in our ICU disclosed a large amount of *Pseudomonas aeruginosa* (33%), while *Staphyloccocus aureus* (10%) and *Escherichia coli* (12%) were found less frequently. In other series different rates have been reported, with *Stapholoccous aureus* the main causative organism in pneumonia (29.5%) followed by *Pseudomonas aeruginosa* (15.1%) and *Escherichia coli* (14,7%). In other series [1, 3] the incidence of pneumonia was significantly reduced by selective decontamination of the digestive tract. Gram-negative bacilli in particular have been reduced by this prophylaxis. During the last 6 months we have also tried to reduce the incidence of *Pseudomonas aeruginosa* by administering gentamicin via the tracheal tube; a first evaluation of this strategy will be possible at the end of 1990. A further aim of this prospective study will be to develop a reasonable prophylactic antibiotic regimen of all patients under long-term ventilation.

No serious difficulties with resistance have been encountered in this study. The Neurosurgical Department will continue in close collaboration with the Institute of Microbiology to register in detail any change in the bacterial spectrum and to avoid the selection of any possibly resistant bacteria.

References

1. Daschner F (1985) Nosocomial infections in intensive care units. Intensive Care Med 11:284–287
2. Hartenauer U, Diemer W, Gähler R, Ritzerfeld W (1990) Nosokomiale Infektionen in der operativen Intensivmedizin – Ergebnis einer fünfjährigen prospektiven Erhebung. Anästh Intensivhter Notfallmed 25:93–101
3. Konrad F, Schwalbe B, Heeg K, Wagner H, Wiedeck H, Kilian J, Ahnefeld FW (1989) Kolonisations-, Pneumoniefrequenz und Resistenzentwicklung bei langzeitbeatmeten Intensivpatienten unter selektiver Dekontamination des Verdauungstraktes. Anaesthesist 38:99–109
4. Lackner F, Wewalka G, Rotter M, Kilian J, Hummel E, Hartenauer U, Gähler R, Scherzer E, Pauser G (1989) Infektionsüberwachung an Intensivstationen: Eine multizentrische Pilotstudie. Anästh Intensivhter Notfallmedinin 24:133–142
5. Ledingham IMcA, Alcock StR, Eastaway At, McDonald JC, McKay IC, Ramsay G (1988) Triple regimen of selective decontamination of the digestive tract, systemic cefotaxime, and microbiological surveillance for prevention of acquired infection in intensive care. Lancet 9:785–790
6. Schimpf SC, Miller RM, Polakavetz S, Harnick RB (1974) Infection in the severely traumatized patient. Ann Surg 179:352–357

Risk During the First Hours After Severe Head Injury

R.A. Frowein[1], U. Stammler[1], R. Firsching[1], G. Friedmann[2], and F. Thun[2]

Survivors of Severe Head Injury

In spite of numerous publications from Gordon, Gothenburg [7], Karimi, Cologne [10], Vigouroux, Marseille [15], and many other authors, objective figures for the survivors of the first hours after severe head injury are rare and differ widely (Fig. 1). In 578 cases of head injury treated in 1984/85 in a large general hospital in Ravenna, Servadei et al. [14] reported 3% (19 cases) deaths at the site of accident and during transport. Another 3% (17 patients) died in the emergency room, and 7 out of 542 patients (1.2%) died in hospital later. In Paris, among 1157 neurosurgical emergency trauma patients, Charpentier et al. [2] recorded a mortality of

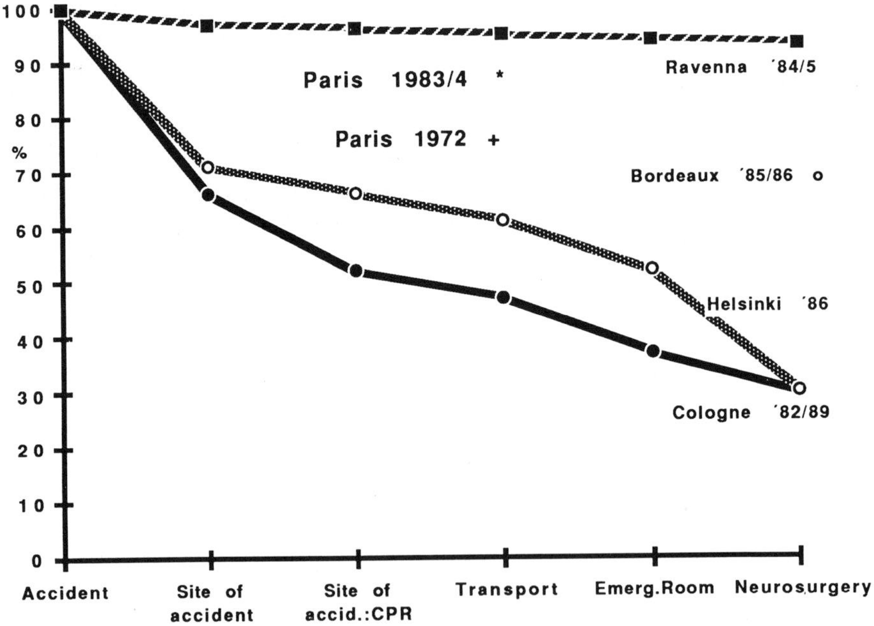

Fig. 1. Survivors after head injuries

[1] Neurochirurgische Klinik, Universität Köln, Geibelstr. 22, W-5000 Köln 41, FRG
[2] Abteilung Radiologie, Universität Köln, Joseph-Stelzmann-Str. 9, W-5000 Köln 41, FRG

Advances in Neurosurgery, Vol. 19
W. J. Bock, Ch. Lumenta, M. Brock, M. Klinger (Eds.)

25% in 1972, which they reduced to 12% in 1983/84. Dautheribes et al. [3] in Bordeaux had 70% survivors. Hernesniemi et al. [9] in Helsinki reported in 1986 that out of 223 severely head-injured patients (excluding suicides) 68 patients, i.e. 30%, died at the site of accident, leaving 70% survivors. Bouillon (1982, personal communication), one of the organizers of first aid in Cologne, reported on 130 comatose head-injured patients at the site of accident. In those who needed cardiopulmonary resuscitation, the mortality even reached 90%, like in patients with other causes of cardiac arrest [4, 11, 13]. Both Hernesniemi et al. [9] and Bouillon found that 10%–20% of initially comatose head-injured patiends died during transport, another 17% in the emergency room, and finally of the remaining patients 30% died in spite of neurosurgical treatment. Thus, the Helsinki and Cologne centers came to the same dramatic finding: that in cases of severe head injuries resulting in coma at the scene of accident, only half of the patients can be treated clinically, and that the proportion of final survivors is only 30%.

Time After Injury of Admittance of Patients with Hematomas

The formation of extracerebral hematomas in the first hours after injury is an important problem. Figure 2 shows the cumulative numbers of 363 patients with epidural hematomas and 440 patients with subdural hematomas admitted during two periods, 1974–1979 and 1980–1988. The numbers of patients per year are corre-

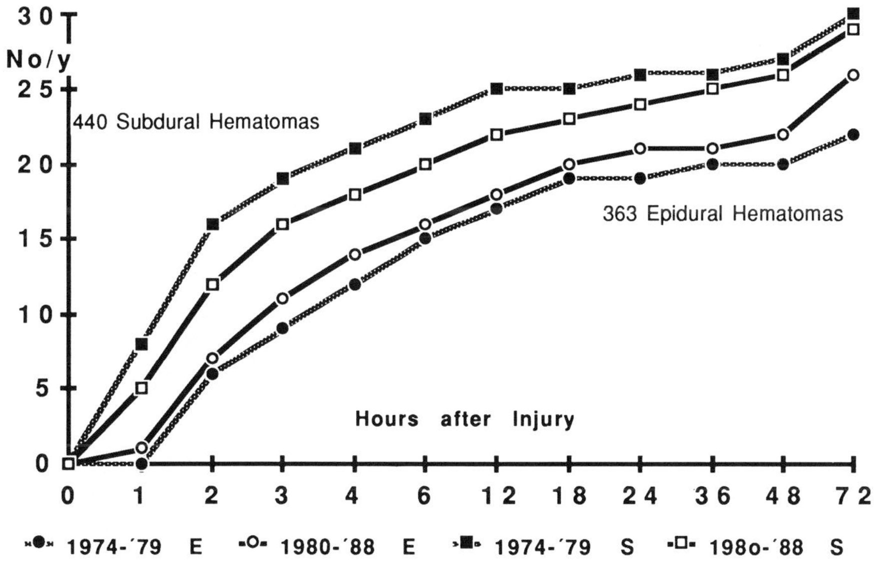

Fig. 2. Time from injury to admission of patients with traumatic epidural and subdural hematomas. Cumulative numbers per year, 1974–1979 and 1980–1988

lated to the amount of time after injury that patients were admitted and to the diagnosis, established by angiography or computed tomography (CT).

About 25 epidural and 30 subdural hematomas were seen per year. The cumulative presentation shows that about half of all patients (with either kind of extracerebral hematoma) were admitted during the first 2–4 h after injury. This may be considered as proof of the high efficiency of the rescue services. The incidence of early admission and diagnosis of epidural hematomas has hardly increased, while the incidence of acute subdural hematoma decreased in the second period, 1980–1988, probably because small subdural hematomas accompanying larger cerebral contusions are not included here.

The number of patients admitted with epidural hematomas within the 1st hour after injury is very low, zero to 1, whereas of the total number of patients with subdural hematomas admitted within 4 h after injury, one-third were admitted in the 1st hour, counting the larger hematoma in cases with extra- and subdural hematoma. The sharpest increase in incidence is clearly seen during the 2nd hour after trauma, before and after 1980.

Mortality in Hematoma Patients

The mortality in patients with early manifesting hematomas is under discussion in the literature [1, 5, 6, 8]. Our patients show a clear difference between the periods before and after 1980 (Fig. 3). Large subdural hematomas in the 1st hour after injury were nearly all fatal. The mortality of more than 90% with these has not changed much over the years, because early large subdural hematomas accompany early

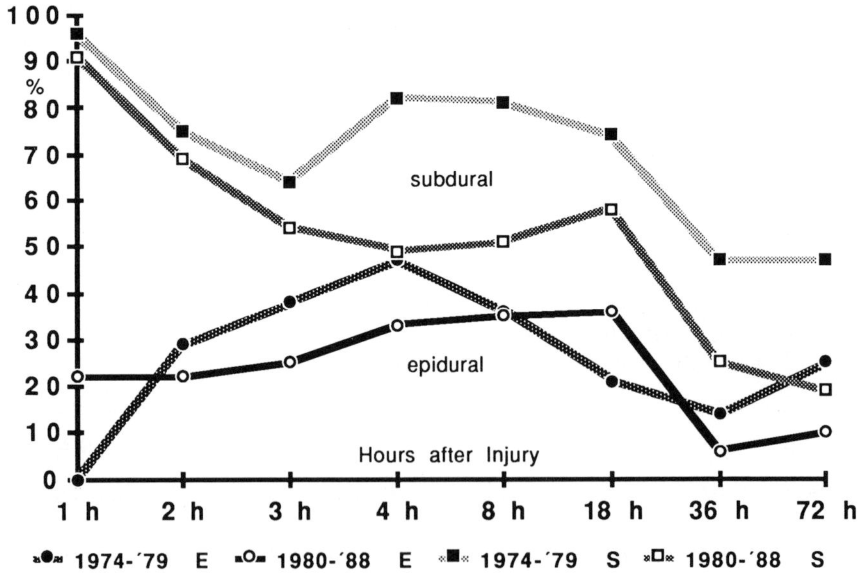

Fig. 3. Epidural and subdural hematomas: mortality 1974–1979 and 1980–1988

large underlying cerebral contusions and lacerations which determine the patient's further clinical course despite surgery. However, subdural hematomas which develop less rapidly and manifest later, up to 3 h after injury, were associated with a lower mortality of about 60%. There was a new rise in mortality with subdural hematomas diagnosed in the second part of the day of injury in the period up to 1979; this peak was no longer visible in the 1980–1988 period, probably due to more efficient management.

The mortality with early epidural hematomas is generally low in the very rare patients admitted during the 1st hour, but increases up to 40% in the following hours. This pattern too was less pronounced after 1980. Diagnosis of epidural hematoma after 4 h seems to be often delayed.

If in the literature, therefore, statistics demonstrate a marked reduction in mortality with epidural and subdural hematomas in the past few years, one must assume that this progress relates to the period of about 4–18 h after injury. This period, however, relates to only one-third of the hematomas while the high mortality associated with subdural hematomas seen in the first 3 h has not actually changed.

Time of Manifestation of Focal Space-Occupying Lesions

In this attempt to assess improvements in diagnosis and treatment, it was necessary to evaluate the incidences, time of manifestation, and degree of risk associated with focal space-occupying lesions during the first few hours after injury.

We analyzed 409 cases of either epidural, subdural, intracerebral hematomas, large or enlarged contusions, according to the timing of initial CT. Only three large contusions had been seen on the initial CT scan. During the first 3 h acute subdural and, to a lesser degree, epidural hematomas predominated, decreasing rapidly in number with the interval after injury. From 6 to 12 h after injury onwards, enlarged contusions became more frequent or secondary intraventricular hemorrhages occurred [12], and these processes continued in the latter part of the 1st and on the 2nd day.

Admission and CT Investigation: Time, Incidence, Mortality

Hematomas and contusions are seen in only one-half of all patients admitted in a comatose state; the other half have diffuse lesions. For this reason, we have presented in Fig. 4 the distribution over time (n/h) of the admissions of all 978 patients received in our hospital between 1980 and 1988 in a comatose state, with initial CT investigations are various intervals after injury, compared with just the admissions of those with acute epidural, subdural, and intracerebral hematomas. The peak in the latter of 126 cases as early as in the 2nd hour after injury is of great significance for diagnosis and operation. The relative high number of 70 hematomas diagnosed out of 83 patients admitted 6 to 18 h after injury is due to delayed diagnosis

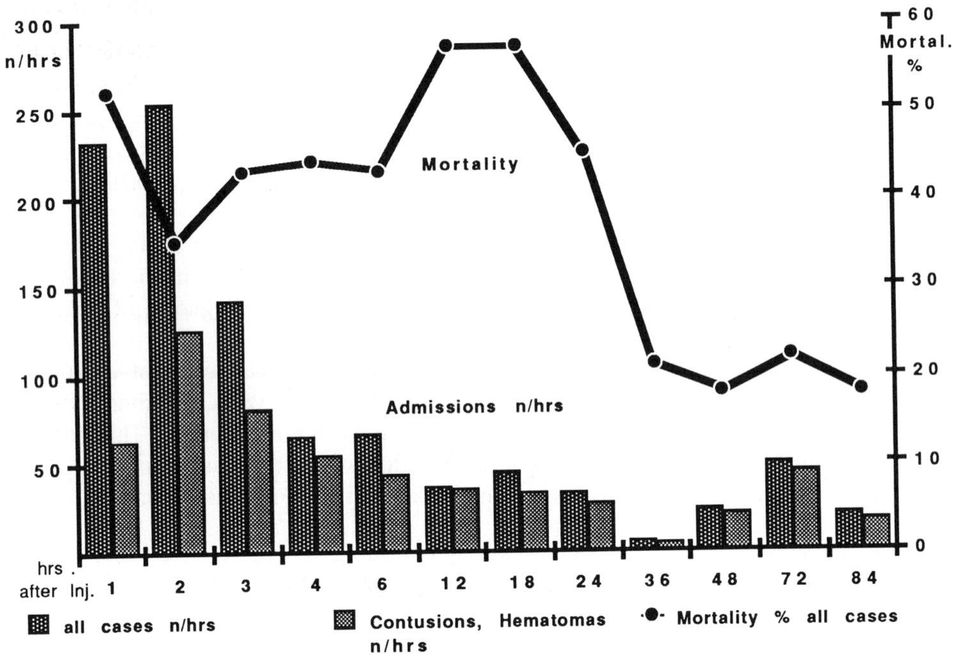

Fig. 4. Risk of death (*black line*) in the first hours after injury: 978 patients with head injuries 1980–1988 distributed over time (n/h) of the admission

of epidural and subdural hematomas and also to the beginning of the enlargement of the contusions and the intracerebral hematomas.

The actual risk during the 1st hours in represented by the mortality, that is the black line, which is derived from the outcome in all patients admitted and investigated at the various intervals after trauma. The important point to notice is that after a first peak of 52% mortality in the patients admitted in the 1st hour after injury, there is a similar peak of 56% mortality due to lesions emerging about 12–18 h after injury.

We have quantified as precisely as possible the timing and extent of risk associated with the manifestation of focal and diffuse posttraumatic lesions during the first hours after injury. Awareness of the periods of highest risk should be a guide to appropriate diagnostic and therapeutic measures after various intervals following trauma.

References

1. Becker DP, Miller JD, Ward JD, Greenberg RP, Young HF, Sakalas R (1977) The outcome from severe head injury with early diagnosis and intensive management. J Neurosurg 47:491–502

2. Charpentier Cl, Roux FX, Cioloca C, Mérienne L, Meder JF, Charpentier E, Chodkiewicz JP (1986) La prise en charge des traumatisés du crâne à lère du samu et du scanner. Neurochirurgie 32:519–522
3. Dautheribes M, Destandau M, Guerin J, Leman P, Boulard G, Marquinaud E, Mehsen M, Thicoipe M, Cochard P, Maurett P, Leger L, Claverie JP (1988) Étude de 200 cas de traumatismes crânio-cérébraux graves. Agressologie 29:445–447
4. Engelhardt GH, Purrmann H, Zapf C (1990) Die kardiopulmonale Reanimation (CPR) im Krankenhausbereich. In: Hierholzer G, Böhm HJ (eds) Reanimation im Rettungswesen, Springer, Berlin Heidelberg New York
5. Frowein RA, Keila M (1972) Bagatelltraumen bei subduralen Haematomen. Beitr Gerichtl Med 29:87–88
6. Frowein RA, Schiltz F, Stammler U (1989) Early post-traumatic intracranial hematoma. Neurosurg Rev [Supl 1] 12:184–187
7. Gordon E (1986) Guidelines for management. Acta Neurochir [Suppl) (Wien) 36:58–59
8. Hernesniemi J (1979) Outcome following acute subdural haematoma. Acta Neurochir (Wien) 49:191–198
9. Hernesniemi J, Valtonen S, Männikkö KA (1986) Kann die Mortalität bei schweren traumatischen Hirnschäden überhaupt mehr reduziert werden? Zentralbl Neurochir 47:99–104
10. Karimi A (1988) Traumatische und nicht traumatische Notfälle. de Gruyter Berlin
11. Obertacke U, Walz M, Schmidt-Neuerburg KP (1990) Die cardiopulmonale Reanimation (CPR) als Aufgabe des NAW-Rettungssystems. In: Hierholzer G, Böhm HG (eds) Reanimation im Rettungswesen. Springer, Berlin Heidelberg New York
12. Piek J, Bock WJ (1986) Secondary intraventricular haemorrhage in blunt head trauma. Acta Neurochir (Wien) 83:105–107
13. Safar P (1988) Resuscitation from clinical death: pathophysiologic limits and therapeutic potentials. Crit Care Med 10:923–941
14. Servadei F, Giucci G, Piazza G, Bianchedi G, Rebucci G, Gaist G (1989) A prospective clinical and epidemiological study of head injuries in nothern Italy: The commune of Ravenna. Neurosurg Rev [Suppl 1] 12:429–435
15. Vigouroux RP (1989) The organization of neurotraumatology in France. Neurosurg Rev [Suppl 1] 12:3–11

Disturbances of Water-Electrolyte Regulation After Surgery of the Hypothalamus and Pituitary Region

G. Hildebrandt and H.W. Mueller[1]

Introduction

Disorders of water-electrolyte balance frequently complicate the postoperative management of neurosurgical patients, mainly after surgery of the hypothalamus and the pituitary region [9]. In order to gain insight into the selection of optimal treatment, we tried to characterize this postoperative water-electrolyte dysregulation in a large patient population using newly available laboratory methods.

Patients and Methods

In 151 patients harboring hypothalamo-hypophyseal lesions, clinical and neuroradiological (CT/MRI) workups were performed preoperatively and 2–4 and 12 weeks postoperatively. There were 53% female and 47% male patients. Ages ranged from 5 to 81 years. The incidences of the different types of hypothalamo-hypophyseal lesions and the surgical approaches are shown in Table 1. Blood and urine samples were collected before operation, on postoperative days 1–10, and 3 and 12 months after operation. These were used to determine plasma antidiuretic hormone (ADH, normal values: 1.4 ± 0.1 pg/ml), serum aldosterone (8.5 ± 1.2 ng/dl), plasma atrial natriuretic factor (ANF, 43.7 ± 5.7 pg/ml), serum and urinary osmolality (S_{osmo}, 288 ± 5.4 mosmol/kg, U_{osmo}, 752 ± 206.2 mosmol/kg), sodium concentration (S_{Na^+}, U_{Na^+}), creatinine (S_{crea}, U_{crea}) and diuresis. In the early postoperative phase diuresis was assessed hourly for up to 72 h, S_{osmo} once and U_{osmo} twice per day up to the 10th postoperative day. To test the functional reserve of the antidiuretic system, osmotic stimulation by a 2-h infusion of hypertonic saline (5%) at a rate of 0.06 ml/kg body weight per minute was performed [11]. Patients over 50 years of age and those with cardiopulmonary risk factors were excluded from this test. Criteria for different types of postoperative diabetes insipidus (DI) are outlined in Table 2. According to Burrows et al. [1] patients were classified as having postoperative "syndrome of inappropriate secretion of ADH" (SIADH), when the following criteria were fulfilled: $S_{osmo} < 277$ mosmol/kg, $U_{osmo} > S_{osmo}$,

[1] Neurochirurgische Klinik der Justus-Liebig-Universität, Klinikstr. 29, W-6300 Giessen, FRG

Advances in Neurosurgery, Vol. 19
W. J. Bock, Ch. Lumenta, M. Brock, M. Klinger (Eds.)

Table 1. Incidence of hypothalamo-hypophyseal lesions and surgical approach in 151 patients

Diagnosis	Number of patients	Surgical Approach Transcranial	Transsphenoidal
Extra-arachnoid lesions			
Inactive adenomas	52	22	30
Active adenomas	33	11	32
Meningiomas	17	17	
Teratoma, chordoma, dermoid	5	5	
Pituitary hyperplasia	1		1
Intra-/extra-arachnoid lesions			
Craniopharyngioma	16	16	
Optic/hypothalamic gliomas	13	13	
Inflammatory lesions	4	2	2
Total	151	86	65

Table 2. Criteria for different types of postoperative diabetes insipidus

Type of diabetes insipidus	Criteria
I	Three-phase course[a]
II	Manifest[b], transition into latent[c] form
III	Manifest, normalization within 3 months
IV	Manifest for more than 12 months (permanent)
V	Manifest, normalization within 7–10 days

[a] Initial polyuria (manifest DI), normo-oliguria on postoperative days 3–7, permanent (manifest) DI subsequently

[b] ADH < 1 pg/ml, $U_{osmo} \leq S_{osmo}$, diuresis ≥ 5000 ml/24 h, no detectable level of ADH during infusion of hypertonic saline

[c] ADN < 1 pg/ml, $S_{osmo} < U_{osmo} = 1$ SD, diuresis < 5000 ml/24 h, at least one detectable level of ADH during infusion of hypertonic saline

renal fractional Na^+ excretion ($FE_{Na}{}^+$)[1] > 1.3% [2]. To assess the prolactin (PRL) secretory reserve of the residual anterior pituitary lobe, basal (b, 7.6 ± 0.06 ng/ml) and maximal (m, 48.8 ± 4.0 ng/ml) PRL levels after intravenous administration of 400 µg thyrotropin releasing hormone (Antepan, Henning) were measured pre- and 10–14 days postoperatively [3, 8]. Patients with PRL-secretion tumors were excluded from the evaluation of PRL. The levels of PRL, aldosterone, and ANF were assessed using commercially availably radioimmunoassays (RIA). ADH was measured in duplicate by a specific RIA (Incstar, IBL, Hamburg) after extraction of plasma with Sep-Pak C_{18} cartridges [3]. The lowest detectable level of ADH was 1.0 pg/ml. The results for S_{osmo}, U_{osmo} and $FE_{Na}{}^+$ were expressed as the mean (M) ± standard deviation (SD) and for all other data as M ± standard error of the mean (SEM). For statistical evaluation the Wilcoxon test, the Wilcoxon matched pairs signed rank test, and the χ^2 test for correctness of fit were used.

Results

The frequency or absence of postoperative DI and the severity and incidence of postoperative DI were determined by the operative approach and extent of tumor removal ($\chi^2 = 18.9$, $p = 0.002$, 5 d.f; Table 3). Decompression via the transsphenoidal route (65 procedures) was associated with a lower frequency of the more severe types of DI (7 patients), whereas the transcranial approach (86 procedures) caused a higher rate (33 patients). The 50 patients with no or only mild DI, as a group, had a significant drop in basal and maximal PRL levels compared with preoperative values (pre-vs. postoperative: PRL_b = 14.3– ± 1.5 ng/ml vs. 9.6– ± 1.1 ng/ml, $p < 0.05$; PRL_m = 31.4 – ± 2.9 ng/ml vs. 24.9 – ± 2.9 ng/ml, $p < 0.05$). In the 40 patients with more severe degrees of DI, PRL levels were significantly increased (prevs. postoperative: PRL_b O 15.3 – ± 3.1 ng/ml vs. 19.7 –± 3.4 ng/ml,

Table 3. Frequency and type of diabetes insipidus in relation to surgical cranial approach (151 patients)

Approach and extent of resection	Patients with no DI	Patients with DI type I	II	III	IV	V
Transsphenoidal						
total resection	15	1	1	3	4	5
subtotal resection	21	1				14
Transcranial						
total resection	9	3	1	4	10	5
subtotal resection	16	3	5	4	11	15

---

[1] $$FE_{Na}{}^+ = 100 \times \frac{U_{Na}{}^+ \times S_{Crea}}{S_{Na}{}^+ \times U_{Crea}}$$

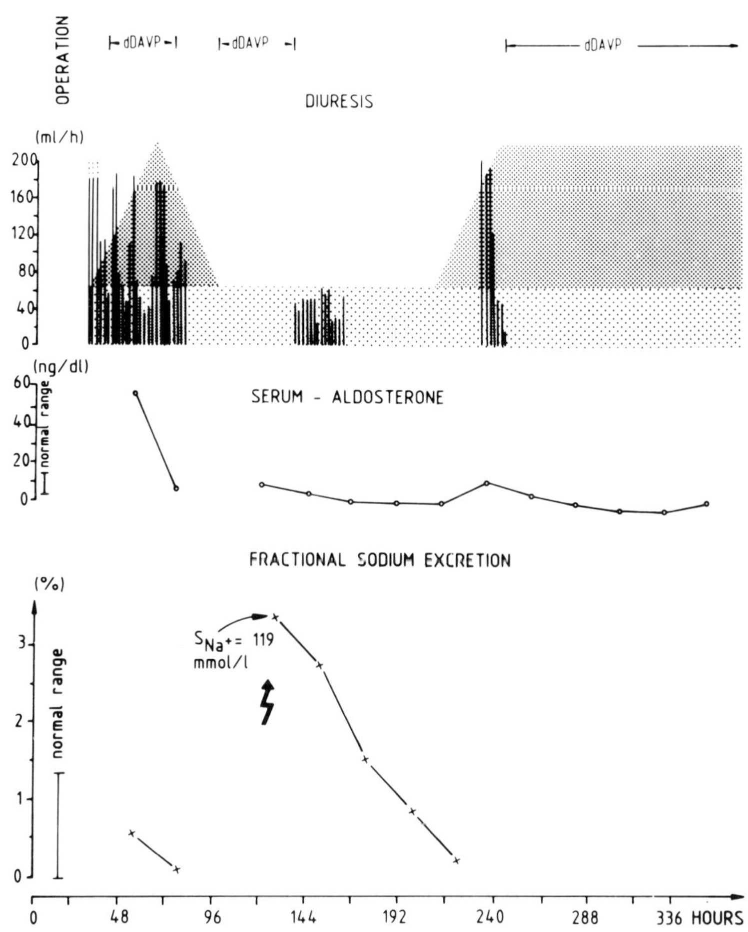

Fig. 1. Illustrative case report. The graphs outline the postoperative course of diuresis, serum aldosterone, and $FE_{Na}{}^{+}$ in an 8-year-old child in whom total decompression of a craniopharyngioma of the third ventricle was performed via the transcallosal approach. The child received dDAVP treatment in the immediate postoperative period because of severe polyuria. During the (normouric) interphase of a three-phase DI (outlined schematically by the *shaded area*), which was not recognized immediately, dDVAP treatment was continued and caused hypotonic hypervolemia, suppression of aldosterone, severe hyponatremia ($S_{Na}{}^{+}$ = 119 mmol/l), increased renal fraction Na^{+}excretion, and a grand mal seizure due to brain edema. The symptoms were reversed by fluid restriction, intravenous furosemide and interruption of dDAVP treatment until DI reappeared; it remained permanent.

$p < 0.05$; PRL_m 23.9 –± 7.6 ng/ml vs. 38.6 –± 7.9 ng/ml, $p < 0.05$). Extra-arachnoidal tumor growth was associated with more frequent absence of or presence of only mild postoperative DI, whereas in tumors with partial or complete loss of the arachnoid membrane as a plane of cleavage in the area of the infundibulum, the ratio was shifted to the more severe degrees of DI (ratio of no DI or types III, or V to types I, II, or IV in inactive adenomas 44:6, $p < 0.01$; in craniopharyngiomas

2:14, $p < 0.01$). Thirteen out of 151 patients fulfilled the laboratory criteria of SIADH, usually during the period from the 2nd to the 10th postoperative day. In eight cases hyponatremia, hypo-osmolality, and increased FE_{Na}^+ were caused by something other than an inappropriate increase of endogenous ADH. These patients all received treatment with an ADH analog (1-deamino-8-D-arginine vasopressin, dDAVP, half-life > 12 h) because of postoperative DI of various degrees (see illustrative case report, Fig. 1). In this group of patients ANF ranged within normal limits (48–62.7 pg/ml), whereas aldosterone had a tendency to decline compared with preoperative values. Only in 3% of cases was endogenous ADN inappropriately increased (1.4–17.5 pg/ml) in relation to adiminished S_{osmo}.

Discussion

According to our results, operative manipulations of tumorous lesions confined to the hypothalamus and the pituitary region are more frequently associated with neurohypophyseal dysregulation than with disturbances of sodium balance. In addition, the severity and incidence of postoperative DI is increased after a transcranial attempt at total removal of a lesion which has no plane of cleavage due to loss of the arachnoid. In addition to the neurohypophyseal system operation via the transcranial route may affect mainly the tuberoinfundibular dopaminergic system or the median eminence–portal venous vessel complex at the supradiaphragmatic level through direct or indirect mechanical injury, e.g. distortion of the pituitary stalk [3, 4]. On the basis of this observation and the fact that transsphenoidal decompression improves hypothalamic dopaminergic inhibitory control over the PRL secretion of the residual anterior pituitary lobe, whereas the transcranial approach worsens it [3, 4], the degree of postoperative DI may be predicted by comparison of pre- and postoperative basal and maximal PRL levels. This may be done even in the very early postoperative period, because stress-induced PRL increases return to baseline levels within 24 h after surgery [6].

In our series of 151 patients the postoperative frequency of true SIADH was as low as that observed by others [7]: 3%. More often it was associated with inappropriate dDAVP treatment, which caused hypervolemic hyponatremia through suppression of the renin-angiotensin-aldosterone system and increased loss of renal sodium [10]. This supports the view of Nelson et al. [5] that there is a spectrum of abnormalities in the hyponatremic, natriuretic patient from true SIADH to a salt-wasting syndrome. ANF has recently been brought into the context of SIADH [2], but this could not be substantiated by our results.

Conclusion

For practical purposes we suggest volume replacement as a first step in the management of postoperative DI, and administration of ADH analogs with shorter half-lives in cases where a severe degree of DI is predicted from PRL measurements

(PRL results may be obtained within 120 min using a microenzyme-linked immunosorbent assay). In dDAVP-induced hyponatremia the medication must be discontinued, with fluid restriction and occasionally the intravenous administration of furosemide. Administration of mineralocorticoids and/or hypertonic saline is of no value. In cases of true SIADH we agree with Reeder and Harbaugh [7] who recommend the intravenous administration of urea, lithium, phenytoin or demeclocycline as ADN antagonists.

References

1. Burrows FA, Shutack JG, Crone RK (1983) Inappropriate secretion of antidiuretic hormone in a postsurgical pediatric population. Crit Care Med 11:527–531
2. Cogan E, Debiève MF, Pepersack T, Abramov M (1986) High plasma levels of atrial natriuretic factor in SIADH. N Engl J Med 314:1258
3. Hildebrandt G (1989) Neuroendokrinologische Funktionsstörungen bei intrinsischen und extrinsischen Prozessen des hypothalamo-hypophysären Systems. Eine Untersuchung aus neurochirurgischer Sicht. *Habilitationsschrift,* University of Giessen
4. Maira G, Anile C, de Marinis L, Barbarino A (1989) Prolactin-secreting adenomas: surgical results and longterm- follow-up. Neurosurgery 24:736–743
5. Nelson PB, Seif SM, Maroon JC, Robinson AG (1981) Hyponatremia in intracranial disease: perhaps not the syndrome of inappropriate secretion of antidiuretic hormone (SIADH). J Neurosurg 55:938–941
6. Noel GL, Shuk HK, Stone IG, Frantz AG (1972) Human prolactin and growth hormone release during surgery and other conditions of stress. J Clin Endocrinol Metab 35:840–851
7. Reeder RF, Harbaugh RE (1989) Administration of intravenous urea and normal saline for the treatment of hyponatremia in neurosurgical patients. J Neurosurg 70:201–206
8. Stracke H, Schröder O, Bleyl H, Schatz H (1984) Assessment of definitive residual pituitary-adrenal function and of hydrocortisone replacement therapy 10 to 14 days after microsurgery for pituitary adenomas. Horm Metab Res 16:157–158
9. Tindall GT, Barrow DL (1986) Disorders of the pituitary. Mosby, St Louis, pp 451–471
10. Valkusz Z, Laczi F, Lászlo FA (1982) Development of the Schwartz-Bartter syndrome after the administration of chlorpropamide and 1-deamino-8-D-arginine vasopressin. Endokrinologie 79:345
11. Zerbe RL, Robertson GL (1981) A comparison of plasma vasopressin measurements with a standard indirect test in the differential diagnosis of polyuria. N Engl J Med 305:1539–1546

CBF Dynamics During Hyperventilation Therapy for Intracranial Hypertension

J. Meixensberger[1], A. Brawanski[1], M. Holzschuh[1], I. Danhauser-Leistner[2], and W. Ullrich[1]

Introduction

Induced hypocapnia is one of the main therapeutic tools in the treatment of intracranial hypertension: the reduction of intracranial pressure is added to a decrease in cerebral blood volume after vasoconstriction of pial vessels and arterioles [4]. On the other hand, the prognosis of head injured patients is certainly affected by secondary ischemic brain damage [3]. The present study was therefore undertaken to evaluate the hemodynamic effects of hyperventilation therapy after brain injury. We were especially interested in the following issues:

1. What is the course over time of cerebral blood flow (CBF) under conditions of induced hypocapnia?
2. Are there any differences in absolute global CBF values and the corresponding CO_2 reactivity of CBF?
3. Is there a risk of inducing a drop in CBF, causing ischemic brain damage? Can this risk vary over the course of time after head injury?

Patients and Methods

Our series comprises 30 patients, 18 male, 12 female. Their ages ranged from 7–79 years, with an average of 32.3 years. Twenty-five patients had a closed head injury with focal or diffuse brain injury and five had a spontaneous subarachnoid hemorrhage with or without intracerebral hematoma. On admission all patients had a Glasgow Coma Scale score of less than 8. After scanning by computed tomography (CT) to rule out the presence of a space-occupying hematoma, all patients were conservatively treated by sedation and automatic ventilation in our intensive care unit. Besides epidural monitoring of intracranial pressure (ICP), serial CT scans were performed to evaluate the nature and extent of brain injury over time.

A mobile unit for bedside measurements (Novo Cerebrograph 10a) with ten detectors, five placed over each hemisphere, was utilized for CBF measurements. Regional CBF was measured after intravenous administration of 10–15 mCi Xenon

[1] Neurochirurgische Klinik und Poliklinik der Universität Würzburg, Josef-Schneider-Str. 11, W-8700 Würzburg, FRG
[2] Anästhesiologisches Institut der Universität Würzburg, Josef-Schneider-Str. 11, W-8700 Würzburg, FRG

Advances in Neurosurgery, Vol. 19
W. J. Bock, Ch. Lumenta, M. Brock, M. Klinger (Eds.)

133. Regional CBF was calculated as the initial slope index (ISI) [7] by a bicompartmental model [5]. At various intervals (days 1–14) we performed two CBF measurements at different $PaCO_2$ levels in order to determine resting CBF under therapeutic conditions and the CO_2 reactivity of CBF. We calculated mean global CBF and determined mean global CO_2 reactivity as change in CBF per 1 mmHg change in $PaCO_2$. We assumed an upper normal limit for global CBF of 35 ml/100 g min (ISI) [2, 6] and a normal limit for CO_2 reactivity of 0.75 ml/100 g min per 1 mmHg change in $PaCO_2$ [1]. Additionally, we continuously monitored arterial blood pressure, determined arterial $PaCO_2$ blood gas content, and measured body temperature. Statistical analysis was done using the paired and unpaired Student's *t* test.

Results

Time Course of Global Resting CBF

Sixty measurements were taken under resting conditions at a $PaCO_2$ of 30.6 ± 2 mmHg (mean ± SD). The CBF data are given in Fig. 1. We found a reduced CBF according to Obrist' classification [6] in 52% of the measurements. In 48% of measurements we detected hyperemia. We calculated a global CBF of 43.6 ± 4.6 ml/100 g min (ISI) in the hyperemia group; the group with reduced CBF had a mean CBF of 29.1 ± 4.1 ml/100 g min (ISI). There were no significant differences between the two groups for $PaCO_2$, mean arterial blood pressure, hemoglobin, body temperature, age, and mean ICP.

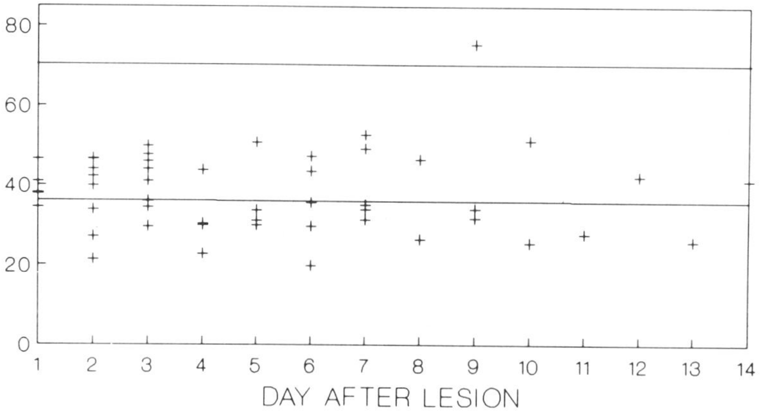

Fig. 1. Global resting CBF after brain injury. Normal range of global CBF 35–69 ml/100 g min (ISI) [2, 6]. Number of measurements = 60

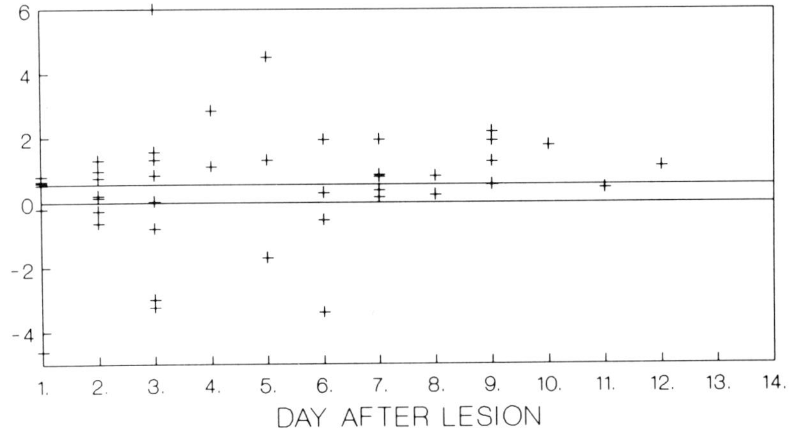

Fig. 2. Global CBF CO_2 reactivity after brain injury. CBF CO_2 reactivity calculated as induced change in CBF per 1 mmHg change in $PaCO_2$. Normal CBF CO_2 reactivity > 0.75 ml/100 g min (ISI) change in CBF per 1 mmHg in $PaCO_2$ [1]. Number of measurements = 52

Time Course of CBF CO2 Reactivity

The CO_2 reactivity of CBF was calculated 52 times. The mean change in $PaCO_2$ amounted to 6.7 mmHg; data are given in Fig. 2. Generally we detected reduced or inverse CBF CO_2 reactivity, usually in the first 8 days after injury, but normal cerebrovascular reactivity was also found in individual cases during this critical period of intracranial hypertension.

Correlation Between Global Resting CBF and CO_2 Reactivity

A total of 42 measurements made under resting and activation conditions were included. The correlation coefficient between the absolute global ISI values at rest and the values of CBF reactivity to induced change in $PaCO_2$ did not reach statistical significance ($r = 0.26$). We were unable to demonstrate any significant difference between the hyperemia group and the group with reduced CBF. In the hyperemia group we found normal CO_2 reactivity in 70.6% of cases and reduced reactivity in 29.4%, whereas in the group with reduced CBF 54.5% of cases had reduced and 45.5% had normal CO_2 reactivity (Fig. 3).

Risk of Inducing Decreased CBF Causing Ischemic Brain Damage

There is a risk of inducing a decreased CBF with hyperventilation combined with intact cerebrovasular CO_2 reactivity, which we found in 52% of our cases. Furthermore, absolute flow values seemed to be of importance. Table 1 summarizes results for patients with intact CO_2 reactivity in the hyperemia group and in the

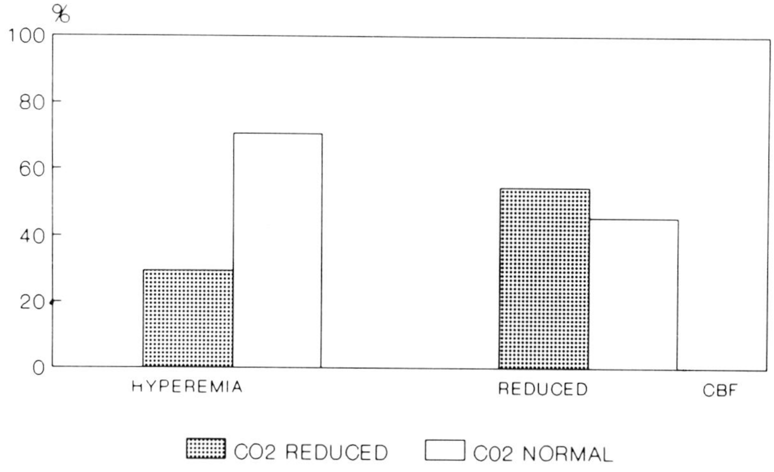

Fig. 3. Global resting CBF and CBF CO_2 reactivity. Percentage of cases of the hyperemia group and group with reduced CBF [1, 2, 6] with reduced and normal CO_2 reactivity

group with reduced CBF under increased hyperventilation to a $PaCO_2$ of 25 mmHg. Only in the group with reduced CBF (25% of our total cases) did we find decreased global CBF values, which may be causing ischemia in damaged brain.

Discussion

The prognosis for severe head injury depends on the primary lesion and on secondary brain damage [3]; intracranial hypertension during the course of brain edema influences cerebral perfusion pressure and finally CBF, causing a risk of secondary ischemic brain damage. On the other hand, a reduction of cerebral blood volume by hyperventilation is part of the conservative treatment of high ICP. In face of these two facts, one may ask whether the hemodynamic effects of hyperventilation increase the risk of ischemic brain damage, and how long hyperventilation should be maintained.

Analyzing our data regarding global CBF under induced hypocapnia to about 30 mmHg $PaCO_2$, we rarely found reduced absolute flow values close to the borderline of ischemia. However, we had already excluded a group of patients who can be at risk of ischemia under such treatment: hyperventilation of patients with reduced CBF and intact CBF CO_2 reactivity can reduce CBF to ischemic levels (Table 1). This risk increases if CO_2 reactivity is normal during the time after injury. We should therefore reflect critically upon the duration and extent of hyperventilation therapy given, in order to avoid additional ischemic brain damage. This is confirmed by the negative results of a clinical study in which prophylactic hy-

Table 1. Effect of increased hyperventilation on global CBF in the hyperemia group and the group with reduced CBF with normal CO_2 reactivity (mean values ± SD)

$PaCO_2$ (mmHg)	Hyperemia group (ml/100 g min)	Group with reduced CBF (ml/100 g min)
30.2 ± 2.4	42.4 ± 4.7	29.8 ± 4
25.2 ± 2.4	35.4 ± 4.7	22.8 ± 4

perventilation did not improve the outcome of patients [8]. Only carefully balanced hyperventilation therapy may possibly be a powerful tool in the treatment of intracranial hypertension.

References

1. Maximilian VA, Prohovnik I, Risberg J (1980) The cerebral hemodynamic response to mental activation in normo- and hypercapnia. Stroke 11:342–347
2. Messeter K, Nordström CH, Sundberg G, et al. (1986) Cerebral hemodynamics in patients with acute severe head trauma. J Neurosurg 64:231–237
3. Miller JD (1985) Head injury and brain ischemia – implications for therapy. Br J Anaest 57:120–129
4. Muizelaar JP, Van der Poel HG, Li Z, et al. (1988) Pial arteriolar vessel diameter and CO_2 reactivity during prolonged hyperventilation in the rabbit. J Neurosurg 69:923–927
5. Obrist WD, Thomson HK Jr, Wang HS, et al. (1975) Regional cerebral blood flow estimated by ^{133}Xenon inhalation. Stroke 6:245–256
6. Obrist WD, Langfitt TW, Jaggi JL, et al. (1984) Cerebral blood flow and metabolism in comatose patients with acute head injury. J Neurosurg 61:241–253
7. Risberg J, Ali Z, Wilson EM, et al. (1975) Regional cerebral blood flow by ^{133}Xenon inhalation. Preliminary evaluation of an initial slope index in patients with unstable flow compartments. Sroke 6:142–148
8. Ward JD, Choi S, Marmarou A, et al. (1989) Effects of prophylactic hyperventilation on outcome in patients with severe head injury. In: Hoff JT, Betz AL (eds) Intracranial Pressure VII. Springer, Berlin Heidelberg New York

THAM in Traumatic Brain Swelling: A Comparative Experimental and Clinical Study

M.R. Gaab, K. Seegers, R.J. Smedema, H.E. Heissler, and C. Goetz[1]

Abstract

The effect of the THAM on the indices of brain edema after trauma was investigated in animal experiments and clinical studies. In rats under artificial respiration, THAM was infused intravenously and its effects compared to those of equivalent doses of sodium bicarbonate and of phenobarbital. Six hours after trauma, brain water and sodium contents (wet–dry weight technique) in both traumatized and contralateral hemispheres had been best reduced by THAM. Potassium remained at almost normal levels with THAM.

In 80 patients with traumatic brain swelling, elevated ICP (> 25 mmHg) was alternately treated by THAM (18–36 g/100–200 ml, 1–2 h), mannitol (20%, 125–250 ml, 20–40 min), or sorbitol (40%, 70–140 ml, 20–40 min). The ICP was rapidly reduced by THAM; the maximum relative falls induced by THAM, mannitol, and sorbitol were identical (approx. 33%). The slopes of fall of ICP with THAM and mannitol were similar: with sorbitol the slope was steeper. The effect of THAM on ICP, however, lasted longer than that of osmotherapy. EEG recovery was more pronounced with THAM, as measured by computer analysis of the EEG. Blood plasma investigation (pH, PCO_2, osmolality, base excess) showed the effect of THAM not to be osmotic. The rise in pH base excess indicates an intracerebral buffering mechanism. The encouraging results of THAM treatment suggest carrying out a randomized clinical trial with this drug in patients suffering severe head injury.

Introduction

A reduction of intracerebral pressure (ICP) bei THAM (also called TRIS buffer, tromethamine, trametamol) was first shown in 1962 by Dos et al. [3] in animal experiments with hypercapnic intracranial hypertension. In 1976, Akioka et al. [1] found a drop in ICP, a recovery of EEG activity, and a restoration of cerebrovascular CO_2 reactivity in dogs with intracranial balloon inflation; in six patients with brain edema around tumors, a similar decrease in ICP was seen with 0.3 mol THAM injected intravenously [1]. In cats with cold brain lesions we found a rapid

---

[1] Neurochirurgische Klinik, Medizinische Hochschule Hannover, Konstanty-Gutschow-Str. 8, W-3000 Hannover 61, FRG

Advances in Neurosurgery, Vol. 19
W. J. Bock, Ch. Lumenta, M. Brock, M. Klinger (Eds.)

fall in ICP and a recovery in EEG activity which was better than with osmotherapy [4, 5, 9]. In patients with head injury, a reduction of ICP, a rise in cerebral perfusion pressure (CPP), and EEG improvement were also found [8, 9]. However, further than in these encouraging pilot studies, THAM has not yet systematically been investigated. We therefore tried to evaluate the possible role for THAM in treatment for head injury by further experimental and prospective clinical studies.

Materials, Patients, and Methods

Animal Experiments

In male SP rats with 250–300 g body weight, a freezing brain injury was induced in the right hemisphere by placing a cold copper stamp (5 x 6 mm) on the intact skull during anesthesia with 6–7 mg ketamine (Ketanest) intraperitoneally. Trauma was standardized using a stereotactic apparatus for identical trauma location and a constant freezing temperature of –73°C for 3 min. Animals were randomized for treatment with sodium bicarbonate (0.33 mmol/ml), with THAM (0.66 mmol/ml, equivalent buffering capacity [11]), or with phenobarbital (1 mg/ml initially, then 2 mg/5 ml per 6 h). Normal rats ("controls"), animals without therapy (respiration/edema) and with vehicle infusion (infusion mixture, 0.45% NaCL + 2.5% glucose = respiration/infusion) served as control groups [6, 7].

Treatment was started by a 1-ml bolus intravenous injection into the tail vein 5 min after injury followed by intravenous infusion (Perfusor) at a constant rate of 5 ml per 6 h. All animals were respirated (THAM depresses respiration [11]) with 70% N_2O and 30% O_2 (four rats simultaneously respirated with the Brackebusch respirator [2]).

Six hours after injury, the animals were decapitated. Water, sodium, and potassium contents of each brain hemisphere were measured (wet–dry weight technique; flame photometry [6, 7].

Clinical Study

Twenty-one patients with traumatic brain swelling documented by computed tomography (CT) and with an ICP of 25 mmHg or more were treated alternately with THAM, mannitol, or sorbitol infused intravenously. A total of drug doses were evaluated: 80 of THAM (18–36 g/100–200 ml, 1–2 h), 82 of 20% mannitol (125–250 ml, 20–40 min) and 40 of 40% sorbitol (70–140 ml, 20–40 min).

ICP was measured continuously with an epidural Gaeltec sensor and arterial blood pressure (SAP) with a temporal artery catheter [5]. In a subgroup of patients (see Fig. 3) EEG activity was continuously recorded (two channels, bipolar $F_3/P_3 - F_4/P_4$). All biosignals were evaluated using a computerized bedside neuromonitor [5]; in addition to time plots and frequency histograms, we calculated:

- Maximum relative fall in ICP (*d*% ICP)
- Maximum relative fall in SAP (*d*%SAP)
- Time at which minimum ICP and SAP occurred ($t\mathrm{ICP}_{min}$; $t\ \mathrm{SAP}_{min}$)
- Slope of ICP fall (*v*ICP, mmHg/min)
- Duration of ICP fall until 50% of preinfusion value regained (t_{fall}, min)

EEG activity was evaluated via fast Fourier transformation (compressed spectral array, chronospectra [5]); the absolute and relative power changes in the alpha, beta, theta and delta ranges were calculated.

For statistical analysis, the SPSS-X package version 3.3 was used.

Results

Animal Experiment

In the animals, 6 h after induction of cold lesions, a highly significant ($p < 0.001$) increase in water and sodium contents in both hemispheres was seen (Fig. 1a–d). The rise in water and sodium was much higher in the traumatized hemisphere than in the other. In animals on restricted fluids intake this edema formation was less than in rats receiving vehicle infusion ($p < 0.01$ on trauma side). The potassium contents decreased in the traumatized hemisphere after trauma, again more pronounced in the animals whose fluid intake was restricted than in those receiving vehicle infusion (Fig. 1e, f).

Administration of sodium bicarbonate did not significantly decrease water and sodium uptake. Only the loss of potassium was less in animals receiving bicarbonate than in those receiving vehicle infusion, but not significantly different to the potassium loss in animals on fluid restriction. A significant improvement in all variables, however, was seen with barbiturate therapy. THAM treatment had the best effect of the drugs investigated: it decreased the water and sodium uptake markedly and significantly. Potassium levels were even kept nearly normal (Fig. 1).

Clinical Study

In all patients but one, THAM, mannitol, and sorbitol all effectively reduced ICP and increased CPP with every infusion. The one exception was a male patient, 18 years old, who had a very high ICP (> 65 mmHg) and a CPP constantly below 30 mmHg; in this patient none of the drugs improved the ICP, indicating the presence of complete vasoparalysis.

The effects of THAM and mannitol on ICP were almost identical (Fig. 2): the maximum fall in ICP (*d*% ICP) was 33%–34% and occurred about 60 min after start of infusion. The drop in SAP too was similar with these two drugs (about 18%, often reduction of a hypertensive Cushing response). However, the mean duration of the reduced ICP was longer with THAM (79 min) than with mannitol (69 min), and the initial increase in SAP after osmotherapy resulting in a transient

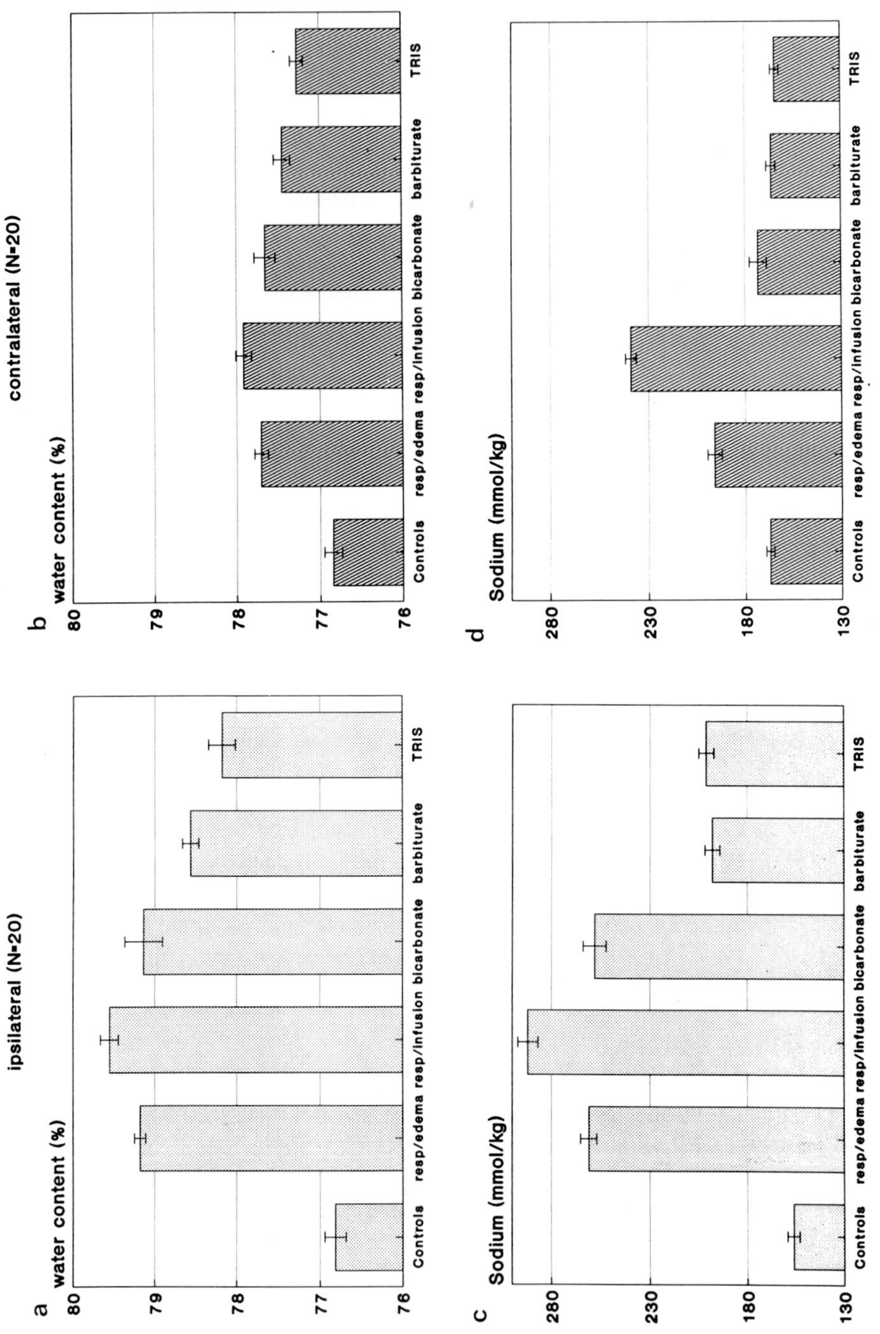
a
ipsilateral (N=20)
water content (%)
80
79
78
77
76
Controls
resp/edema
resp/infusion
bicarbonate
barbiturate
TRIS
b
contralateral (N=20)
water content (%)
80
79
78
77
76
Controls
resp/edema
resp/infusion
bicarbonate
barbiturate
TRIS
c
Sodium (mmol/kg)
280
230
180
130
Controls
resp/edema
resp/infusion
bicarbonate
barbiturate
TRIS
d
Sodium (mmol/kg)
280
230
180
130
Controls
resp/edema
resp/infusion
bicarbonate
barbiturate
TRIS

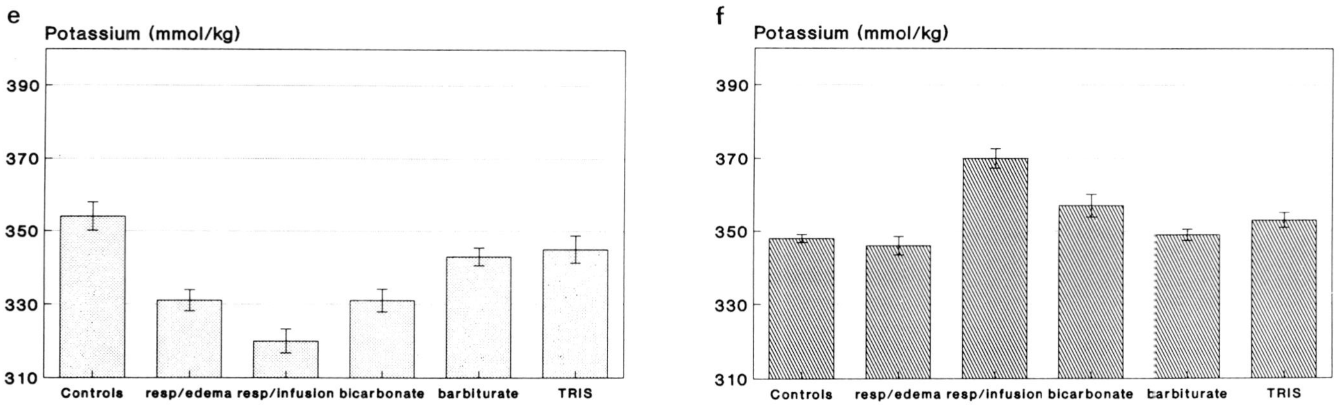

Fig. 1 a–f. Sodium bicarbonate, THAM, and phenobarbital in experimental brain edema. Best effect on sodium and water uptake produced by THAM (**a–d**), potassium preserved at almost normal levels. *Controls*, normal animals; *resp/edema*, trauma, fluid restriction; *resp/infusion*, trauma with infusion mixture

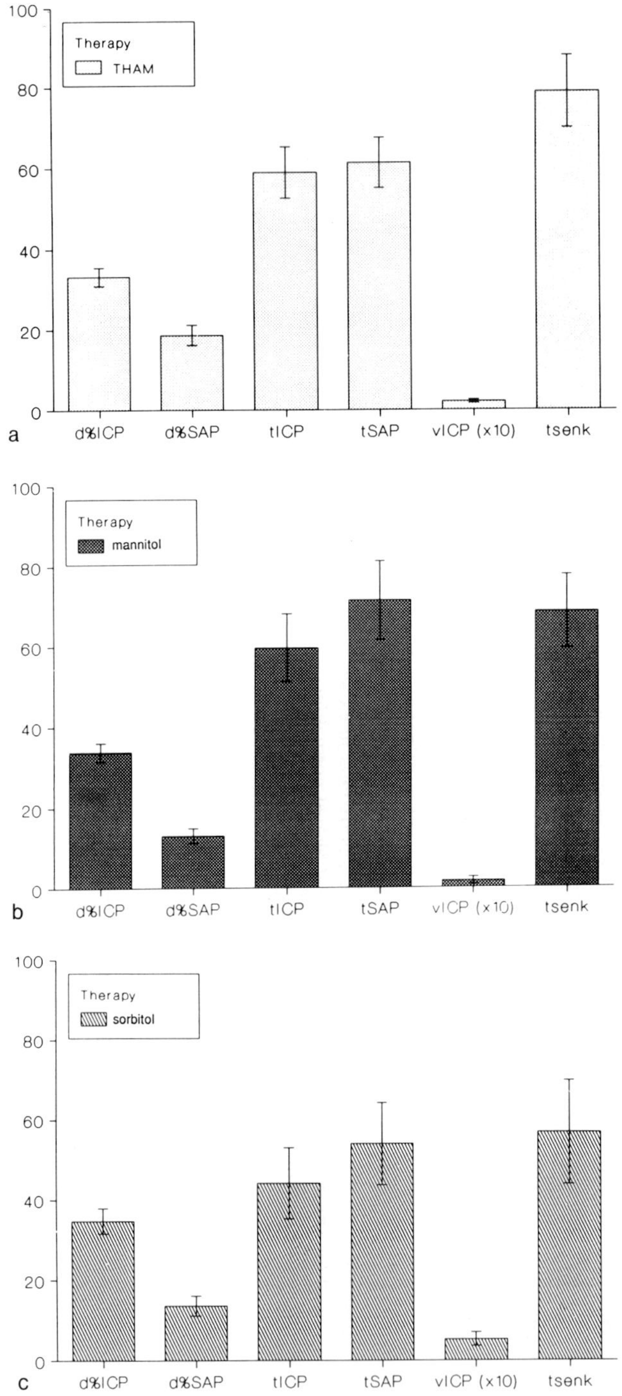

Fig. 2 a–c. Effect of THAM, mannitol, and sorbitol on ICP and SAP in patients with traumatic brain edema: THAM and mannitol have almost identical effect; fall in ICP steeper but shorter with sorbitol fall in CPP for about 10 min was not seen with THAM. The effect of sorbitol on ICP was shorter (mean 57 min) than those of THAM and mannitol. However, due to the high osmolality of sorbitol, the ICP fell about twice as steeply (0.52 mmHg/min) than with THAM (0.21 mmHg/min) or mannitol (0.17 mmHg/min).

In spite of this more dramatic effect on ICP of sorbitol, however, EEG improvement was faster and more pronounced with THAM (Fig. 3): Alpha- and beta wave power increased immediately after the start of THAM infusion, when ICP was still high, while, in contrast to the effect of sorbitol, slow wave activity significantly decreased.

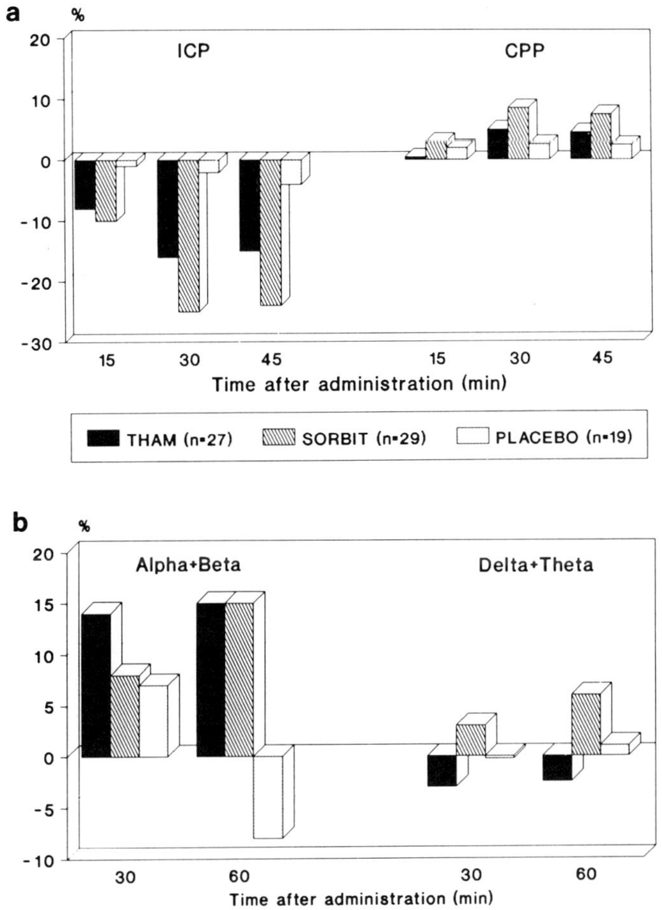

Fig. 3 a, b. Effect of THAM and sorbitol on **a** ICP and CPP and **b** EEG. Although the fall in ICP was steeper with sorbitol, the effect of THAM on ICP was more rapid and more pronounced. *Placebo*, infusion mixture

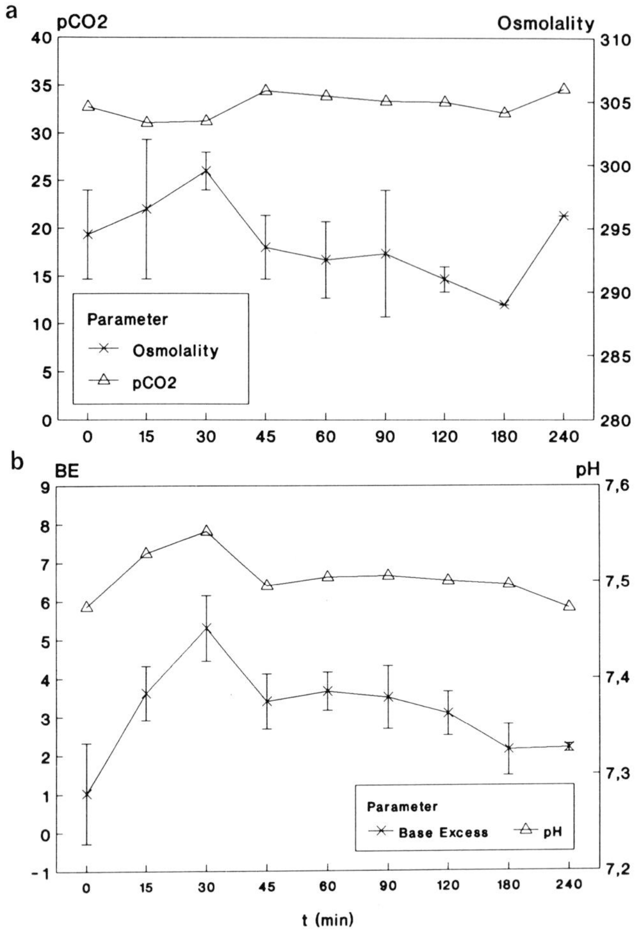

Fig. 4 a, b. THAM and blood parameters. **a** No significant change in osmolality or PCO_2. **b** Increase in pH and base excess

This effect of THAM cannot be attributed to osmotic dehydration, as is shown by the course of plasma osmolality (Fig. 4a). Blood PCO_2 was not significantly changed by THAM either, excluding CO_2-mediated vasoconstriction as the reason for the decrease in ICP. Apart from an already known hypoglycemic effect [11], we found only considerable changes in blood pH and base excess after administration of THAM (Fig. 4b). The significant increase in pH and more pronounced increase in base excess occurred parallel to the fall in ICP.

Discussion

According to our experimental and clinical results, THAM is a potent drug in the therapy of elevated ICP after trauma and also in preventing the formation of edema after head injury. Not only in our cold lesion model, which is not directly comparable to clinical brain contusion, but also after a fluid percussion trauma [13] THAM significantly improves the indices of edema such as water and sodium content. The preservation of almost normal potassium levels even in the directly traumatized hemisphere may indicate a protective effect on the neurons after injury [4, 6–8].

Clinically, THAM is at least equal to mannitol or sorbitol in the therapy of ICP after trauma. Compared to mannitol, it effects an almost identical improvement in ICP, often lasting longer, and in contrast to mannitol, the effect of THAM on ICP can be prolonged by continuing the infusion at a low rate (controls of blood base excess are essential). The reduction in ICP achieved with sorbitol is steeper but lasts for shorter than with THAM, while THAM has the better effect on the EEG, as an index of neuronal nutrition and activity. The rapid fall in ICP is not correlated to increasing blood osmolality, and especially the rapid EEG improvement suggests that THAM has a direct effect on the traumatized tissue. According to the increase in blood pH and the rise in base excess, a direct buffering action of THAM in the brain and especially in the edematous area is assumed. In contrast to bicarbonate, THAM rapidly crosses the blood-brain barrier [11, 12); recently Korn and coworkers succeeded in directly measuring brain tissue pH during THAM infusion, using implanted microelectrodes [10]; they found a steep increase in pH in the initially acidotic edematous brain tissue during THAM infusion, running parallel to the increase in blood pH. This direct intracerebral buffering also explains the depressive effect of THAM on respiration [11].

In a first pilot study, Rosner et al. [12] found not only a significant fall in ICP, but also an increased survival rate among head injury patients treated with THAM. The data on THAM treatment in head injury cases suggest that a larger prospective clinical trial should be carried out; we are presently preparing one with a multicenter group.

References

1. Akioka T, Ota K, Matsumoto A, Iwatsuki K, Doi A, Okao S, Nimomiya K, Nishimoto A (1976) The effect of THAM on acute intracranial hypertension. An experimental and clinical study. In: Beks JWF, Bosch DA, Brock M (eds) Intracranial pressure III. Springer, Berlin Heidelberg New York, pp 219–233
2. Brackebusch HD, Cunitz G, Lidl H, Weis KH (1974) Simultaneous ventilation of small animals by way of a time-controlled pressure generator. Pharmacology 11:241–246
3. Dos SJ, Nahas GG, Pappen EM (1962) Experimental correction of hypercapnic intracranial hypertension. Anesthesiology 23:46–50
4. Gaab MR, Knoblich OE, Spohr A, Böneke H, Fuhrmeister U (1980) Effect of THAM on ICP, EEG and tissue edema parameters in experimental and clinical brain edema. In:

Shulman K, Marmarou A, Miller JD, Becker DP, Hochwald GM, Brock M (eds) Intracranial Pressure IV. Springer, Berlin Heidelberg New York, pp 664–668
5. Gaab MR (1986) Routine computerized neuromonitoring. In: Miller JD, Teasdale GM, Rowan JO, Galbraith SL, Mendelow AD (eds) Intracranial pressure VI. Springer, Berlin Heidelberg New York, pp 240–247
6. Kerscher-Habbaba I (1984) Die Therapie des Hirnödems mit Phenobarbital und Dexamethason im Experiment. MD Thesis, Medical Faculty, University of Würzburg, Germany
7. Kesting U (1984) Therapie des experimentellen Hirnödems mit Natriumbikarbonat und THAM. MD Thesis, Medical Faculty, University of Würzburg, Germany
8. Knoblich OE, Gaab MR (1978) Comparison of the effects of osmotherapy, hyperventilation and THAM on brain pressure and EEG in experimental and clinical brain edema. In: Frowein RA, Wilcke O, Karimi-Nejad A, Brock M. Klinger M (eds) Advances in neurosurgery, vol. 5. Springer, Berlin Heidelberg New York, pp 336–345
9. Knoblich OE, Gaab MR (1978) Wirkung von Hyperventilation und THAM-Behandlung auf Hirndruck und elektrische Hirnaktivität im experimentellen Hirnödem. Neurochirurgia (Stuttg) 21:109–119
10. Korn A, Kepplinger F, Czech T, Urban G, Schuster H (1990) Continuous pH and potassium monitoring in brain parenchyma and blood. Eigth international symposium on brain edema, Berne, 17–20 June 1990
11. Nahas GG (1986) The clinical pharmacology of THAM. Clin Pharm Ther 4:784–803
12. Rosner MJ, Elias KG, Coley I (1989) Prospective, randomized trial of THAM therapy in severe brain injury: preliminary results. In: Hoff JT, Betz AL (eds) Intracranial pressure VII. Springer, Berlin Heidelberg New York, pp 611–616
13. Yoshida K, Corwin F, Marmarou A (1990) The effect of THAM on brain edema in experimental brain injury. Eigth international symposium on brain edema, Berne, 17–20 June 1990

Effects of the Antihypertensive Drug Ketanserin on Intracranial Pressure in Patients with Head Trauma

L. Heytens[1,2], J. Verlooy[2], C. De La Porte[2], M. Van Vyve[2], P. Selosse[2], and L. Bossaert[1]

Introduction

Neurotraumatized patients are often hypertensive. Their elevated blood pressure generally results from increased activity of the autonomic nervous system – i.e. a hyperadrenergic state – and is most often accompanied by an increased heart rate and elevated cardiac output. Other clinical patterns such as the Cushing's response of bradycardia and hypertension also occur.

Sudden and serious hypertension has to be avoided in patients with severe head trauma, as autoregulation may be impaired so that compensatory arteriolar constriction in response to elevated blood pressure does not occur. The excessively elevated cerebral perfusion pressure in turn can lead to the exacerbation of edema formation, vascular engorgement, and increased intracranial pressure [3].

The widely used vasodilating antihypertensive drugs such as nitroprusside and hydralazine can cause cerebral vasodilation with subsequent increase in cerebral blood volume and possibly intracranial pressure. These drugs are therefore best avoided in patients with head trauma. Adrenergic blocking drugs such as propranolol (β blocker) and labetalol (α and β blocker) are considered safer. As the number of these drugs usable in this setting is still very limited, however, it seems worth evaluating the use of the newer antihypertensive drugs for treatment of hypertension after head trauma.

The aim of this study was to evaluate whether ketanserin – a serotonin S_2-antagonist and short-acting antihypertensive drug – can be safely used in patients with and without intracranial hypertension after neurotrauma. This idea was based on a study by Van Aken et al. [5] published in 1984 in *Critical Care Medicine* in which ketanserin was shown not to influence intracranial pressure or compliance in dogs and was thus considered to be probably safe in neurosurgical patients.

Patients and Methods

Fifteen patients with head injury admitted to our Neurosurgical Intensive Care Unit were included in the study. Their ages ranged between 12 and 75 years, but most

[1] Department of Intensive Care, University Hospital Antwerp, Wilrijkstraat 10, B-2520 Antwerp, Belgium
[2] Department of Neusorugery, University Hospital Antwerp, Wilrijkstraat 10, B-2520 Antwerp, Belgium

Advances in Neurosurgery, Vol. 19
W. J. Bock, Ch. Lumenta, M. Brock, M. Klinger (Eds.)

($n = 9$) were between 12 and 17 years old. They were all comatose (Glasgow Coma Scale scores between 4 and 9) and hemodynamically stable at the time of the study, which was carried out on the 2nd–4th days after the injury. Patients with space-occupying intracranial hematomas that needed to be evacuated were excluded. Intracranial pressure monitoring by intraventricular catheter had already been instituted because of clinical or radiological suspicion of posttraumatic intracranial hypertension. Consent was obtained from next of kin.

Intracranial pressure had to have been stable for at least 1 h before patients were entered in the study. All patients were breathing spontaneously, usually through an endotracheal tube. Pretest PCO_2 values were between 34 and 40 mmHg. Temperature ranged from 36.4° to 38°C. A bolus of ketanserin 0.1 mg/kg body weight was injected intravenously over 10 s. Heart rate, mean arterial pressure, central venous pressure and intracranial pressure were measured just prior to and 1, 2, 3, 4, 5, 6, 10, 15, 30 and 60 min after injection. Cerebral perfusion pressure was calculated by subtracting intracranial pressure from mean arterial pressure.

All measurements after the administration of ketanserin were statistically compared to the pretest values using Student's t test; p values below 0.05 were taken to indicate a significant difference.

Results

The 0.1 mg/kg dosage resulted in a decrease in mean arterial pressure from a baseline value of 102.7 ± 8.0 mmHg to 84.6 ± 6.3 mmHg at 1 min (all results expressed as mean ± SD); the difference was statistically significant at all time intervals ($p < 0.0001$). This decrease in mean arterial pressure was accompanied by a small increase in heart rate from 94.1 ± 15.6 to 101.3 ± 17.7 bpm; this difference was statistically significant at 1 min only ($p < 0.05$). There was also a slight decrease in central venous pressure, from 4.5 ± 2.9 mmHg to a minimum of 3.5 ± 2.6 mmHg at 1 h ($p < 0.01$).

Intracranial pressure (range 4–30 mmHg) rose from 11.3 ± 7.1 to 13.6 ± 6.9 mmHg ($p < 0.05$) at 1 min. The difference was statistically significant at 1 min only and not thereafter. The increase in intracranial pressure, however, was of different magnitude in the individual patients; an increase of more than 5 mmHg was seen in four patients and lasted between 5 and 60 min. The mean baseline intracranial pressure in these four patients was not significantly different from the reference intracranial pressure of the other 11 patients (9.3 ± 2.9 versus 12.0 ± 7.1 mmHg).

Cerebral perfusion pressure was also significantly reduced from a baseline mean of 91.7 ± 11.2 to a minimum of 71 ± 10.4 mmHg after 1 min, and leveled out at around 7 mmHg thereafter ($p < 0.0001$ for all intervals).

Discussion

Ketanserin, the first selective serotonin S_2-antagonist, has been shown to be an effective antihypertensive drug that can be suitable combined with diuretics or β blockers. A single intravenous dose reduces systolic and diastolic blood pressure within a few minutes, the magnitude of the effect being dependent upon the severity of the hypertension. Ketanserin lowers blood pressure by reducing systemic vascular resistance and has some α_1-adrenoceptor blocking effects [4]. Intravenous administration of ketanserin was found to be useful in controlling perioperative hypertension and also in treating postoperative shivering [2].

Many authors recommend the treatment of hypertension after head injury in order to minimize edema formation and brain swelling. However, considerable controversy exists concerning the ideal blood pressure in this setting, and some investigators in fact tolerate elevated cerebral perfusion pressures (83].

The use of vasodilating drugs such as nitroprusside, nitroglycerin, and hydralazine for treatment of hypertension after head injury may in itself be deleterious, as cerebral vasodilation leads to an increase in cerebral blood volume and this in turn may lead to elevated intracranial pressure. As mean arterial pressure decreases and intracranial pressure increases cerebral perfusion pressure can drop to an unacceptably low level. Antihypertensive drugs therefore have to be carefully evaluated before they can be recommended for general use – e.g., in patients without intracranial pressure monitoring – after head trauma.

Ketanserin has vasodilating properties but has been shown not to influence intracranial pressure in two animals studies. In 1984 Van Aken et al. [5] demonstrated that ketanserin 1 mg/kg body weight reduced blood pressure without influencing intracranial pressure or intracranial compliance in two groups of dogs, one without and one with intracranial hypertension. From this study it was concluded that ketanserin might be a safe antihypertensive drug in neurosurgical patients.

In a study in cats, Auer et al. [1] demonstrated that serotonin itself has a dual effect on cerebral arteries, i.e., dilatation of the small arteries and constriction of arteries wider than 2000 μm. In the same study ketanserin – the serotonin antagonist – induced dilatation of the larger arteries but did not induce the expected vasoconstriction in the smaller pial arteries. It was concluded from further experiments with ketanserin and/or its solvent alone that part of the theoretically expected constriction of the small pial arteries was antagonized by a dilatatory effect of the solvent and/or by the autoregulatory dilatation in answer to the fall in blood pressure. In this study, too, intracranial pressure did not increase after injection of ketanserin.

In the present study ketanserin was found to be an effective antihypertensive agent in these patients, with a statistically significant drop in mean arterial pressure during the whole 1-h observation period. The baseline mean arterial pressure was only moderately elevated, a fact mainly due to the very young age of most patients. In each individual patient, however, we considered correction of the hypertension to slightly supranormal values necessary. An increase in heart rate was also observed but certainly not such as to give rise to clinical concern. The drop in central venous pressure was probably the result of the vasodilatory effects of the drug.

At first sight the small increase in intracranial pressure – by a mean of only 2.3 mmHg – does not seem to be of clinical relevance. It is important, however, to note that 4 of the 15 patients tested showed an increase in intracranial pressure greater than 5 mmHg, an effect lasting up to 60 min. This was considered to be clinically relevant, and we in fact interrupted the study because of this finding: originally we had planned to investigate a total of 20 patients but because of this result we only evaluated 15. Since we did not measure intracranial compliance – a technical act in itself not devoid of potential deleterious effects in patients with head trauma – we cannot speculate on the possible influence of differences in baseline compliance on the effect of the injection of ketanserin on intracranial pressure.

Obviously, as mean arterial pressure decreased and intracranial pressure slightly increased, cerebral perfusion pressure also decreased significantly. In a few patients with high baseline intracranial pressure, to which we thought that the hypertension might contribute, cerebral perfusion pressure dropped to around 60 mmHg, a value we consider to be too low.

We conclude that ketanserin is an effective antihypertensive agent in patients with head trauma. It can, however, probably via its vasodilatory effects, induce an increase in intracranial pressure, at least in some patients, and should therefore be used very cautiously in patients with head trauma.

References

1. Auer LM, Leber K, Sayama I (1985) Effects of serotonin and its antagonist ketanserin on pial vessels. J Cereb Blood Flow Metab 5:517–521
2. Nalda MA, Gomar C, Luis M (1985) The effect of ketanserin on post-anaesthetic vasoconstriction and shivering. Eur J Anaesthesiol 2:265–277
3. Simard JM, Bellefleur M (1989) Systemic arterial hypertension in head trauma. Am J Cardiol 63:32C–35C
4. Symoens J, Janssens M (1986) Ketanserin: a novel cardiovascular drug. Drug Dev Res 8:159–172
5. Van Aken H, Anger C, Puchstein M, Thijs J, Lawin P (1984) Influence of ketanserin, an antihypertensive agent with specific 5-HT_2-receptor blocking activity, on intracranial pressure. Crit Care Med 12(1):4–7

A Comparison Between Mannitol and Glycerol Therapy for Intracranial Hypertension

R.J. Smedema and M.R. Gaab[1]

Introduction

The treatment of intracranial hypertension is still the subject of discussion [4]. In our neurosurgical intensive care unit intracranial pressure (ICP) is routinely monitored with a miniaturized epidural transducer (Gaeltec ICT/b transducer) [6]. After surgically treatable causes of intracranial hypertension have been ruled out, basic therapy consists of elevation of the upper part of the body and artificial ventilation with moderate hyperventilation (arterial PCO_2 between 30 and 35 mmHg). When ICP can not be kept below 25 mmHg, additional drug therapy is started. We use osmotic diuretics and TRIS buffer [4].

The aim of this study was to compare the effectiveness of two different osmotic diuretics in the treatment of intracranial hypertension.

Patients and Methods

Fourteen patients from our intensive care unit, all intubated and under sedation, were studied. Seven of them had head injuries and seven had undergone supratentorial craniotomy and tumor extirpation. There were nine male and five female patients; ages ranged from 21 to 55 years.

ICP was continuously monitored, in 12 patients via a miniaturized epidural pressure transducer and in two via a ventricular catheter connected to a pressure transducer. Drift in both systems, which was quite small, was corrected twice a day.

Together with ICP, systemic blood pressure was monitored, either continuously or at 15-min intervals. Arterial blood gases were frequently evaluated to maintain arterial PCO_2 between 30 and 35 mmHg. Serum electrolytes and glucose were intermittently measured and corrected, if necessary. Fluid balance was corrected several times a day. Treatment with an osmotic diuretic was started when ICP exceeded 25 mmHg for 10 min or more.

The following regimens were compared:

1. Mannitol 20% 0.5 g/kg intravenously in 30 min
2. Glycerin 10% 0.5 g/kg intravenously in 60 min
3. Glycerol 85% 0.7–0.75 g/kg through a nasogastric tube

[1] Neurochirurgische Klinik, Medizinische Hochschule Hannover, Konstanty-Gutschow-Str. 8, W-3000 Hannover 61, FRG

Advances in Neurosurgery, Vol. 19
W. J. Bock, Ch. Lumenta, M. Brock, M. Klinger (Eds.)

The 85% glycerol solution was mixed with an equal volume of an 0.9% saline solution. Absence of bowel sounds was not a contraindication to the use of this regimen. The regimens were employed randomly. In all, 102 treatments were given that could be further analyzed, which was done using SAS statistic procedures (SAS Institute Inc., version 6.03). The criterion of significance was p value below 0.05.

Results

Figure 1 shows the results for the time from the start of treatment to the first visible reduction in ICP. The mean time lags were 8.1 min for intravenous glycerol, 9.5 min for intravenous mannitol, and 11.4 min for oral glycerol. There was no significant difference between these. In some cases ICP occurred much later than the average, especially the case in the oral glycerol group.

Figure 2 depicts the results for the delay between the start of treatment and the lowest recorded pressure. The mean values varied between 45.9 min for intravenous mannitol and 57.5 min for oral glycerol, which was not significantly different.

In Fig. 3 the maximum reduction of ICP is shown as a percentage reduction of the initial pressure. The greatest reduction (by a mean of 51%) was obtained in the oral glycerol group. In the intravenous glycerol group a mean reduction of 48.3% was calculated. Both these values differed significantly from the mean value in the intravenous mannitol group (32.6%).

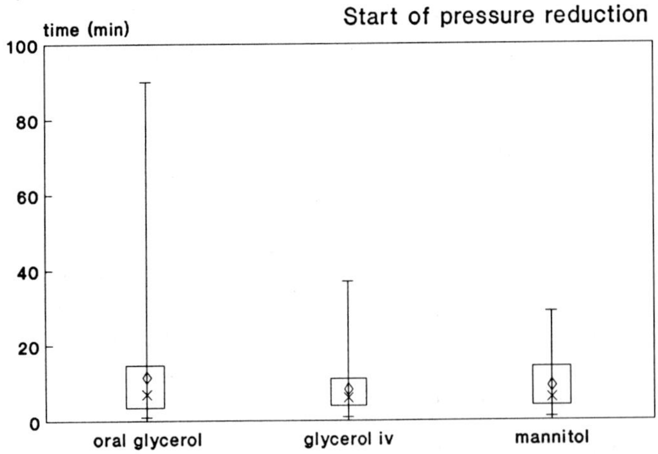

Fig. 1. Start of ICP reduction. No significant differences. In these box and whisker graphs (Figs. 1–4) the mean is represented by a *diamond* and the median by an *x*. The *box* represents the range from the first to the third quartile. The *whiskers* cover the range from the minimum to the maximum value

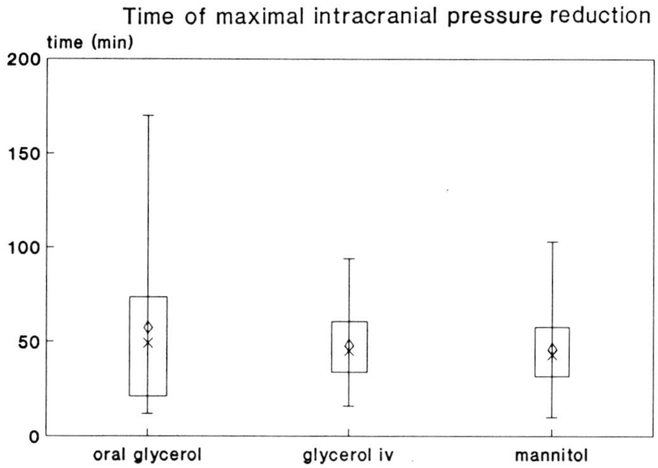

Fig. 2. Time from start of treatment to lowest recorded ICP. No significant differences

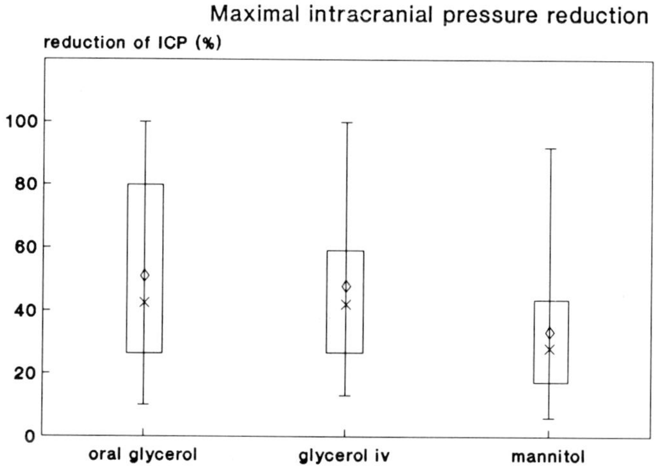

Fig. 3. Maximum ICP reduction. Significantly better results for orally and intravenously administered glycerol

Figure 4 represents the time from the start of treatment to the point at which ICP regained its initial level. The effect of treatment in the oral glycerol group (mean time 201.2 min) lasted significantly longer than the effect in the intravenous glycerol and intravenous mannitol groups (mean times 147.3 and 134.1 min respectively). In some patients in the oral and intravenous glycerol groups, pressure reduction lasted up to 6 h.

In the 102 treatments, ICP increased three times, once in each treatment group. In the oral glycerol group the increase in ICP was the result of the patient's vomiting after the mixture was administered through the nasogastric tube.

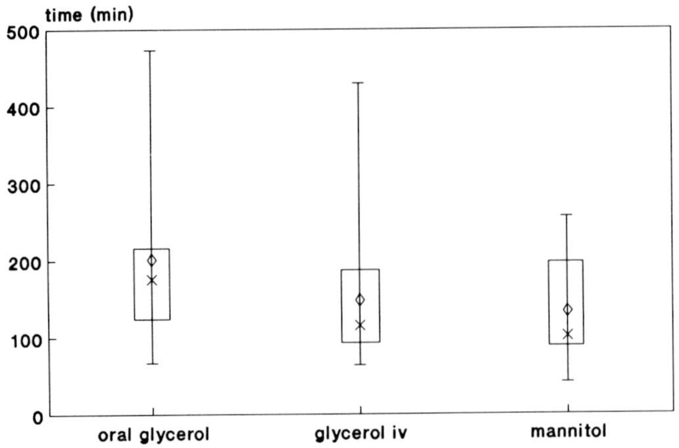

Fig. 4. Duration of ICP reduction. Significant results for orally administered glycerol only

We also recorded cases in which ICP did not change at all: there were five in the mannitol group (21%), two in the intravenous glycerol group (6%) and three in the oral glycerol group (9%).

Discussion

Osmotic diuretics decrease ICP and cerebral edema through dehydrating normal brain tissue by establishing an osmotic gradient across the blood–brain barrier. In addition, a possible decrease in blood viscosity resulting in vasoconstriction and decrease in cerebral blood volume is under discussion [12]. Mannitol is the main representative of this group of diuretics [13]. To reduce ICP it must be given intravenously [16]. It is inert, causes almost no toxic reactions, and is eliminated by renal excretion [8]. Alternatively, glycerol can be used [4, 8, 13]. Its value in reducing ICP has often been described [1, 5, 14, 15). Glycerol can be given orally and intravenously and is largely metabolized [9]. Rapid rates of administration and high concentrations can lead to hemolysis [13]. Neither of these two substances crosses the intact blood–brain barrier [2, 3].

The precise dosage requirements of osmotic diuretics are still matter of debate [8, 11, 13]. We prefer small dosages, e.g. 0.5 g/kg body weight over 30 min [4], except in acute situations.

In this study we compared the effects of equivalent intravenous doses of mannitol and glycerol; to prevent hemolysis the infusion time for glycerol was set at double that for mannitol.

Unlike MacDonald and Uden [10], who concluded that a 20% mannitol solution and a 20% glycerol solution were equally effective in lowering ICP, we found a significantly better reduction of pressure in the intravenous glycerol group, even with the lower glycerol concentration of 10%. However, we agreed with these authors in finding the duration of effect equally long with both.

In comparison with the intravenous regimens, glycerol given by the oral route caused a significantly greater reduction of pressure within the same time interval. The duration of action was significantly longer.

These results may be explained by the amount of osmoles given in each therapy regimen, as has been proposed by Hase and Reulen [7].

Only minor changes in fluid balance and serum electrolytes were observed in the three groups. The intravenous administration of glycerol was not complicated by hemolysis.

Conclusion

1. Comparing the effects of 10% glycerol given intravenously, 85% glycerol given orally, and 20% mannitol given intravenously, we observed a greater and/or longer lasting pressure reduction with the glycerol solutions.
2. Orally administered glycerol proved to be potent in reducing intracranial hypertension in brain-injured patients or after craniotomy.

Acknowledgment. The autors thank H.E. Heissler for his statistical analysis.

References

1. Cantore G, Guidetti B, Virno M (1964) Oral glycerol for the reduction of intracranial pressure. J Neurosurg 21:278–283
2. Crone C (1965) The permeability of brain capillaries to non-electrolytes. Acta Physiol Scand 64:407–417
3. De los Reyes RA, Ausman JI, Diaz FG (1980) Agents for cerebral edema. Clin Neurosurg 28:98–107
4. Gaab MR (1985) Einfluß der Intensivbehandlung auf das zerebrale Verhalten bei Schädel-Hirn-Trauma. In: Henschel WF (ed) Organfunktion unter Intensivtherapie. Zuckschwerdt, Munich, pp 34–60
5. Gaab M, Pflughaupt KW (1977) Experimentelle und klinische Untersuchungen zur intravenösen Glyzerintherapie beim Hirnödem. Acta Neurochir (Wien) 37:17–31
6. Gaab M, Knoblich OE, Fuhrmeister U (1979) Miniaturisierte Methoden zur Überwachung des intrakraniellen Druckes. Langenbecks Arch Chir 350:13–31
7. Hase U. Reulen HJ (1980) Wirkung von Sorbit und Mannit auf den intrakraniellen Druck. Neurochirurgia (Stuttg) 23:205–211
8. Heinemeyer G (1987) Clinical pharmacokinetic considerations in the treatment of increased intracranial pressure. Clin Pharmacokinet 13:1–25
9. Lin ECC (1977) Glycerol utilization and its regulation in mammals. Annu Rev Biochem 46:765–775
10. MacDonald JT, Uden DL (1982) Intravenous glycerol and mannitol therapy in children with intracranial hypertension. Neurology (NY) 32:437–440
11. Marshall LF, Smith RW, Rauscher LA, Shapiro HM (1978) Mannitol dose requirements in brain-injured patients. J Neurosurg 48: 169–172
12. Muizelaar JP, Lutz HA, Becker DP (1984) Effect of mannitol on ICP and CBF and correlation with pressure autoregulation in severely head-injured patients. J Neurosurg 61:700–706

13. Quandt CM, de los Reyes RA (1984) Pharmacologic management of acute intracranial hypertension. Drug Intell Clin Pharm 18:105–112
14. Tourtelotte WW, Reinglas JL, Newkirk TA (1972) Cerebral dehydration action of glycerol. I. Historical aspects with emphasis on the toxicity and intravenous administration. Clin Pharmacol Ther 13:159–171
15. Wald SL, McLaurin RL (1982) Oral glycerol for the treatment of traumatic intracranial hypertension. J Neurosurg 56:323–331
16. Warren SE, Blantz RC (1981) Mannitol. Arch Intern Med 141:493–497

Decompressive Craniectomy After Severe Head Injury: Useful Therapy in Pathophysiologically Guided Indication

M. Rittierodt, M.R. Gaab, and M. Lorenz[1]

Introduction

The indication for and operative technique and efficiency of decompressive craniectomy after severe head injury are still matters of controversy [1, 4–7). Operative decompression is often performed only on the basis of computed tomography (CT) and the patient's clinical course, without definite proof of the presence of uncontrollable intracranial hypertension [1, 5, 6]. Poor outcomes are often the result of extremely severe primary brain injury, e.g., with primary bulbar syndrome [1, 5]. Regarding operative technique, small subtemporal craniotomies are often used, following Cushing's method [2]. Small bone flaps, however, do not reliably reduce the intracranial pressure and may produce local brain incarceration with bridge vein compression. We therefore use a large bifrontal or frontal-parieto-temporal decompressive craniectomy with a wide dura opening. The indication is based on clinical status, continuous ICP monitoring, and on additional electrophysiological data. The results are encouraging.

Patients and Methods

From 1978 to 1990 cranial decompressive craniectomy was carried out in 37 patients aged 4–34 years (26 male, 11 female; interval between injury and operation 5 h to 10 days; 18 unilateral and 19 bilateral decompressive craniectomies). The indication for operation was based on the following:

- Younger age (at first ≤ 30 years, now ≤ 40 years)
- No deleterious primary brain damage
- No space-occupying lesion (hematoma, focal contusion, hygroma, ventricular enlargement) which could be directly operated upon
- No large infarction areas visible on CT
- ICP not controllable by conservative methods and cerebral perfusion pressure (CPP) falling below 40–50 mmHg
- Intracranial hypertension *associated with* clinical and electrophysiological deterioration (CT, Glasgow Coma Scale, mydriasis, EEG, sensory evoked potentials, brain stem auditory evoked potentials); in recent years also deterioration on

[1] Neurochirurgische Klinik, Medizinische Hochschule Hannover, Konstanty-Gutschow-Str. 8, W-3000 Hannover 1, FRG

Advances in Neurosurgery, Vol. 19
W. J. Bock, Ch. Lumenta, M. Brock, M. Klinger (Eds.)

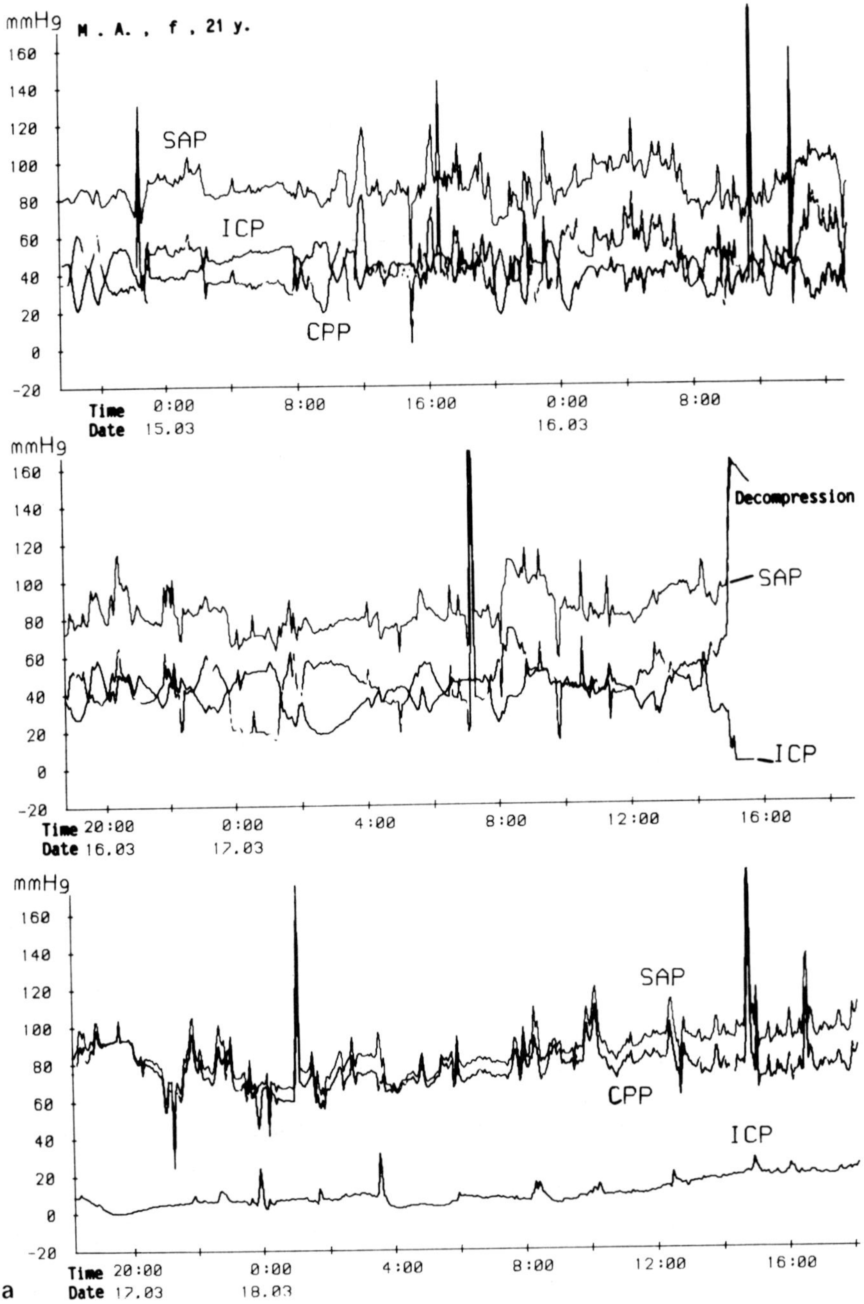
mmHg
M. A., f, 21 y.
160
140
120
100
80
60
40
20
0
-20
SAP
ICP
CPP
Time 0:00 8:00 16:00 0:00 8:00
Date 15.03 16.03
mmHg
Decompression
SAP
ICP
Time 20:00 0:00 4:00 8:00 12:00 16:00
Date 16.03 17.03
mmHg
SAP
CPP
ICP
Time 20:00 0:00 4:00 8:00 12:00 16:00
Date 17.03 18.03

a

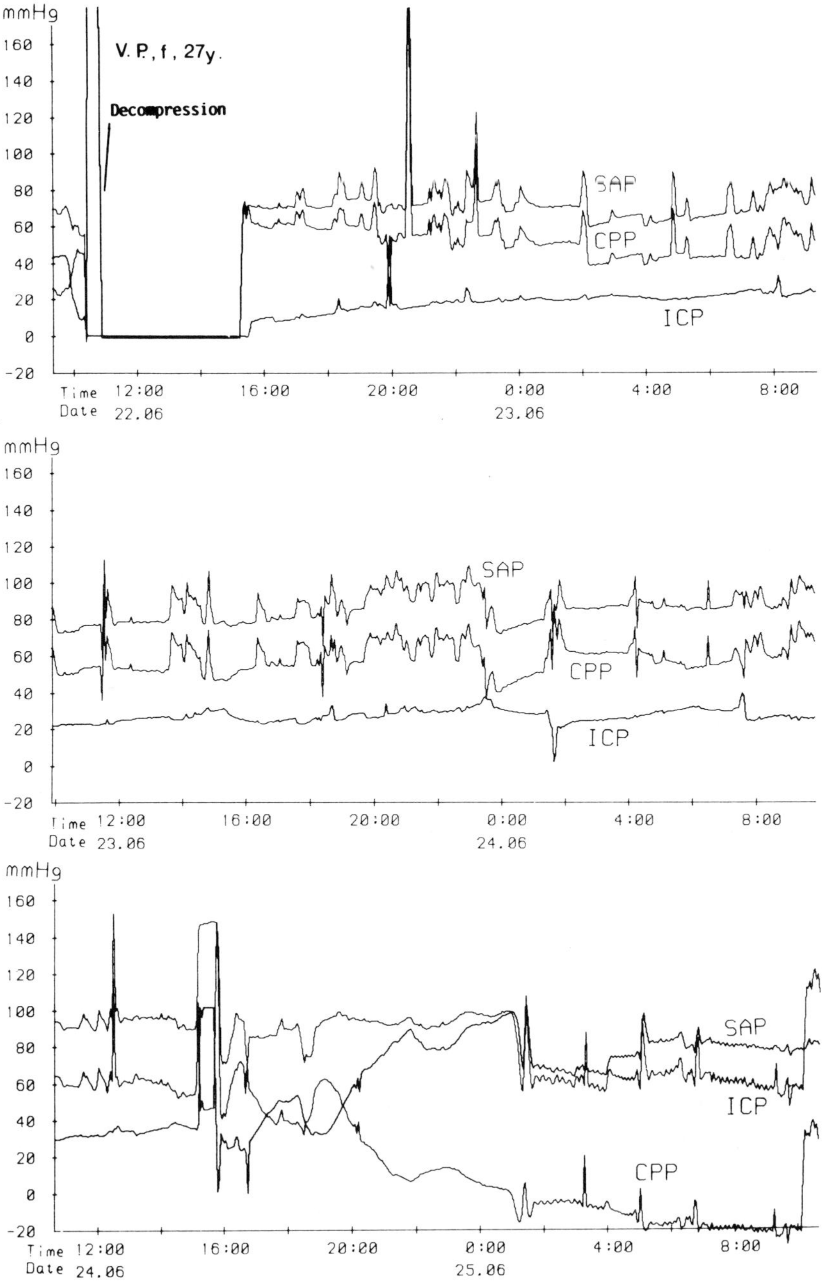

b

Fig. 1. a Permanent normalization of ICP and CPP after timely operative decompression; full rehabilitation. **b** ICP decompensation and complete cerebral ischemia despite decompression – operation too late and patient died

transcranial Doppler sonography (TCD) (increase in pulsatility index, fall in diastolic flow)
– No irreversible brain stem herniation of terminal bulbar brain syndrome.
The monitoring protocol was standard for all patients.

ICP was continuously monitored with an epidural Gaeltec sensor or a ventricular catheter [3]. Simultaneously, the CPP was calculated from the ICP and the arterial blood pressure (SAP, Neuromonitor; [3]). CT scans were performed at intervals. For the last 4 years middle cerebral arterial (TCD) flow velocity, EEG activity (Fourier analysis), SEP, and BAEP have been recorded additionally, at least twice daily.

Clinical status was assessed using an extended Glasgow Coma Scale and outcome after 1 year using the Glasgow Outcome Scale (1 = death, 2 = vegetative state, 3 = severely disabled, 4 = moderately disabled, 5 = rehabilitated). The operative concept for the decompressive craniectomy is based on a large unilateral (in patients with unilateral swelling) or bilateral (patients with diffuse swelling) fronto-parieto-temporal bone flap. A wide gap is made in the dura, and dural defect is covered with the temporal muscle and its fascia.

After between 4 weeks and 12 months the craniectomy is closed with a Palacos implant or by autologous bone flap – our preference is subcutaneous preservation of the bone in the thigh or abdomen.

Results

Out of 37 patients five died: three due to brain damage, the other two as a consequence of adult respiratory distress syndrome. Three remained in a vegetative state (all had had a poor clinical status to begin with). Fourteen achieved full social rehabilitation, 12 remained moderately disabled. One patient had a wound infection with secondary healing. Thirteen patients had subdural effusions; eight hygromas disappeared spontaneously or after puncture. In five cases hydrocephalic ventricles developed and were treated by ventriculoperitoneal shunting.

In all but three patients ICP was completely controlled by the decompressive craniotomy (Fig. 1a); in some patients some smaller increases in ICP in the days following the operation (e.g., B-waves) required single doses of osmotherapy. In all surviving patients the ICP was normalized by at most 6 days after operation; later increases in ICP were never attributable to brain edema but were caused by hygromas or CSF circulation disorders.

In the three patients who died from further brain swelling in spite of large-scale operative decompression, the final ICP decompensation occurred within 48 h after operation. The intracranial hypertension finally equalled the SAP, indicating complete vasoparalysis (Fig. 1b). All three patients were already in poor clinical condition immediately after injury (GCS ≤ 4; see Fig. 4) and had bulbar brain syndrome (GCS 3, dilated and fixed pupils) at the time of operation. In these patients the decision to operate was based on the continued presence of BAEPs (wave V, Fig. 2b); however, the absence of SEPs and the clinical signs of bulbar brain syndrome al-

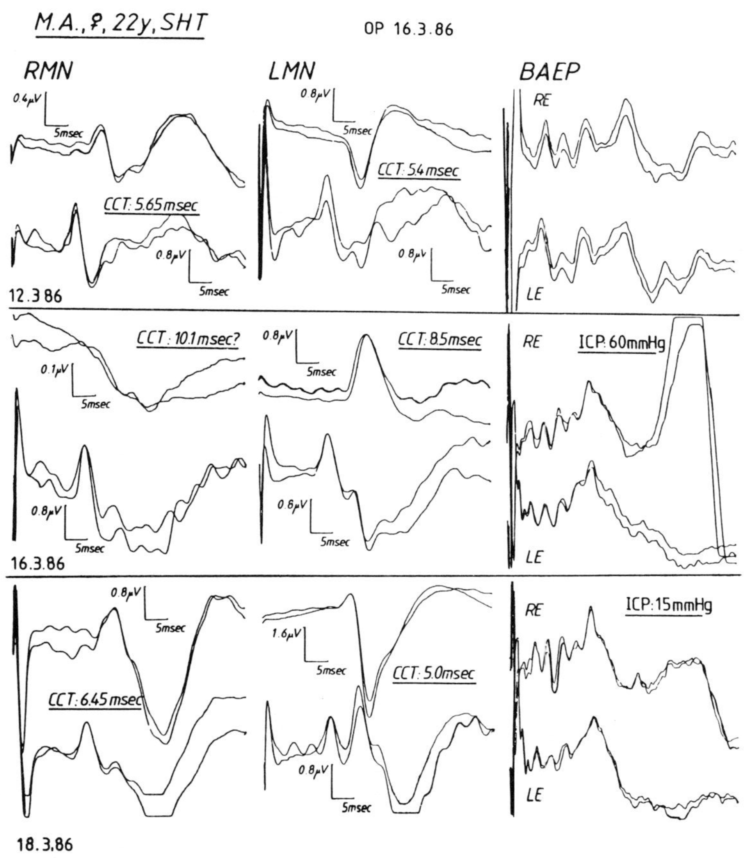

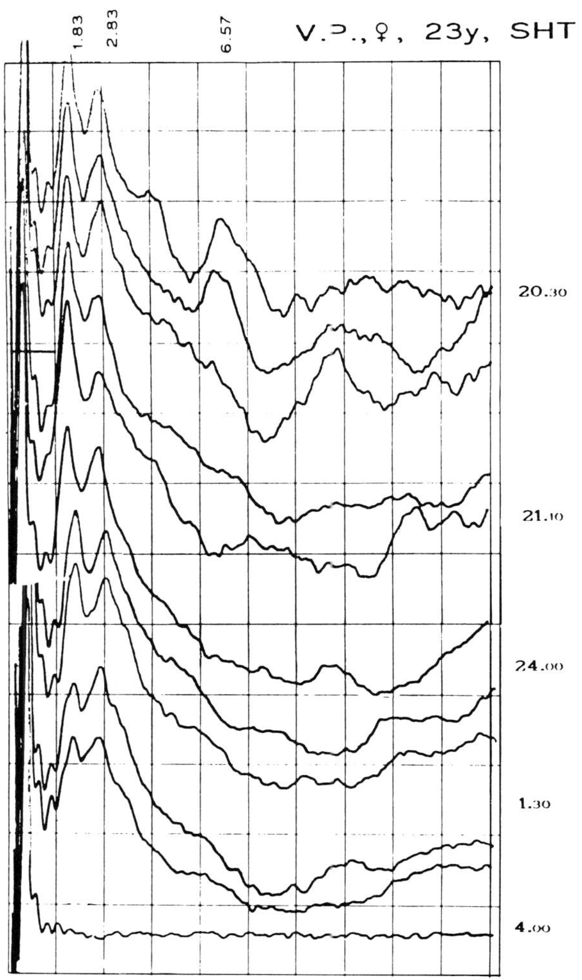

Fig. 2. a Only mild primary brain damage, secondary brain compression shown by intact BAEPs and deteriorating SEPs (CCT), rapid recovery after craniectomy. **b** Irreversible brain stem compression despite craniectomy. Same patients as in Fig. 1

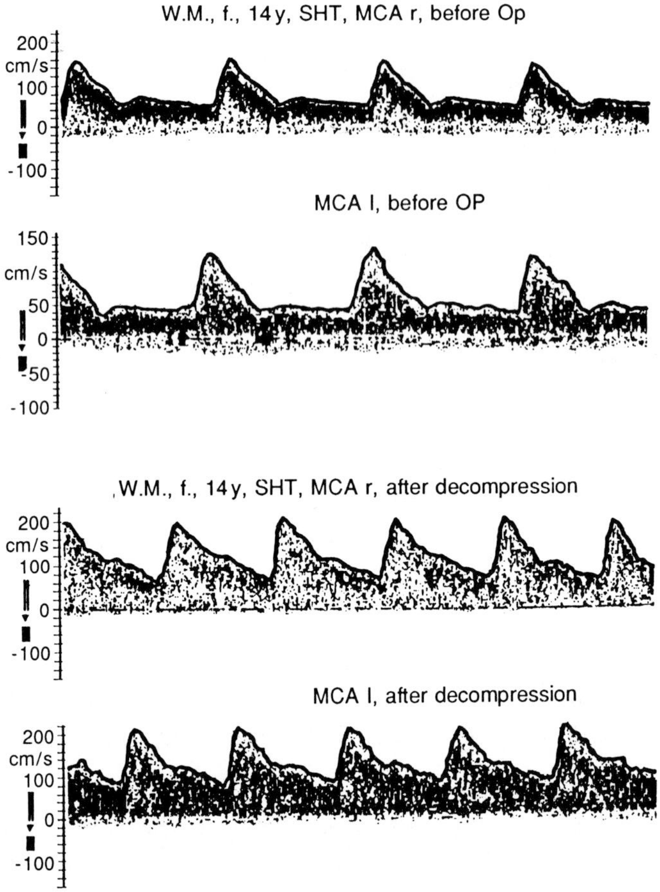

Fig. 3. TCD and decompressive craniectomy: increase in pulsatility and fall in diastolic flow normalized after operation

low the assumption that supratentorial circulatory arrest had already taken place at the time of operation. Operative decompression could not then prevent the subsequent complete ischemic brain necrosis (Figs. 1b, 2b).

All patients with a secondary deterioration after initially well preserved SEPs and BAEPs indicating only mild primary brain injury achieved good rehabilitation (GOS 4 or 5), if the decompression was performed before SEPs and BAEPs were lost completely (Fig. 2a). The rapid normalization of electrophysiological parameters after operative decompression was often striking (Fig. 2a). In these patients the ICP decompensation and electrophysiological deterioration were associated with a rise in the pulsatility index (TCD; Fig. 3). The decrease in diastolic flow on TCD and the increase in pulsatility index were immediately normalized by operative decompression. In addition to continuous ICP recording, monitoring of SEPs,

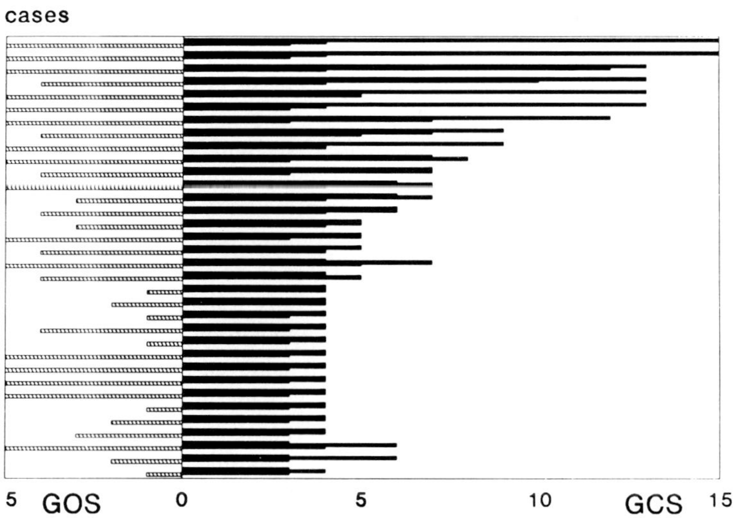

Fig. 4. Prognosis after operative decompression: good outcome (GOS, *left*) in patients with GCS ≥ 8 immediately after trauma (*long line, right*) or GCS ≥ 5 on day 1 (*intermediate line, right*), despite GCS 3–4 at time of decompression (*short line, right*)

BAEPs, and the TCD signal of the MCA is very helpful for a proper and timely indication for operative decompression, allowing reliable assessment of the severity of primary brain injury and giving clear warning of imminent secondary tentorial herniation (Fig. 2a).

The best *predictor of prognosis after decompressive craniectomy* is the initial severity of brain injury (Fig. 4). All patients with a GCS ≥ 8 immediately after trauma or GCS ≥ 6 on day 1 after injury achieved a good result. In these patients with only mild or moderate primary brain injury, the outcome is determined by the development of secondary brain swelling and intracranial hypertension, which can definitely be controlled by operative decompression.

Discussion

Our results, with approximately 40% full rehabilitation and an additional 30% of patients with a satisfactory quality of survival, indicate that decompressive craniectomy performed in accordance with our pathophysiological criteria is an effective and beneficial form of treatment.

The pathophysiological criteria of decompressive craniectomy are uni- or bilateral brain swelling – as demonstrated by CT – associated with uncontrollably elevated ICP and a deterioration in clinical condition. In addition EEG, SEP and BAEP recording, and TCD are helpful in timing the operation. The operative technique must include a large bone flap – uni- or bilateral – and a wide dura opening.

We believe that bad results such as those desribed in the literature [81, 5] are due to delaying the operation until too late, when there is already irreversible brain stem herniation, or operating on patients with very severe primary brain injury which cannot be influenced by any treatment.
In the last 12 years we have performed decompressive craniectomies in only 37 patients out of more than 500 who had severe head injury requiring complex neuromonitoring [3]. The indication for operative decompression is thus rather rare. A good outcome can probably only be expected in younger patients; however, no clear age limits can be defined for this operation. There is no correlation between duration and level of intracranial hypertension. The only reliable predictor of a good outcome is the Glasgow Coma Score on admission and on first day after injury. In our series, all patients with an initial GCS ≥ 8 achieved full rehabilitation. A bad outcome will result from an irreversible primary brain injury with an initial GCS ≤ 4. Operative decompression is therefore only effective in delayed secondary brain damage with brain swelling which can not be controlled by conservative means. In cases of primary decompression immediately after trauma with early signs of brain stem failure there is no indication for operation.

Summary

Since 1978 only 37 patients have fulfilled our indication criteria for decompressive craniectomy, which are: age below 40 years, no serious primary brain injury, clinical deterioration correlated to intracranial hypertension and to deterioration of electrophysiological parameters. Eighteen patients underwent unilateral and 19 patients bilateral decompressive craniectomy with a large bone flap and a wide dura opening.

The results are very encouraging: of the 37 patients 14 achieved full social rehabilitation (GOS 5), 12 are moderately disabled, 3 remained in a vegetative state, and only 5 died (2 due to adult respiratory distress syndrome). A reliable predictor of outcome is the severity of primary brain injury: patients with only mild or moderate primary injury (initial GCS ≥ 8) and secondary brain swelling not controllable by conservative means have a good prognosis (GOS 4–5). In addition to clinical observation, repeated CT scanning and ICP monitoring are mandatory. In addition EEG, SEP and BAEP monitoring, and TCD are helpful in assessing the timing of operative management.

References

1. Alkarico AM, Ward JD, Choi SC, Marmarou A, Young HF (1987) Outcome after severe head injury. Relationship to mass lesions, diffuse injury and ICP course in pediatric and adult patients. J Neurosurg 67:648–656
2. Cushing H (1905) The establishment of cerebral hernia as a decompressive measure for inaccessible brain tumors, with the description of intramuscular methods of making the bone defect in temporal and occipital regions. Surg Gynecol Obstet 1:297–314

3. Gaab MR (1986) Routine computerized neuromonitoring. In: Miller JD, Teasdale GM, Rowan JO, Galbraith SL, Mendelow AD (eds) Intracranial pressure VI. Springer, Berlin Heidelberg New York, pp 240–247
4. Gaab MR, Knoblich OE, Fuhrmeister U, Pflughaupt KW, Dietrich K (1979) Comparison of the effects of surgical decompression and resection of local edema in the therapy of experimental brain trauma. Childs Brain 5:484–498
5. Karlen J, Stular D (1987) Dekompressive Kraniotomie bei schwerem Schädelhirntrauma nach erfolgloser Behandlung mit Barbituraten. Neurochirurgia 30:35–39
6. Kjellberg RM (1971) Bifrontal decompression craniotomy for massive cerebral edema. J Neurosurg 34:488–493
7. Sörensen N, Gaab MR, Gruss P, Halves E, Miltner F (1982) Decompressive craniectomy, an ultimate therapy in cranio-cerebral trauma. In Monograph Paediatr 15:96–99

Safety of Fraxiparine Administration in Neurosurgical Patients: Preliminary Report

F. Martens, T. Bruyns, T. Vandekerckhove, J. Caemaert, O. Kalala, and L. Calliauw[1]

Introduction

Deep venous thrombosis and pulmonary embolism are feared complications in surgical patients during the postoperative period. These thromboembolic complications are a source of postsurgical morbidity and mortality which cannot be ignored. In neurosurgical patients the frequency of postoperative venous thrombosis in the calf is estimated to be 29%–43% on the basis of studies with ^{125}I-fibrinogen [3]. This high frequency can be attributed to the lengthy operations, prolonged postoperative bedrest, and motor deficits. Preventive measures have been investigated, among them administration of heparin derivatives.

Fraxiparine (CY 216) is a low-molecular-weight heparin fraction which has a specific activity against factor Xa and only a moderate action against factor IIa. It has a prolonged action of at least 18 h.

Several prospective, randomized, double blind studies have demonstrated the value of preoperatively administered Fraxiparine in the prevention of thromboembolic complications after general orthopedic surgery complications [1, 2, 4]. Nevertheless, in neurosurgery there has been some reluctance to follow this practice, because of the possible disastrous effects of bleeding within the confines of the skull.

The aim of the present study was to establish whether preoperative administration of Fraxiparine was a safe procedure in respect of postoperative blood loss.

Material and Methods

Fifty patients consecutively admitted for elective intracranial surgery were randomized into two groups. The first group received Fraxiparine 12 h before surgery, the second 24 h after. The dosage was 100 IU/kg body weight. Afterwards Fraxiparine continued to be administered daily to all patients. The surgeons did not know to which group patients had been randomized and were therefore not biased. Blood samples were obtained on admission and 2 h before and 24 h after surgery. Hematocrit, hemoglobin, platelet count and clotting indicators (thrombin time, partial thrombopolastin time, activated partial thromboplastin time, fibrinogen) were

[1] Department of Neurosurgery, University Hospital Gent, De Pintelaan 185, B-9000 Gent, Belgium

Advances in Neurosurgery, Vol. 19
W. J. Bock, Ch. Lumenta, M. Brock, M. Klinger (Eds.)

measured. The postoperative blood loss was calculated from the drainage fluid volume and its hematocrit and from the arterial hematocrit.

Exclusion criteria were contraindications for Fraxiparine administration: blood clotting disorders, duodenal and gastric ulcers, etc.

Results

The two groups were comparable ($p \leq 0.05$) as to age, sex, distribution, height, weight and type of surgery.

There were no statistical differences between the two groups in the different blood samples for platelet count, partial thromboplastin time, thrombin time, and fibrinogen during surgery. Activated partial thromboplastin time was significantly higher in the preoperatively treated patients 2 h before surgery and this difference was still significant 24 h later (Fig. 1). Nevertheless, although postoperative blood loss was less in the preoperatively treated patients, the difference was not significant (Fig. 2).

There were no bleeding complications or wound hematomas in either group.

Conclusion

This study indicates that preoperatively administered Fraxiparine has no influence on postoperative blood loss. However, since the number of patients in this preliminary study was limited, this should not be regarded as a definitive conclusion.

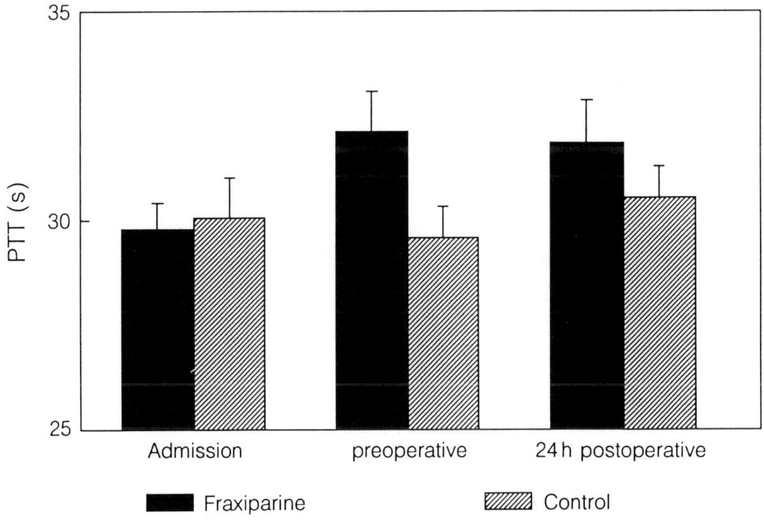

Fig. 1. Activated partial thromboplastin time

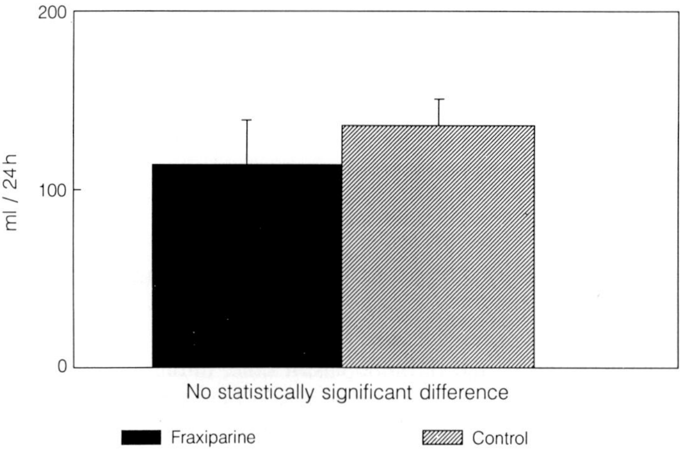

Fig. 2. Postoperative blood loss

References

1. Kakkar VV, Murray WJG (1985) Efficacy and safety of low molecular weight heparin (CY 216) in preventing postoperative venous thrombo-embolism: a co-operative study. Br J Surg 72:786–791
2. Samama M, Boissel JP, Combe-Tamzali, Leizorovicz A (1989) Clinical studies with low molecular weight heparins in the prevention and treatment of venous thromboembolism. Ann NY Acad Sci 556:386–404
3. Swann KW, Black PM (1984) Deep vein thrombosis and pulmonary emboli in neurosurgical patients: a review. J Neurosurg 61:1055–1062
4. The European Fraxiparin Study (EFS) Group (1988) Comparison of a low molecular weight heparin and unfractionated heparin for the prevention of deep vein thrombosis in patients undergoing abdominal surgery. Br J Surg 75:1058–1063

Subject Index

acrylates 42
acute
- care 191
- heart distress 100
adenocystic carcinoma 30
adjuvant irradiation therapy 31
ALMO Statistik-System 85
alpha-chloralose 24, 27
amaurosis 154
amino acids 216
anaplastic astrocytoma 146
angioarchitecture 35, 81
angiography 137
- selective 36
- superselective 36, 37
angioma-feeding arteries 78
angioma(s)
- cavernous 103, 116
— pontine 119
- intracranial 74
- nonoperable 44
- simple 44
angiomatosis, diffuse 43
angiotensin II 24, 27
anosmia 29
anterior
- communicating artery 85
- cranial fossa 29
- cranial skull base 29, 32
antibiotic regimen, prophylactic 226
antihypertensive drug 255, 257, 258
aphasia 91
arteriovenous malformations (AVM) 61, 66
- brain 35
- cerebral 39, 55, 84, 100, 103
- fistula 41
- infratentorial 71
- intracranial 81
- large 63
- multiple 81
- posterior fossa 81
- supratentorial 71
astrocytoma(s) 137, 142
- anaplastic 146
- low grade 144
- malignant 142, 144
attentiveness stress test 203
autosomal dominant mode 130
avitene 38

bacterial spectrum 222
ballon-directed system 41
basal ganglia 123
B-cell lymphoma 144
Benton Visual Retention Test 104, 105
beta-radiation-emitting isotopes 161
bleeding episodes 103
bone flap 268
- infected 31
Bourneville glioma 144
brachium pontis cavernoma 119
brain
- arteriovenous malformations 35
- compression, secondary 269
- damage
— assessment 205
— delayed secondary 272
- edema 24, 26
— cytotoxic 20
— experimental 249
— formation 27
— vasogenic 26
- tumors
— adults 171
— children 135, 171
— children, neurological grades 173
— malignant supratentorial 146

brainstem 123
- cavernomas 110
- cavernous hemangiomas 123
bromodexyuridine (BUdR) 156
butylacrylate 67

calorimetry, indirect 211, 215
caudate nucleus 117, 119
- cavernoma 119
cavernoma 103, 130
- anomalies 81
cavernous
- angiomas 103, 116
— cerebral 110
— hemangiomas 110, 122, 123
— spinal 123
— supratentorial 123
- sinus 110
— cavernoma 112
CBF
- CO_2 reactivity 243
- decreased 242
- dynamics 240
- global resting 241, 243
- measurements 240
- regional 240, 241
central
- conduction time (CCT) 205, 206
- motor conduction time (CMCT) 196
cerebellar
- peduncles 117
— inferior 119
— superior 119
- venous angiomas 98
cerebellopontine angle 123
cerebral
- arteriovenous malformations (see also arteriovenous malformations -AVM-) 61, 66
- glioma 151
- hyperemia 24
- trauma 108
cerebral AV fistulas 100
cerebrocranial arteriovenous shunts (CAVS) 100
chemo- and radiotherapy, combined 148
chemotherapy 138, 144
- systemic 155
cholesterol crystals 159
chondrosarcoma 31
circle of Willis 70
CO_2 laser 112, 119
coma
- grade 207
- nontraumatic 194
- outcome 207
- traumatic 194
comatose patients 197, 215
- follow-up times 167
computed tomography (CT) 30, 35, 68, 74, 90, 101 111, 116, 119, 122
- contrast-enhanced 95
- scanning 272
computerized stereotactic operation 151
congestive cardiac failure 100
consciousness, impaired 137
cranial
- fossa, middle 122
- nerve
— deficit 137
— dysfunction 119
- palsies 123
craniopharyngioma 137, 142, 143, 158
- cystic 158
„cryptic“ malformations 122
CSF samples 226
cyanoacrylates 38

death, causes 192
decompressive craniectomy 265, 272
- bilateral 265, 268
- pathophysiological criteria 271
- predictor of prognosis 271
- TCD 270
- unilateral 268
depression 108
deterioration in clinical condition 271
Deutsche Interdisziplinäre Vereinigung für Intensiv- und Notfallmedizin (DIVI) 187
„developmental venous anomaly“ 92
diabetes insipidus
- postoperative 235, 238
- surgical cranial approach 235
dilated artery, media 70
dimensions depression 104
draining veins 36
„drop-by-drop“ method 42

Dulbecco's modified minimal essential medium (DMEM) 21
dural fistulas 81, 100
dysgerminoma 144

ectodermal tumors 135
edema formation 253
elastic lamina 70
electrical stimulation 196
elevated ICR 253
embolization 37, 38, 41, 44, 54
- arterial 100
- curative 39
- „emergency" 101
— endovascular 57, 66
- intraoperative 60
- intravascular techniques 66
- palliative 39
- partial 47
- preoperative 60
- superselective 46
embryogenesis 94
embryonal tumors, classification 169
emotional behavior 107
endocrinological disturbances 164, 166
endogenous infection 225
- ascending 226
endoscopic biopsy 30
endovascular
- occlusion, permanent 38
- procedures 55
- techniques 63
— superselective 46
- therapy 50
— delayed 101
energy expenditure 215
ependymomas 137, 142
epidermal growth receptor 180, 181, 182
epidural hematomas, mortality 230
epilepsy 50, 103
epistaxis 29
esthesioneuroblastomas 29
European Associations of Neurosurgical Societies (EANS) 5
event-related potential (ERP) 202
- latency 202
EWL (Eigenschaftswlrterliste) 104
extra-arachnoid lesions 235

facial
- AV fistula 100
- capillary hemangiomas 100
feeding arteries 36
- lenticulostriate 85
- terminal type 37
- transit type 37
fentanyl 24, 27
fibrosarcoma 144
focal
- cerebral injury 27
- cold lesion 24, 26
foramen magnum 81
foreign-body giant cells 49
fourth ventricle 123
fraxiparine administration 274

gamma knife 69, 96
γ-radiation 161
gangliocytoma 135
ganglioma uncus 144
gastrointestinal bleeding, massive 102
Glasgow
- Coma Score on admission 272
- Outcome Scale 57
glioma 135
gliosis 36
glucose loads, high 215
glycerol therapy 259, 263
- oral 260, 263
gold Au 198 161
Gollin's Incomplete Figures Test 104

H_2 clearance 24, 27
hamartoma 144
head injuries 240
- diffuse 201
— electrophysiological studies 201
— information processing 201
- hypertension 257
- risk of death 232
- severe 205, 228, 243, 265
- trauma, treatment of hypertension 255
headache, recurrent 50
hemangioblastoma 103, 104
hematoma patients, mortality 230
hemiparesis 91
hemispheric tumors, neurological grading 172

hemodynamic stress 70
hemorrhage 36, 39
- aneurysmal subarachnoid 88
- intracranial 50, 53, 75
- recurrent 50
- spontaneous intracranial 71
- subarachnoid 17, 92
hemorrhagic infarction 91, 92
hemosiderin 113
heparin derivatives 274
hepatic failure, acute 102
high voltage therapy 163
hormone dysregulation 154
human brain tumors
- EGF receptor 180
Hunt and Hess grade 18, 76, 88
hydrocephaly 100, 138
hyperventilation 242
- therapy, CBF dynamics 240
hypomania 104, 107, 108
hypophyseal adenoma 144
hypotension, systemic 101
hypothalamo-hypophyseal lesions 235
- surgical approach 235
hypothalamus surgery 234

ICP see intracranial pressure
idobutyl 2-cyanoacrylate (IBC) 56
immunohistochemistry 169
implanted
- iodine 125
- isotopes 151
infarction 36, 39
infection rate 222
infratentorial approach 119
intensive care
- medicine 188
— mortality 192
- units, general 222
interhemispheric approach 66, 68
International Society for Pediatric Neurosurgery (ISPN) 136
interstitial irradiation 151, 153, 155
intra-extra-arachnoid lesions 235
intracavitary brachytherapy (IB) 158, 161
intracerebellar angioma 96
intracerebral
- hematoma 31, 230
- pressure
— reduction 245
— sorbitol 251
— THAM 247
intracranial
- arteriovenous malformations 46, 50, 74
— coexistence aneurysms 70
— microsurgical treatment 50
- bleeding 66, 68
- hemorrhage 50, 53, 102, 107
— recurrent 107
- hypertension 240, 259
— brain-injured patients 263
— osmotic diuretics 259
— treatment 259
- pressure (ICP) 205, 207, 255, 261
— decompensation 270
— increased 29
— monitoring 205, 272
— reduction maximum 261
- venous angiomas 94
intravascular techniques 66
irradiation 31, 151
ischemic brain damage 242, 243
isobutyl-2-cyanoacrylates 38, 101
isoflurane 24, 27

K^+-induced glial swelling 20
Kaplan and Meier method 153
Karnofsky performance status 153
Kernohan classification 153
ketanserin 255, 257, 258
Ki-67-positive cells 177
- histopathological characteristics 178
- different gliomas 177

labeling index 178
lamina quadrigemina 110
leptomeningeal recanalisation 49
linear accelerator 103
Luessenhop and Generalli's scheme 87
lymphocytic reaction 49
lymphopenia 219

Mab 425 181
macrocephaly 100
magnetic resonance images (MRI) 35, 90, 101, 111, 116, 119, 122, 127
- gadolinium-enhanced 95, 97

- T1- and T2-weighted 35
magnetoelectric stimulation 196
mannitol 260
maxillary sinuses 30
medulloblastoma 135, 137
memory functions 104
meningitis 224
mesencephalon 117, 119
mesodermal tumors 135
microaneurysms 37
microarteriovenous malformations 130
microballoon 41
microcoils 38
microhemorrhages 123
- multiple intralesional 120
- recurrent 113
Minnesota Multiple Choice Personality Inventory (MMPI) 104
MMC (Horizon Metabolic Computer) 211
mnemonic deficits 107
monoclonal antibody Ki-67 176
mortality 230, 232
motor evoked potentials (MEP)
- patterns 195
- prognostic value 194, 197
— comatose patients 197

n-butyl-cyanacrylate 38, 101
Na^+/K^+-ATPase 20, 22
nasal breathing, impaired 29
neuro-rhinosurgical operation 29
neuroectodermal tumors 135
neurologic deficit, permanent 39
neuropsychological abnormalities 103
neuroradiology, superselective endovascular 61
neurosurgeon, doctor in charge 192
neurosurgical
- intensive care 187, 193, 222
— admission 190
— unit/ward 189, 190, 192, 193
— unit/ward, causes of death 193
— unit/ward, tasks 189
- patients 274
- training 5
neuroticism 104, 108
neurotraumatized patients, body temperature 218
nitrogen balance 214, 215
nursing staff, shortage 189
nutritional
- regimen 212
- study 215

„occult malformations" 116
oligodendroglioma 142
operative decompression, 271, 272
- electrophysiological parameters 270
optic
- glioma 142, 163
- nerve gliomas, subtotally removed 165
oral glycerol 261
osmotic diuretics 259

paraglioma 135
paranasal sinuses 29
paraparesis 127
paraplegia, acute 123
parenteral nutrition 211
patients, thiopentone-treated 217
pediatric brain tumors 135
phosphorus 32 161
physiological processing, temporal progression 201
pilocytic astrocytomas 153, 154, 163
- follow-up times 165
- localization 164
- proliferative activity 176
pineal
- region 123
- tumors 138, 142, 143
pinealoblastoma 143
pituitary
- gland 123
- region 234
plain radiography 30
plexus papilloma 137, 144, 148
pneumencephalography 137
pneumonia 223
- organisms 224
polarized light microscopy 159
polyvinylalcohol (PVA) 38, 41, 101
post-traumatic
- condition 190
- hyperemia 26
postembolization radiosurgery 61
posterior fossa 123
postoperative

- blood loss 275
- diabetes insipidus 235, 238
primitive neuroectodermal tumors (PNET) 137, 146, 168, 169, 182
- EGF receptors 182
PRL
- levels 236, 238
- stress-induced 238
proptosis 29
protein level, body 216
proton beam therapy (PBT) 69, 74
- stereotactic 75
psychasthenia 104, 107
psychomotor
- retardation 139
- seizures 154
psychopathic deviation 104, 107, 108
psychosyndromes, organic 103
pulmonary embolism 274
pulsatile index 205

radiation
- necrosis, delayed 63
- therapy 54, 138
radio- and chemotherapy, combined 148
radiosurgery 68, 69
radiotherapy 56, 163
- efficacy 165
- follow-up times 167
- pilocytic astrocytomas 163
regional cerebral blood flow (rCBF) 24, 27
rehabilitation, early 191
renal nitrogen loss 214
revascularization malformation 67
rhabdomyosarcoma 31
rhenium 186 161
Riechert-Mundinger stereotaxic frame, modified CT-compatible 152
risk
- of death, head injuries 232
- factors, main 37

saccular aneurysms 36, 37
schizophrenia 104, 107, 108
- scale 106
schwannoma, malignant 144
seed implantation 155
seizures 53, 66, 123, 137
- focal 111
- generalized 111
- grand mal 93
- psychomotor 154
septicaemia 223
serotonin S_2-antagonist 257
severe head injuries 265
- comparative analysis 205
- decompressive craniectomy 265
- prognosis 243
- risk 228
- survivors 228
Shi and Chen's system 88
SIADH 238
silk sutures 38
single photon emission computed tomography (SPECT) 74
social rehabilitation 272
sodium 249
somatosensory evoked potentials (SEP) 17, 205, 206
- CCT 207
- coma grade 208
sorbitol 251
Spearman's rank correlation coefficient rho 85
Spetzler-Martin grading system 51, 53, 87, 88
sphenoidal sinuses 30
spinal cavernous hemangiomas 123
spontaneous intracranial hemorrhages
- basal metabolic rate 215
- comatose patients 215
- energy requirements of patients 211
- resting energy expenditure 213, 215
squamous carcinoma 31
staphylococcus
- *aureus* 226
- *epidermidis* 226
stereotactic
- biopsies 123, 148
- intracavitary irradiation 158
- irradiation 103, 107
- radiosurgery 50, 63
Stroop Test 104
subarachnoid hemorrhage (SAH) 17, 92
subdural hematomas 230
subtemporal approach 119

subtonsillar approach 119
superior sagittal sinus 94
supracerebellar approach 119
supratentorial
- cavernomas 110
- gliomas 171, 174
— cerebral 151
— childhood 174
— prognosis 174
- tumors 137, 141
— children 180
— children, anti-epidermal growth factor receptor antibody 180
— children, immunohistochemical investigations 180
— malignant 146
surgical extirpation 148
survivors after head injuries 228
systemic chemotherapy 155

teleangiectasias, capillary 130
tentorial herniation 271
THAM 245, 246, 251, 253
- CCP 251
- intracerebral pressure 247, 251
- treatment 247
thiopental 24, 27
thiopentone therapy
- high dose treatment 220
- immunosuppression 220
- immunsuppressive effect 217
- incidence of infection 220
- lymphopenia 219
- susceptiblity to infection 217
- therapy-resistant raised ICP 220
thromboembolic complications 274
thromboplastin time, partial 275
Trailmaking Test 104
transcranial
- Doppler sonography (TCD) 17, 74, 205, 207
- magnetoelectric stimulation 196
transcranial-transbasal approach 32
transsylvian approach 119
transtemporal approach 68
transtonsillar approach 119
traumatic brain swelling 245, 246
treatment, organizational consequences 192
tumor(s)
antigens, specific 180
- classification, histological diagnoses 172
- grading scheme, prognostic indicator 171
- midline 174

U tests 105
ultrasonography (US) 101
undifferent carcinoma 31
unit-acquired infections 224
urinary infections 224, 226

vascular
- hamartomas 129
- malformations, asymptomatic cryptic 127
- steal syndromes 103
vein of Galen aneurysm malformations (VGAM) 100
venous
- angiomas 90, 97, 99 130
— infratentorial 94
— intracranial 94
- thrombosis 82
— deep 274
ventricular system 123
visual defects 164
von Recklinghausen's disease 144

water uptake 249
water-electroylyte balance, disorders 234
Wechsler Adult Intelligence Scale (WAIS) 104
WHO
- astrocytoma grade I 163
- grade 148
wire-guided catheter 41

yttrium 90 158, 161

M. Brock, H. M. Mayer, K. Weigel,
Free University of Berlin (Eds.)

The Artificial Disc

1991. X, 102 pp. 51 figs. 11 tabs.
Hardcover DM 80,– ISBN 3-540-51857-6

The development of new biocompatible implant materials as well as the advances in operative techniques in spinal surgery raise the question as to the prosthetic replacement of degenerated, herniated or injured intervertebral discs. Although "disc-surgery" accounts for the vast majority of all surgical procedures of the spine, the idea of an artificial disc has not yet found a final and satisfying solution. The purpose of this book is to give a survey of the state of the art concerning the concept, design, experimental investigations and, in some cases, clinical application of different kinds of disc prostheses.
Only a few scientific groups are dealing with this problem. Protagonists and representatives of all these groups have made contributions to this book, presenting their individual views, experimental approaches and clinical experience with different kinds of artificial discs.

Springer-Verlag
Berlin
Heidelberg
New York
London
Paris
Tokyo
Hong Kong
Barcelona